FUNDAMENTALS
OF PSYCHIATRY

- TASMAN
- MOHR

FUNDAMENTALS
OF PSYCHIATRY

Allan Tasman, MD
Professor and Chairman
Department of Psychiatry and Behavioral Sciences
University of Louisville School of Medicine, Louisville, Kentucky, USA

and

Wanda K. Mohr, PhD, APRN
Professor of Psychiatric Nursing
University of Medicine and Dentistry of New Jersey, Stratford, NJ, USA

WILEY-BLACKWELL

A John Wiley & Sons, Ltd., Publication

Library of Congress Cataloging-in-Publication Data

Tasman, Allan
 Fundamentals of psychiatry / Allan Tasman and Wanda K. Mohr.
  p. ; cm.
 Includes index.
 ISBN 978-0-470-66577-0 (paper)
 1. Psychiatry. I. Mohr, Wanda K. 1947- II. Title.
 [DNLM: 1. Psychiatry. 2. Mental Disorders. 3. Mental Health. WM 100]
 RC454.M62 2010
 616.89–dc22

A catalogue record for this book is available from the British Library.

This book is published in the following electronic formats: ePDF 9780470975183; ePub 9780470976258

Set in 9.5/11.5pt Times Roman by Thomson Digital, Noida, India
Printed and bound in Singapore by Fabulous Printers Pte Ltd

First Impression 2011

To my family with love and thanks for your love and support

Allan

In loving memory of my parents, "Paczuszka" i "Litek,"
and to Brian for then, now, and always.

Wanda

Contents

Preface

The treatment of patients with psychiatric or neurobehavioral problems continues to evolve as we increase our knowledge about pathophysiology and translate these findings into new and refined clinical approaches. Such ongoing changes demand ongoing education and a strategy that includes and supports multidisciplinary practice. Despite the fact that the care of psychiatric patients requires teamwork and a shared vision, it is not often that we see collaboration between authors of different educational backgrounds and from different disciplines. In this book, we have tried to pioneer and champion such a partnership and teamwork, recognizing that complex mental health problems cannot be understood or treated solely by one discipline.

The idea for this book came about when we recognized the need for a resource in which the massive knowledge base in psychiatry was condensed in a user-friendly way, suitable for use as an introductory clinical text. Our intent was not to be exhaustive or comprehensive, but to distill the content to a "need to know" form. We carefully edited the comphrensive two-volume *Psychiatry, Third Edition* (edited by Tasman, Kay, Lieberman, First, and Maj), selecting from each chapter the information essential for a thorough but compact first textbook for those in training in a mental health discipline or a practitioner interested in a clinical reference. Some of the chapters may seem truncated but all the requisite elements of each topic and subject matter are present. The vision for this book includes our keen recognition that such a text will provide a foundation upon which readers at the start of their clinical careers can build. Moreover, we recognize that change occurs so rapidly and exponentially in the area of mental health that what is considered best practice today may change based on newly acquired information. Hence, the present text is meant to be a springboard for readers who wish to further research topics as more data become available through ongoing studies. To that end, we provide a list of suggested print and online resources at the ends of chapters so that readers can augment what is in each chapter.

This work is guided by an integrative approach to patient care that acknowledges the complexity and uniqueness of the whole person within his or her contexts, making use of many means of understanding them. The nature of psychiatric disorders is such that understanding the person who has the illness, with all their pre-existing personal strengths and weaknesses, is essential to optimal understanding of the patient and for implementing a treatment plan. Our philosophical approach affirms the collaborative relationship between patients, their families, and caregivers from different disciplines.

Our intended audience includes several groups. Students and practitioners in training as well as instructors will find this a useful beginning text. Primary-care practitioners, who are the front-line caregivers encountering many mental health problems in daily practice, will also find this a useful basic clinical reference guide.

In writing this book, we recognize that there is great diversity in the assortment of clinicians licensed to diagnose and treat mental illnesses, and substantial differences in their training, knowledge and skills. These individuals include a wide range of practitioners – psychologists, psychiatrists, primary care and specialist physicians, social workers, advanced psychiatric nurses, marriage and family therapists, addiction therapists, and a wide variety of counselors (e.g., psychosocial rehabilitation, school, addiction, and pastoral counselors). We acknowledge that professionals work with patients to develop appropriate individualized therapeutic approaches informed by the best evidence in their fields. The text is intended to provide trainees and practitioners in all disciplines a solid base upon which they can build and tailor their therapeutic approaches, both within the unique perspective of their own discipline and within interdisciplinary treatment situations.

The text provides a complete reference for each DSM disorder and includes screening and assessment measures, differential diagnosis, laboratory tests needed in diagnosis, and treatment. We have emphasized the major treatment modalities for each disorder and special issues practitioners may face in treating patients with each disorder, including consultation and referral concerns. Our book also provides information on therapeutic communication, diagnostic methods, psychiatric emergencies, and ethical/legal issues the practitioner may confront in day-to-day practice.

We are indebted to our editors, including Joan Marsh and Fiona Woods, and the team at Wiley. They shared their expertise in a patient and collaborative manner, working through the process of turning ideas into a finished manuscript. We are also grateful to our families who watched the gestation of this book and cheered us on through the months of writing and re-writing.

Allan Tasman
Wanda K. Mohr

Acknowledgments

We gratefully acknowledge the following contributors to *Psychiatry, Third Edition*, from which material for this book was adapted. The relevant chapters in this volume are indicated [].

Henry D. Abraham [18]
Adekunle G. Ahmed [39]
Sonia Ancoli-Israel [12]
Martin M. Antony [15]
Gordon J. G. Asmundson [15]
Thomas F. Babor [18]
Jennifer R. Baker [18]
Mark S. Bauer [13]
Fred Beauvais [18]
Jean C. Beckham [15]
David M. Benedek [10]
Heather Berlin [22]
Robert J. Boland [34]
Alan Breier [25]
Timothy A. Brown [15]
Gerard E. Bruder [30]
Deborah L. Cabaniss [30]
Joseph R. Calabrese [34]
Chia-Hui Chen [33]
Francine Cournos [30]
Jonathan R. T. Davidson [15]
Darin D. Dougherty [30]
Deidre M. Edwards [36]
Jane L. Eisen [15]
Stuart J. Eisendrath [24]
Richard S. Epstein [9]
Milton Erman [12]
Ayman Fanous [15]
John P. Federoff [39]
Morgan Feibelman [20]
Roberto Lewis-Fernández [7]
Michael B. First [4]
Anne M. Fleming [24]
W. Wolfgang Fleischacker [35]
Amanda M. Flood [15]
Robert L. Frierson [17]
Paul J. Fudala [18]
Anthony J. Giuliano [30]
Thomas A. Grieger [10]
Heinz Grunze [14]
Jaswant Guzder [7]
Jeffrey M. Halperin [11]
John H. Halpern [18]
Kathryn L. Hale [36]

Carlos A. Hernandez-Avila [18]
Kevin Ann Huckshorn [38]
Zahinoor Ismail [33]
Iliyan Ivanov [11]
G. Eric Jarvis [7]
Charles Y. Jin [18]
Courtney Pierce Keeton [11]
Martin B. Keller [34]
David E. Kemp [34]
Laurence J. Kirmayer [7]
Ami Klin [11]
Kim Klipstein [21]
William M. Klykylo [30]
Thomas R. Kosten [18]
Amy E. Lawrence [15]
Douglas S. Lehrer [30]
Frances R. Levin [18]
James L. Levenson [28]
Stephen B. Levine [29]
Jeffrey A. Lieberman [35]
Keh-Ming Lin [33]
Margaret T. Lin [33]
Sarah H. Lisanby [37]
David A. Lowenthal [30]
Christopher P. Lucas [11]
Rachel E. Maddux [36]
José R. Maldonado [27]
Rif S. El-Mallakh [18]
Stephen R. Marder [35]
Kim J. Masters [38]
Randi E. McCabe [15]
Elinore F. McCance-Katz [18]
James McPartland [11]
Glenn A. Melvin [38]
David B. Merrill [35]
Juan E. Mezzich [7]
Seiya Miyamoto [35]
David P. Moore [23]
Stephanie N. Mullins-Sweatt [19]
David J. Muzina [34]
Jeffrey H. Newcorn [11, 21]
Benjamin R. Nordstrom [18]
Ahmed Okasha [9]
Maria A. Oquendo [38]

Brooke S. Parish [26]
Jayendra K. Patel [25]
Michele T. Pato [15]
Katharine A. Phillips [15]
Debra A. Pinals [25, 39]
Bruce G. Pollock [33]
Kelly Posner [38]
Mark Hyman Rapaport [36]
Scott L. Rauch [30]
Neil Rosenberg [18]
Cécile Rousseau [7]
Stefan Rowny [37]
Maria Angeles Ruiperez [7]
Fabian M. Saleh [39]
Cornelius Schüle [14]
Kurt Schulz [11]
Larry J. Seidman [30]
Kevin A. Sevarino [18]
Charles W. Sharp [18]
David Shaffer [11]
Vanshdeep Sharma [11]
Daphne Simeon [22]
Michael W. Smith [33]
Stephen M. Sonnenberg [2]
Matt W. Specht [11]
David Spiegel [27]
Barbara H. Stanley [38]
James J. Strain [21]
Steven Taylor [15]
Jane A. Ungemack [18]
Amy M. Ursano [2]
Robert J. Ursano [2]
Fred R. Volkmar [11]
B. Timothy Walsh [16]
John T. Walkup [11]
Alexander Westphal [11]
Christina G. Weston [30]
Thomas A. Widiger [19]
George E. Woody [18]
Sean H. Yutzy [26]
Shu-Han Yu [33]
Charles H. Zeanah [20]

Unit 1
Foundations

Introduction

This chapter introduces the concepts of mental health and mental illness. It provides an overview of the contexts within which mental illnesses are prevented, diagnosed, and treated and the many problems such conditions pose for patients and their families. The topics discussed in this chapter will be relevant throughout the entire book.

1.1 Mental health and mental illness

Mental health refers to the successful performance of mental function, resulting in productive activities, fulfilling relationships, and the ability to adapt to change and cope with adversity. Mental health provides people with the capacity for rational thinking, communication skills, learning, emotional growth, resilience, and self-esteem. People experiencing emotional well-being or mental health function comfortably in society and are satisfied with their achievements. Mental health is one of the leading health indicators that reflect the major public health concerns in the United States. Related indicators of interest to the mental health community include substance abuse, injury and violence, and access to healthcare.

The American Psychiatric Association (APA) defines mental illness as a clinically significant behavioral or psychological syndrome experienced by a person and marked by distress, disability, or the risk of suffering, disability, or loss of freedom. The symptoms of the disorder must be above and beyond expected reactions to an everyday event. The behavioral or psychological condition must result from brain functioning or malfunctioning, and it must cause the person distress, impairment, or both. It cannot be a cultural practice to which the majority culture in a society objects or that might cause distress to non-members of a cultural group. For example, some cultures believe that women should be subservient to men and expect the behavior of both sexes to reflect this idea. People of Western cultures might view such women as dependent or co-dependent, yet the behavior of these women is perfectly normal within the parameters of their own culture.

1.2 Incidence and prevalence of mental illness

Psychiatric illnesses are common in the United States and internationally. The prominence of mental disorders in the total pattern of worldwide morbidity and mortality has been reported by the World Health Organization (WHO). According to their 2002 estimates, mental illnesses account for 25% of all disability across major industrialized countries. Mental illness ranks first in terms of causing disability in the US, Canada, and Western Europe.

In the US an estimated 26.2% of people (57.7 million) suffer from a diagnosable mental disorder in a given year. Data from the National Comorbidity Survey suggests that an estimated 13 million US adults (approximately 1 in 17) have a seriously debilitating mental illness. The main burden of

Fundamentals of Psychiatry, First Edition. Allan Tasman and Wanda K. Mohr.
© 2011 John Wiley & Sons, Ltd. Published 2011 by John Wiley & Sons, Ltd.

illness is concentrated in this smaller population. Mental disorders are the leading cause of disability in the US and Canada for ages 15–44. Nearly half of people having any mental disorder meet the criteria for two or more disorders. In terms of mortality, suicide alone is the eleventh leading cause of death in the US, with approximately 30 000 deaths per year, and this is an issue of concern worldwide as well. Determining the costs associated with mental illness is challenging, but estimates suggest annual treatment costs in the US of $100 billion, with significantly more for indirect costs; $193 billion per year is estimated for lost earnings alone.

At least 20% of children in the United States have a diagnosable mental disorder; only 5% of these children have severely impaired functioning. In adults aged 18–54 years, 14.9% have anxiety disorders, 7.1% have mood disorders, and 1.3% have schizophrenia. Depression, a serious mental health problem in any age group, is particularly problematic in older adults. Between 8% and 15% of older adults have depression, but the condition is often undiagnosed and untreated in this age group because depression is mistakenly thought of as part of "normal aging." People aged 65 years or older have the highest suicide rates of any age group. According to the Alzheimer's Association, Alzheimer's disease occurs in 8–15% of those older than 65 years (4.5 million cases) and that number is expected to increase to 11–16 million in the US by 2050. Approximately 125 000 people age 22–64 with mental illness live in nursing homes, 283 800 are incarcerated. Of 2 million individuals who are homeless over the course of a year, 50% have a mental illness and/or substance abuse disorder.

Table 1.1 contains National Institute of Mental Health statistics on the prevalence of some of the more common mental illnesses.

Table 1-1 Prevalence of mental illnesses in the United States	
Disorder	**Prevalence**
Mood disorders (major depressive disorder, dysthymic disorder and bipolar disorder)	Approximately 20.9 million US adults, or about 9.5% of the population aged 18 and older, have a mood disorder in a given year
Major depressive disorder	Major depressive disorder affects approximately 14.8 million US adults, or about 6.7% of the population aged 18 and older in a given year
Dysthymic disorder	Dysthymic disorder affects approximately 1.5% of the US population aged 18 and older in a given year (this translates to about 3.3 million US adults)
Bipolar disorder	Bipolar disorder affects approximately 5.7 million US adults, or about 2.6% of the population aged 18 and older in a given year
Suicide	In 2006, 33 300 (approximately 11 per 100 000) people died by suicide in the US
Schizophrenia	Approximately 2.4 million US adults, or about 1.1% of the population aged 18 and older, have schizophrenia in a given year
Anxiety disorders	Approximately 40 million US adults aged 18 and older, or about 18.1% of people in this age group, have an anxiety disorder in a given year
Panic disorder	Approximately 6 million US adults aged 18 and older, or about 2.7% of people in this age group, have panic disorder in a given year
Obsessive–compulsive disorder (OCD)	Approximately 2.2 million US adults aged 18 and older, or about 1.0% of people in this age group, have OCD in a given year
Post-traumatic stress disorder (PTSD)	Approximately 7.7 million US adults aged 18 and older, or about 3.5% of people in this age group, have PTSD in a given year
Generalized anxiety disorder (GAD)	Approximately 6.8 million US adults, or about 3.1% of people aged 18 and over, have GAD in a given year
Social phobia	Approximately 15 million US adults aged 18 and over, or about 6.8% of people in this age group, have social phobia in a given year

Source: National Institute on Mental Health

1.3 Etiology of mental illness

The specific causes of mental illnesses are largely unknown. The pathways leading to mental disorders involve an enormously complex set of interactions. Multiple factors involving genetic predispositions and environmental influences contribute to the development of mental disorders. *Mental Health: A Report of the Surgeon General* identifies the roots of mental illness as some combination of biologic and environmental factors; however, the document cautions against thinking that any one gene is responsible for any mental disorder. In all likelihood small variations in many genes disrupt healthy brain functioning, and under certain environmental conditions this disruption can result in mental illness.

1.4 The burden of mental illness

Given the significant numbers of people with a mental illness, nearly two-thirds of affected individuals fail to seek treatment. Several factors contribute to this reality; they are part of the world within which people with mental illnesses and their families contend.

1.4.1 Stigma

Mental illnesses are exceedingly stigmatized, evoking fear and prejudice based on misunderstanding and misconceptions of these conditions. This stigma is not limited to the public itself but to professionals as well. Misconceptions have ranged from attributing mental illnesses to demonic possession to blaming victims for their problems. This stigmatization has led to discrimination and intolerance based on ignorance of mental illness itself. Stereotyping has had profound consequences for individuals with mental illnesses and their families. It has discouraged public sympathy for the traumatic life dislocation of people with brain disorders, and has prevented public policy from allocating resources (such as medication parity) that would meet their needs. For example, many health plans cover the costs of psychotropic medications at far lower rates than they do for other medications.

Of great concern is the role that stigma plays with children in that it can lead parents to avoid seeking treatment that could dramatically improve their children's condition. Children with psychiatric disorders are stigmatized as much as their adult counterparts by both other children and adults. In a large study of US parents, 30% said they would not want their child to become friends with a child who had depression, and 25% said the same about a child with attention-deficit hyperactivity disorder. Almost 20% of the sample said they would not want a child with either disorder to live next door. Responses to the same questions substituting a "physical" illness were much more generous and understanding. Similar levels of stigmatization have been found repeatedly across other studies with others, such as adolescents, adults, and geriatric populations.

In the policy arena, research funding for the treatment of mental illnesses is often far lower than funds allocated for funding of other disease states. At an individual level, people with mental illness must deal with a painful level of rejection, isolation, and discrimination that erodes their self-assurance and can systematically undermine their self-confidence. People with mental illness are often discounted and invalidated. In the late 1990s when patients and families reported to state officials that they were being mistreated in private mental hospitals, they were dismissed by their third-party payers and regulators until investigative journalists exposed very real instances of systematic abuse. The very label of a mental illness can lead patient behavior to be needlessly pathologized. Stigma builds or reinforces interpersonal, financial, employment, and social barriers to accessing care.

1.4.2 The context of treatment

The President's New Freedom Commission on Mental Health was charged with studying the mental-health care delivery system, identifying the problems and gaps, and recommending changes that would facilitate better outcomes for adults and children with serious mental and emotional conditions. Spanning 12 months of document review, interview with patients, families, providers, and experts, the Commission declared that the mental health delivery system in the US is fragmented and in disarray and that fragmentation too often lead to unnecessary and costly disability, homelessness, school failure and incarceration. Particularly devastating was its conclusion that the US mental health system was not oriented to the most important goal of the people it serves: the hope of recovery.

The fragmented mental-health care delivery system in the US often provides inadequate, inappropriate, or no care. It is very difficult for clients and their families to determine what services are needed and where to find them. The majority of inpatient mental health settings provide services based on a traditional model of care that is often uninformed by recovery-oriented principles or research. This traditional approach is often characterized by paternalistic attitudes, staff-to-patient power differentials, homogenized treatment practices, a lack of voice from the individuals being served, outdated programming, and blatant discrimination as to language practices and policies in inpatient settings.

Common practices include talking about people as if they are their disease ("schizophrenics"), documentation in the medical record that is pejorative ("needy," "attention-seeking" or "manipulative"), arbitrary wake-up and bedtime rules, and expectations that patients and their families will passively accept treatment team recommendations that they may not have been involved with developing. These conventions can be experienced as patronizing, shaming, and disrespectful, and they can contribute to lack of trust, lack of treatment adherence, and poor outcomes.

Poor outcomes also result from the lack of resources for effective care. While the effectiveness of psychotropic medications has reduced the need for hospitalization when hospitalization is necessary, lengths of stay in hospitals have decreased. Managed care companies often mandate certain types of treatment, favoring short-term time-limited approaches, even when a person's needs are for longer, more intensive treatment. For these and other reasons, many patients are being discharged from hospitals and long-term facilities when they lack the skills to survive or live adaptively outside institutionalized settings.

To recover and become completely well, patients must be reintegrated into their communities. The money for treatment must follow them back into their community to be used for appropriate and accessible care. Coordination and collaboration among agencies providing services are needed but, as the New Freedom Commission concluded, they are lacking.

1.5 The recovery movement

Historically, people with serious and persistent mental illness have generally been viewed as a marginalized population of human beings who suffered from a chronic, unremitting illness for which there was no "cure." This widely accepted belief destined people with severe and persistent mental illness (SMI) to live without hope of ever attaining the usually expected adult roles in society, such as student, spouse, employee, parent, or homeowner. This pervasive belief also assumed that a person with SMI could expect a life characterized and defined as a "patient" and by "hospitalizations" and that the diagnosis of SMI was akin to a death sentence. People with these illnesses, their families, and the professional licensed and non-licensed staff who were providing healthcare services for them were both directly and subtlety trained to accept this view and to believe that the best outcome that could be hoped for was longer remissions of florid symptoms and a lifelong need for professional care.

In the last three decades, this pessimistic view has been radically challenged and a new theoretical model postulated. Beginning with the emergence of the consumer movement, people labeled with a SMI diagnosis have tried to communicate to us what works for them and what does not. These early pioneers and advocates identified, documented and lived their truths; that recovery from SMI was possible and was occurring, often with very little help from the public mental healthcare establishment. These courageous people were recovering from schizophrenia, bipolar illness, major depressions, and from labels of personality disorder. They spoke and wrote about a phenomenon of recovery that did not seem to be predicated on symptoms, but rather on social supports, adequate medical care when needed, the provision of hope and opportunities that involved real choices and real life. From the 1930s to the early 1980s this grassroots movement received little attention and its proponents often were seen as anomalies.

The *Mental Health: A Report of the Surgeon General* published in 1999 included a comprehensive description of the phenomenon of recovery and described it as having a tremendous impact on "consumers," their families, mental health research, and service delivery. The report credited this turnaround in attitudes as a result of the consumer movement. Recovery had become a rallying cry and a demanded outcome by consumers, their families and advocacy organizations, even while current philosophies, treatments and attitudes continue unchanged in many settings.

1.6 Vision of a transformed mental health system

The New Freedom Commission's report clearly identified the vision of a transformed mental health system when it stated that a successful transformation rested on two principles: (a) services and treatments must be consumer and family centered, geared to give individuals real and meaningful choices about treatment options and providers – and not oriented to the requirements of bureaucracies, and (b) care must focus on increasing the individual's ability to successfully cope with life's challenges, on facilitating recovery, and on building resilience, not just managing symptoms.

In addition to the vision of recovery as a guiding theme, priority goals include: the need to make mental-health care services consumer and family driven, to reduce discrimination and coercion, to eliminate disparities in service provision, to adopt and use promising and evidence-based practices, and to use technology to improve access to care and to information. These goals reflect strong philosophical and value-laden statements that clearly separate the current system of care from the transformed system envisioned by the Commission.

Further Reading

Anthony, W.A., Cohen, MR., Farkas, M.D., and Gagne, C. (2002) *Psychiatric Rehabilitation*, 2nd edn, Boston University, Center for Psychiatric Rehabilitation, Boston, MA.

Centers for Disease Control and Prevention, Atlanta, GA (2008) National Center for Injury Prevention and Control, Centers for Disease Control and Prevention. Web-based Injury Statistics Query and Reporting System (WISQARS). Available at: www.cdc.gov/ncipc/wisqars.

Fink, P.J. and Tasman, A. (1992) *Stigma and Mental Illness*, American Psychiatric Press, Washington, DC.

Kessler, RC., Chiu, WT., Demler, O. *et al.* (2005) Prevalence, severity and comorbidity of twelve-month DSM-IV disorders in the National Comorbidity Survey Replication (NCS-R). *Archives of General Psychiatry*, **62** (6), 617–627.

Lefley, H.P. (1989) Family burden and family stigma in major mental illness. *American Psychologist*, **44**, 556–560.

Mental Health: A Report of the Surgeon General. Available at: http://www.surgeongeneral.gov/library/mentalhealth/home.html.

Mohr, W.K. (1994) The private psychiatric hospital scandal: a critical social approach. *Archives of Psychiatric Nursing*, **8** (1), 4–8.

Murray, C.J.L. and Lopez, A.D. (1996) *The Global Burden of Disease: A Comprehensive Assessment of Mortality and Disability from Diseases, Injuries and Risk Factors in 1990 and Projected to 2020*, Global Burden of Disease series, vol. **1**, Harvard School of Public Health, Cambridge, MA.

National Institute on Mental Health (2008) The numbers count: mental disorders in America. Available at: http://www.nimh.nih.gov/health/publications/the-numbers-count-mental-disorders-in-america/index.shtml.

Rosenhan, D.L. (1973) On being sane in insane places. *Science*, **179**, 250–258.

The President's New Freedom Commission on Mental Health. Available at: http://www.mentalhealthcommission.gov/reports/reports.htm.

World Health Organization (2004) *The World Health Report 2004: Changing History. Annex Table 3: Burden of Disease in DALYs by Cause, Sex, and Mortality Stratum in WHO Regions, Estimates for 2002*, World Health Organization, Geneva, Switzerland. Available at: http://www.who.int/whr/2004/annex/topic/en/annex_3_en.pdf.

The Therapeutic Relationship

2.1 Introduction

Patients who are experiencing psychiatric problems are often frightened and they are vulnerable. This vulnerability is a function of more than their individual emotional distress; it exists within a context of cultural stigma and a mental health system that the President's New Freedom Commission in America asserts is a maze that is fragmented and in disarray. Building a relationship and communicating with them presents challenges for all clinicians. While such a relationship can be highly rewarding, meeting these challenges requires skills, knowledge, and perceptiveness in order to discern what will be most helpful to psychiatric patients and their families.

This chapter focuses on the importance of the therapeutic relationship and effective rapport with patients and their families. It explores dimensions of caregivers' attitudes and behaviors that can enhance or detract from the development and maintenance of a working relationships. The main goal of this chapter is to provide a guide for productive interaction with patients and their families.

2.2 Rapport

Rapport can occur in any social situation. The type of rapport developed in therapeutic situations has its own special characteristics and serves as the building block upon which the relationship rests and it is one means by which a patient achieves therapeutic outcomes. Rapport involves the interpersonal influences arising between patient and clinician that can support the patient's desire to be involved in therapy and to participate with the clinician in constructing a new vision of possibilities. Early in the relationship the patient communicates a need for help with pain, the clinician acknowledges the pain and offers help.

In this early stage of rapport development, shared recognition of the patient's pain helps to establish the working relationship and serve as the foundation for planning and initiating interventions. A clinician's ability to empathize, to understand in feeling terms every patient's subjective experience, is important to the development of rapport. Empathy is particularly important in complex interpersonal behavioral problems in which the environment (family, friends, schools, caretakers) may wish to expel the patient, and the patient has therefore lost hope. For example, suicidal patients and adolescents involved in intense family conflicts can often be convinced to cooperate with an evaluation only when the clinician has shown accurate empathy early in meeting with the patient. When the clinician acknowledges the patient's pain, the patient feels less alone and inevitably more hopeful. This rapport establishes a set of principles of – and expectations for – future

Fundamentals of Psychiatry, First Edition. Allan Tasman and Wanda K. Mohr.
© 2011 John Wiley & Sons, Ltd. Published 2011 by John Wiley & Sons, Ltd.
This chapter is based on Chapter 2 (Amy M. Ursano, Stephen M. Sonnenberg, Robert J. Ursano) of *Psychiatry, Third Edition*

interaction. More elaborate goals and responsibilities of the patient can be developed on this basic building block.

2.3 Listening to the patient

Professionals working with people whose illnesses are expressed through disturbances of thought, perception, emotion, and behavior are called upon to have special expertise in establishing the therapeutic relationship which, along with rapport, is heavily dependent on the ability to listen.

Therapeutic listening defies straightforward definition. However one defines the process it requires exquisite sensitivity to the storyteller and the ability to integrate a humanistic orientation with that of a diagnostician and problem-solver. The listener's intent is to uncover what is wrong and at the same time find out who the patient is, employing tools of asking, looking, testing, and clarifying. Patients are active informers and partners in this process. Listening work takes time, concentration, imagination, a sense of humor, respect, and an attitude that places patients as the heroes of their own stories. Clinicians of all disciplines and theoretical persuasions must learn and use the skill of listening.

Listening is not the same as hearing. Therapeutic listening involves hearing and understanding the speaker's words, attending to inflection, metaphors, imagery, sequence of association, and interesting linguistic selections. It also involves seeing movements, gestures, facial expressions and looking for subtle changes in these, comparing what is being said and seen with what was previously communicated and observed. Not only must the skilled listener attend to what is said, but it is crucial to observe what is omitted or what is evaded, as important meanings can be embedded in what is left out of a patient's story or narrative. Key listening skills are listed in Table 2.1.

2.4 The therapeutic relationship

The therapeutic relationship is a collaborative social process based on reciprocal trust, respect and professional intimacy. This relationship is a mini-ecology within which the work of healing takes place. It requires the appropriate use and balance of knowledge, empathy, and power. In its generic form, it is characterized by the collaboration between expert clinicians and help-seekers to identify, understand and solve problems. The therapeutic relationship is the central medium through which all psychiatric care is provided.

Table 2-1	Listening skills
Skill	**Description**
Hearing	Connotative meaning of words
	Idiosyncratic language
	Figures of speech that tell a deeper story
	Voice tones and modulation
	Stream of association
Seeing	Posture
	Gestures
	Facial expressions
	Other outward expressions of emotion
Comparing	Noting what is omitted or evaded
	Dissonances between modes of expression
Intuiting	Attending to one's own internal reactions
Reflecting	Thinking it all through outside the immediate pressure to respond during the interview

Certain key elements must exist for a therapeutic relationship to develop. These elements include trust, mutual respect, caring, self-awareness and partnership.

2.4.1 Trust

As in all close relationships, the foundation of a therapeutic relationship is trust. People with mental health problems may be particularly reluctant to trust others because they are in emotional pain and may fear being misunderstood. Clinicians must earn patients' trust through their caring presence and sensitive interactions. Some behaviors that foster the development of trust include predictability, consistency, and clear expectations.

Trust is also based on the knowledge that one is accepted without judgment. Mental health problems are often accompanied by shame about socially alienating symptoms (e.g., hallucinations, flashbacks, withdrawal) and an inability to manage relationships with others. Patients need to know that clinicians will not blame, fear, or look down on them. This means that clinicians must gain a level of comfort with psychiatric symptoms so that they can fully accept patients regardless of their level of functioning.

2.4.2 Mutual respect

A therapeutic relationship is based on mutual respect. Although the stigma surrounding mental illness has decreased with greater awareness of the biologic and genetic factors that contribute to patients' conditions and wider use of mental health services, patients and their families still encounter negative and condescending attitudes.

Families of people with mental illnesses often fear being criticized or blamed for causing their loved one's problems. This fear may be rooted in the long history of psychological theories that attributed psychiatric disorders to childhood traumas and family dynamics. Mental illness places a great strain on families who cope daily with such problems as mood swings, unpredictable behavior, and continual dependence on others. In most cases families are doing the best they can to help their loved ones while also coping with their own, often stressful circumstances.

In a therapeutic relationship, respect must be both given and received. Clinicians will need to set limits when patients are disrespectful so that the boundaries of the relationship remain intact. A calm, non-defensive, and respectful demeanor will help to set the tone for professional interaction and reduce unproductive and potentially relationship-destroying emotional outbursts.

2.4.3 Caring

Creating a therapeutic relationship involves expending time and energy. Caring means having the energy and optimism to keep trying to help patients, even in the face of discouragement. Caring also involves showing empathy for patients by listening to their points of view and trying to understand their experiences. Rogers identified three major ingredients of effective helping relationships: empathy, genuineness, and unconditional positive regard.

Empathy can be defined as emotional knowing of another person, going beyond only data about the patient's history, symptoms or disease state; it means feeling what it must be like to be that person. Empathy involves listening carefully, being in tune with what others are saying, and having insight into the meaning of their thoughts, feelings, and behaviors.

Genuineness involves being a real person, truly engaged in knowing and being with the patient in an open, human exchange.

The third key component of helping relationships, *unconditional positive regard*, recognizes that patients are worthy of respect, attention and acceptance regardless of their behavior and despite their flaws and setbacks.

2.4.4 Partnership

Historically, relationships between mental health clinicians and patients have been unequal. The professional was seen as the healer, and the patient was viewed as a relatively passive recipient of treatment. Current approaches across all areas of healthcare, however, emphasize the role of the patients and families as active partners in care. Therapies focus on mutual problem-solving, planning treatments jointly, and empowering patients to care for themselves. The process of partnership involves power sharing and negotiation. Families and loved ones are viewed as an invaluable resource for patients, who are now cared for mostly in community settings, often depending on their families for daily support. While it is true that, in the therapeutic relationship, the professional exercises a certain amount of power over the patient through the use of language and techniques of persuasion and by assuming control of the agenda, the aim of the relationship should be to create a collaborative and open affiliation in which the patient feels free to identify needs, desires, and goals.

2.5 Mediating factors affecting the therapeutic relationship

2.5.1 Self-awareness

Interacting with people who are in emotional pain requires a certain level of maturity and self-awareness. Psychiatric clinicians consider self-awareness to be a precondition for establishing therapeutic relationships; they must be able to monitor and contain their own anxiety when patients discuss frightening incidents or relate tragic events that generate feelings of hopelessness and despair. Being able to listen to patients without mentally or physically fleeing from the situation or offering impersonal platitudes is a key ingredient to a therapeutic relationship. The patient must feel safe with the helping professional and free from the burden of the clinician's own reactions.

Developing self-awareness is a lifelong process that requires continual work. It necessitates disciplined attention to one's own feelings and needs, as well as insight about how to meet those needs. Knowing one's own limits, detecting signs of becoming exhausted or less tolerant, and being able to nourish oneself physically, mentally, and spiritually is essential to becoming a therapeutic agent for others.

2.5.2 Cultural sensitivity

Clinicians should strive to exhibit sensitivity to a patient and his or her family's cultural background and religious beliefs. An awareness of how the patient's cultural background influences values, family functioning, and beliefs helps clinicians to interact effectively and avoid offending patients. For example, in many traditional Hispanic families, acknowledging the father as the head of the family is important. In many African-American families, extended family members such as grandparents and aunts are often key figures, viewed as central to the family's everyday life. Clinicians should attempt to set aside their own concepts of family structure and learn more about how each patient's family relates so that they do not exclude or minimize the importance of people who can influence the patient's recovery and assist with planning care in the community.

Religious beliefs are an important resource for coping with emotional problems. Sometimes they serve as the most important source of strength from the patient's perspective. Patients need to be able to share their beliefs without fear of offending the clinician or provoking judgment. If patients are afraid that their feelings or behavior conflicts with their religious faith or that they have alienated themselves from their religions, a referral to a chaplain may be helpful.

2.5.3 Transference and counter-transference

Transference is the tendency humans have to see someone in the present as being like an important figure from our past. This process occurs outside our conscious awareness and may be a way for the brain to make sense of current experience by seeing the past in the present and limiting the input of new information. Transference is more common in surroundings that provoke anxiety and provide few cues as to how to behave, such as hospital settings. It can influence a patient's behavior and can distort the therapeutic relationship therapeutically or as an impediment. Although transference is a distortion of the present reality, it is usually built around a kernel of reality that can make it difficult for the inexperienced clinician to recognize rather than react to the transference.

Transference is ubiquitous and is part of clinicians' day-to-day experience. Recognizing transference in the therapeutic relationship can aid the clinician in understanding the patient's deeply held expectations of help, shame, injury, or abandonment that derive from childhood experiences.

Transference reactions are not confined to patients; clinicians also superimpose the past on the present, a process called *counter-transference*. Counter-transference is believed to be inevitable and, like transference, it can be damaging or can play an important role within the relationship context. The emotional responses evoked by a patient may provide clinicians with some sense of who patients are, how they relate to others, what their internal world is like, and what a relationship with this patient may involve.

Counter-transference can be manifested in many ways. A clinician's feelings of failure in the face of difficult-to-treat patients can evoke feelings of hopelessness. The wish to rescue a patient is commonly experienced by clinicians. Such wishes indicates a need to look for counter-transference responses. More subtle factors, such as the effects of being overworked, can result in unrecognized feelings of deprivation leading to unspoken wishes for a patient to quit treatment. When these feelings appear in subtle counter-transference reactions, such as being late to appointments, or being unable to recall previous material, they can have powerful effects on the patient's wish to continue treatment. Major developmental events in clinicians' personal lives can also influence their perceptions of their patients. For example, a clinician with a dying spouse may be unable to empathize with a patient's concerns about loss of a job, feeling that it is trivial. Clinicians are encouraged to pay close attention to their feelings of counter-transference, and to seek peer review and supervisory guidance as needed. Rather than eliminating counter-transference altogether, the goal is to use those feelings productively rather than harmfully.

2.5.4 Phases of the therapeutic relationship

The treatment phase – early, middle, or late – affects the structure of the therapeutic relationship with respect to issues to be addressed and the tasks to be negotiated by clinician and patient.

The early stage of treatment involves developing a rapport, formulating goals, and initiating the working alliance. It is important that patients know what they can expect, hence patient education is important to the success of the therapeutic relationship in this early stage. During the introductory phase of the relationship, patients may test the clinician's commitment by acting out or missing appointments. They may exhibit their worst behavior (e.g., challenging, withdrawal) in an attempt to see whether the clinician can handle the intensity of their problems. When this happens, clinicians should remain consistently available, caring, and respectful toward the patient.

The middle stage is marked by refinement of goals and attempting various interventions. While this is happening, transference and countertransference are likely to emerge. Their recognition and management is critical to an ongoing and therapeutic process.

As a part of the termination process, clinicians and patients review what they have learned, discuss what changes have taken place in patients and their lives, and acknowledge the feelings that leave-taking evoke. The termination process involves a loss, even if therapeutics have been brief or unpleasant. If substantial work has been done, both parties may feel the loss of the helping relationship. If goals have not been realized because of time constraints or the limitations of the relationship, the termination may seem less significant.

Patients often regress during the termination phase. Anxiety over the loss of the relationship contributes to reverting to previous maladaptive behaviors. The patient's historical way of dealing with losses may manifest itself during the termination phase. Some patients feel rejected, others withdraw prematurely to protect themselves from the pain of grieving, and others try to end the relationship angrily and abruptly.

During the termination phase, the clinician's job is to remain consistent, caring, and hopeful about the patient's progress. This is the time to review the work that has been done, discuss any remaining questions, clear up misconceptions, and applaud the patient's progress in making changes. On a more human level, it is a time for remembering the high points in the relationship, acknowledging and letting go of the low points, and appreciating the time that the clinician and patient have spent together.

2.6 Other issues affecting the therapeutic relationship

2.6.1 Treatment settings

The clinician–patient relationship takes place in a variety of treatment settings. These include the private office, community clinic, emergency room, inpatient psychiatric ward, teaching hospital clinic, and general hospitals. These are described more fully in Chapter 6. Each setting uniquely affects the clinician–patient relationship. For example, the limits of confidentiality are necessarily extended when practice takes place outside of a private office setting. A private office setting may enable the clinician to establish rapport more rapidly with a patient, but it can also be isolating for the clinician. Working with a team of professionals can enhance or impede therapeutic progress.

Although troubling ecologies exist, few textbooks discuss the toxic environment and its insidious effect on clinicians and patients. The history of mental health has not always been pretty, despite the progress that has been made. In psychiatric settings, people with mental illness are vulnerable. Clinicians and clinical staff are in a position of power. This power comes from not only their position, but also their status as members of a profession with specialized knowledge that patients and their families may not have. The power differential is even greater in locked units to which patients have been involuntarily committed. In the past, patients have been unnecessarily incarcerated simply because they have lucrative insurance policies, or they have been subjected to capricious punishment by staff members, or they have been secluded for hours, and death and injury have happened proximal to restraint use that may or may not have been a necessary intervention. The individual clinicians practicing in these environments were not evil persons, but strong social forces were in operation in each case and people assumed certain roles and behaviors that were inconsistent with their codes of ethics.

Social scientists have concluded that human beings have a tendency to overestimate the importance of dispositional factors or qualities and to underestimate the importance of situational qualities when trying to understand behaviors. Otherwise good people are capable of callousness and cruelty toward their fellow human beings. Moreover, such actions tend to be tolerated and even reinforced by the hierarchy and by peers. The take-home point of this section is that practice environments are not immune to toxicity. Although we may think of ourselves as having a consistent and stable personality across time and space, we are not always the same people working alone as we are working in a group. It is not sufficient to be aware of only one's internal dynamics. Clinicians must be as aware of the ecologies in which they find themselves and be prepared to deal with these powerful forces.

2.6.2 Third-party payer system

Managed care, broadly defined as any care of patients that is not determined solely by the provider, currently focuses on the economic aspects of delivering medical care, with little attention to its potential effects on the clinician–patient relationship. Discontinuity of care and the creation of unrealistic expectations on the part of patients have been raised as likely deleterious effects on that relationship. Other issues that can affect the physician–patient relationship include the erosion of confidentiality, shrinkage of the types of reimbursable services, and diminished autonomy of the patient and clinician in decision-making about treatment.

Many managed care systems dictate a split treatment model, with a psychiatrist or advanced practice nurse prescribing psychopharmacologic treatment and a separate clinician providing psychotherapy. In such a system, there are complicated challenges faced by both clinician and patients. With neither party in complete control of decisions, the therapeutic relationship can become increasingly adversarial and subservient to external issues such as cost, quality of life, political expediency, and social efficiency. Clinicians can best serve their patients by continuing to conduct thorough diagnostic assessments covering the biological, psychological, and social aspects of the patients' conditions to determine the most effective plan for treatment. This plan should be openly shared with patients regardless of whether economic considerations render it infeasible. The clinician and patient may then work together to make the best of what is possible, both aware of the societal and individual factors influencing their actions.

2.6.3 Stress and burnout

Some behaviors of patients are more stressful to deal with than others, including suicidal threats or actions, violence, and passive aggression. They drain clinicians, leaving them personally and professionally depleted, especially when dealing with acutely ill patients and challenging behaviors. Burnout is a problem in all of the helping professions, including medicine, social work, psychology, and teaching. Some warning signs of burnout are loss of energy and enthusiasm, fatigue, and insomnia. Increasing burnout leads to more severe consequences: physical illness or exhaustion, withdrawal, mood changes, depression, hopelessness, and increased use of alcohol and drugs.

Positive coping with job-related stress and burnout requires a concerted effort. Clinical supervision, support systems at home and work allow clinicians to express feelings and keep situations in perspective. Clinicians need to cultivate realistic expectations from their practice, from their jobs, and from themselves. Frequent, brief vacations may be more relaxing and refreshing than infrequent, longer ones. Paying attention to one's health needs brings great returns in stress reduction and increased satisfaction with life. Stress and burnout can be minimized through self-awareness: early detection of stress symptoms, self-care measures, involvement in non-work activities, and setting and maintaining professional and personal priorities.

Clinical Vignette

A young man sought treatment for ill-defined reasons: he was dissatisfied with his work, his social life, and his relationship with his parents. He was unable to say how he thought the psychiatrist could help him, but he knew he was experiencing emotional pain: he felt sadness, anxiety, inhibition, and loss of a lust for living. He wanted help. The psychiatrist noted the patient's tentative style and heard him describe his ambivalence toward his controlling and directing father. With this in mind, the psychiatrist articulated the patient's wish for help and recognized with him his confusion about what was troubling him. She suggested that through discussion they might define together what he was looking for and how she might help him. This description of the evaluation process as a joint process of discovery established a rapport based on shared work that removed the patient's fears of control and allowed him to feel heard, supported, and involved in the process of regaining his health.

KEY POINTS

- The therapeutic relationship is a collaborative social process based on reciprocal trust, respect and professional intimacy necessitating the establishment of rapport.

- Therapeutic rapport involves the interpersonal influences arising between patient and clinician that can support a patient's desire to be involved in therapy and to participate in the therapeutic process.

- Rapport is heavily dependent on the ability to listen, a skill involving time, concentration, imagination, a sense of humor, and respect – among other qualities.

- The foundation of a therapeutic relationship is trust.

- Mutual respect, caring, empathy, genuiness, and partnership are crucial elements of the therapeutic relationship.

- Other factors mediating the therapeutic relationship are self-awareness, cultural sensitivity, transference and counter-transference, treatment setting, third-party payer issues, stress, and burnout.

- The treatment phase – early, middle, or late – affects the structure of the therapeutic relationship with respect to issues to be addressed and the tasks to be negotiated by clinician and patient.

Further Reading

Egan, G. (2009) *The Skilled Helper: A Problem Management and Opportunity Development Approach*, 9th edn, Cengage Learning, Florence, KY.

Farrow, T. and Woodruff, P. (2007) *Empathy in Mental Illness*, Oxford University Press, London.

Hicks, S.F. and Bien, T. (2008) *Mindfulness and the Therapeutic Relationship*, Guilford, New York.

More, E.S. and Milligan, M.A. (1994) *Empathic Practitioner: Empathy, Gender and Medicine*, Rutgers University Press, New Brunswick, NJ.

Trout, J.D. (2009) *The Empathy Gap: Building Bridges to the Good Life and the Good Society*, Penguin, New York.

Zimbardo, P.G. (2008) *The Lucifer Effect*, Random House, New York.

3

An Integrative Approach to Developmental Psychopathology

3.1 Introduction

An integrative approach to patient care as understood in this text acknowledges the complexity and uniqueness of the whole person within his or her contexts, and makes use of many means of understanding them. Affirming the collaborative relationship between patient and caregiver, this approach assumes that professionals work with patients to develop appropriate individualized therapeutic approaches that are informed by evidence in order to achieve optimal health and healing. The chapter concerned with the biological bases of psychopathology (Chapter 5) discusses genetics and other ontogenic mediators of psychiatric illness in more depth. Although it is an oversimplification to separate biology from environment, as they have reciprocal influences on each other, we have chosen to break out the topics while underscoring that any separation of nature from nurture is artificial.

This chapter presents a conceptualization of developmental psychopathology, the multidimensionality of individuals who present for treatment, and briefly discusses normal development. It also includes an examination of the concept of resiliency, and contextual variables that present risk to individuals during different stages of their lives, and how psychiatric illness might present itself across the lifespan.

3.2 Toward a comprehensive, multidisciplinary understanding of psychopathology

With ongoing research, psychiatric professionals continue to develop a better understanding of the roles of biologic, psychosocial, and sociocultural factors in the development of psychopathology. It has become increasingly apparent that explanations based on only one of these factors are likely to be incomplete. Today, the field supports the belief that an interaction of several causal factors produces disorders.

One framework providing a useful heuristic for an integrative approach to psychopathology was developed by Dante Cicchetti and his colleagues. This framework incorporates several different theories and perspectives into an all-inclusive conceptual framework known as the *developmental ecological perspective* (DEP). This perspective is useful for conceptualizing the influences of risk

Fundamentals of Psychiatry, First Edition. Allan Tasman and Wanda K. Mohr.
© 2011 John Wiley & Sons, Ltd. Published 2011 by John Wiley & Sons, Ltd.

and protective factors on a person's development. It simultaneously addresses individual and environmental characteristics, emphasizing the interactive and reciprocal influences of the person, family, culture, and community. It is integrative, including the broader contexts of development and functioning. Additionally, it is informed by the genetic and neurophysiological ontogenic variables that each individual possesses. Underscoring the idea that the child's context affects his or her development, this perspective posits that contextual characteristics and events may enhance or impede a person's development and contribute to his or her adaptation or the emergence of psychopathology.

While developed originally to explain maladaptation in children, the DEP is equally valid in its application to adults. Cicchetti's perspective evolved from the work of ecology theorist Uri Bronfenbrenner, although it does not precisely reflect every aspect of Bronfenbrenner's ideas. Brofenbrenner asserted that people's contexts are crucial to understanding their development and behaviors. Cicchetti's ideas also evolved from the work of various developmental theorists who wrote that, during the course of their development, human beings must achieve *critical competencies* (such as attachment or the development of prosocial behaviors) to successfully meet the challenges of later developmental stages. Research has shown that children who do not master competency-specific tasks (e.g., prosocial behavior) are at increased risk for later social maladjustment.

The DEP draws on and integrates a number of ecological and transactional models to explain how risk and protective factors at multiple levels of an individual's ecology and prior development contribute to our understanding of the developmental consequences of exposure to certain environmental toxins and the processes that underlie maladaptive and resilient outcomes. In this conceptualization, risk and protective factors can be present at all system levels of the person's ecology. Four distinct system levels describe influences operating in the person's environment. The two most distal levels of the environment are the *macrosystem*, which includes the beliefs and values of the culture, and the *exosystem*, which includes aspects of the community in which the individual and family lives.

The more proximal levels of the environment are the *microsystem* and *ontogenic development*, and these systems exert the most direct influences on development. The microsystem includes the immediate settings in which the individual exists, most notably the family home and school. Ontogenic development consists of individual characteristics connected to the person's own development and adaptation. This developmental ecological framework addresses both individual and environmental characteristics, simultaneously emphasizing the interactive and reciprocal influences of the individuals, their family, the community, and the greater sociocultural arena in which they develop and live. It includes the broader contexts of development and functioning, and it is solidly informed by the genetic and neurophysiologic variables inherent within each unique human being (see Chapter 5).

In addition, this perspective hypothesizes that certain contextual characteristics and events may enhance or hinder an individual's development and adaptation. These contextual events can be either risk factors or protective factors. *Risk factors* are those variables that impede development and cause greater hardship. An example would be being born into extreme poverty. *Protective factors* are those variables that constitute buffers and have a helpful effect on individuals. An example would be being born into a supportive family. Examples of risk and protective factors at different levels are described in Table 3.1.

In addition to what they bring by way of their unique ontogenic characteristics (e.g., genetic endowments, temperament) within their contexts, humans continuously are exposed to a multitude of both risk and protective factors across systems that are either proximal or distal to them. *Proximal factors* are those variables that exert the strongest influence on children and to which they are more immediately exposed (e.g., parents to children). *Distal factors* are less adjacent to individuals and

Table 3-1   Examples of risk factors and their effects

Risk Factor	Biologic Effect	Psychologic Effect	Social Effect
Poverty	Malnutrition	Attachment problems	Environmental threats (e.g., community violence)
Maltreatment (abuse/neglect)	Failure to thrive, trauma effects	Disturbed affective responsiveness, attachment problems	Potential risk for suicide and/or antisocial behavior
Maternal substance abuse	Impaired prenatal central nervous system development	Inconsistent, unpredictable parenting, attachment problems	Family dysfunction
Premature birth	Increased developmental disorders or delayed/disrupted central nervous system development	Increased demands on caregivers, parental stress	Environmental destabilization

exert less powerful effects (e.g., school systems to children). Much of how persons will respond and develop is contingent on this complex web of past experiences.

This ecological and developmental view is based on theories with empirical validation, and the perspective has been advanced as a valuable way in which to frame problems of childhood psychopathology and maladaptation. Moreover, it represents the true complexity of people in their contexts. It also serves as a foundation for the kind of interagency collaboration and integration that have been promoted as a holistic and cost-effective way to deliver comprehensive care to those with serious and persistent mental illnesses and their families.

3.3 Theories of development

People and their behavior must be understood in a developmental context. When working with an individual, providers should have an awareness of the point where the person is at in his or her developmental trajectory and what influences are affecting that development. Understanding development is crucial for practitioners in that the life histories of patients demand developmental formulations to achieve a sense of understanding of the origins of the presenting symptoms and disturbing behaviors that bring the patients to psychiatric treatment.

There are many theories of human development, and new ones are emerging constantly, questioning and building on earlier discoveries. There are two classical approaches to the study of human development: the stage model and the longitudinal lines of development model. Each has distinct advantages and disadvantages. The more traditional approach is to examine each stage of development, reviewing how each capability or domain of functioning is unfolding chronologically. An alternative strategy used to teach development is to choose a particular aspect of human development and track it from birth until death. This is a helpful strategy for understanding the process of development and is useful for researchers who are searching for the antecedents of characteristics that occur during later developmental periods. Thinking about development as a series of stages, albeit a conceptually simplistic approach to the complex evolution of the human condition, nevertheless is a useful heuristic for clinicians. It also reflects how practice has unfolded traditionally, with practitioners focusing on specific areas of specialization and interest: pediatric, young adult, and older adult.

There are several domains of human development in which clinicians should be thoroughly grounded in order to understand deviations from "normal" development and the effects of risk/protective factors on these domains. These include biological considerations (including genetic, neurological, and endocronological), and cognitive, emotional, social, and moral development.

3.4 Biological considerations

3.4.1 The role of genes and environment in development

The genes a person possesses contain all of the information required to define the individual. The development of the nervous system depends on environmental as well as genetic factors. At each level and stage of development, the microenvironments and macroenvironments of the human organism play a critical role. But unfolding the genetic program with complex sequences and patterns of expression makes it difficult to separate out the relative contribution of genetic and epigenetic influences. Genes influence the environment through the production of proteins, and the environment, in turn, alters the expression of genes. This reciprocal relationship is played out over the entire course of development.

3.4.2 The role of genes and environment in psychopathology

Genes do not encode mental illnesses, nor behavior. Genes encode proteins, and in psychopathology and the development of mental illnesses individual genes code for a subtle molecular abnormality caused by a genetically altered protein. This could include proteins that regulate neurodevelopment (neuronal migration, selection, differentiation, or synaptogenesis). It could also include proteins ranging from enzymes to transporters, signal transduction molecules, synaptic plasticity factors and many more.

Current thinking about the pathway from gene to mental illness asserts that mental illnesses are not caused by a single gene, nor a single subtle genetic abnormality, but by multiple small contributions from several genes, all interacting with environmental stressors.

3.4.3 Neurological considerations

Brain growth is one of the most basic indicators of neurological development. The brain is already at approximately one-third of its adult size at birth, and it grows rapidly, reaching 60% of its adult weight by approximately 1 year and 90% of its adult weight by 5 years of age. The final 10% of growth occurs during the next 10 years with attainment of full weight by 16 years of age. The processes of myelinization, synapse proliferation, and synaptic pruning occur in the course of the lifespan, but they are particularly active in the first years of life when the functional structure of the brain is becoming defined. Maximum synaptic density is reached at different development time points in different brain regions.

The establishment of biological rhythms occurs in early infancy, as sleep becomes more organized and of shorter nocturnal duration. A stable pattern of temperament gradually becomes established during the second year. Neurons and neuronal networks are use-dependent and, during the preschool period, individual neurons and neural networks are preferentially preserved if they receive stimulation. Motor skills emerge as a reflection of the underlying neuronal development of the central nervous system. By the age of 7 years, considerable sensory integration has occurred. Handedness has been clearly established, and brain plasticity has decreased. In the years of adolescence, full brain weight is achieved, but myelinization continues well into the fourth decade. By the end of the fifth decade, there is often evidence of the beginning of decline in specific neuronal functions, with vision and memory being particularly vulnerable. However, integrative capacities may reach a peak during the later decades.

3.4.4 Endocronological considerations

Hormonal development occurs from the first years of life, but the most dramatic changes in both physical and emotional functions are triggered by the hormonal shifts associated with puberty. In girls, estradiol and progesterone production results in the onset of breast development, followed by the onset of pubic hair growth and vaginal elongation, and finally development of axillary hair. Although there is wide variability in different cultural environments, menarche is usually attained 2 years after the onset of breast development with the average age reported at 12.8 years.

In boys, puberty begins when rising levels of pituitary hormone result in enlargement of the testes and subsequent increases in circulating testosterone. Spermatogenesis occurs after testicular enlargement at approximately 14 years. Pubic hair development is triggered by adrenal androgens and progresses over the course of about 2.5 years. Facial hair tends to develop at between 14 and 15 years of age.

Growth hormone and gonadal hormones are both necessary to initiate the adolescent growth spurt. This occurs earlier in girls. Both an acceleration of bone growth and a maturation of the skeletal structure as reflected by increased bone density and closing of epiphyses occur during this process.

Sexual function peaks early in the adult years in men, but there is only a gradual decline in sexual function throughout adulthood. Women have consistent sexual functioning throughout the child-bearing years and frequently become more orgasmic in their 30s. However, decreases in estrogen levels associated with menopause usually occur at between 45 and 54 years of age. Men have no comparable menopausal change in hormonal levels.

3.5 Cognitive development

Examining cognitive development provides a perspective on the evolution of the capacity to think. Increased cognitive abilities are an integral component required for the onset of language. Changes in thinking ultimately shape the course of emotional, social, and moral development.

Jean Piaget has had the greatest historical influence on the field of child cognitive development. According to Piaget's *cognitive-developmental theory*, children are driven by heredity and environment. They construct knowledge actively as they manipulate and explore their worlds; their cognitive development occurs in stages. Children move through four broad stages, beginning with the infant's sensorimotor activity and ending with the adolescent's elaborate, abstract reasoning system. It is important to understand that Piaget's idea of "stage" is not descriptive but theoretical. It does not refer to some overt behavior but to a constellation of processes underlying a particular behavior.

Piaget's theory has been challenged with critics asserting that he underestimated the competencies of infants and preschoolers. Some adherents to Piaget's theory have modified their views of cognitive stages to suggest that changes in children's thinking are less sudden and more gradual than Piaget suggested. Some researchers recognize distinct stages of qualitative reorganization during the first three years of life, while others have abandoned the idea of cognitive stages in favor of a continuous "information-processing" approach.

The *information-processing perspective* views children as active, sense-making beings who modify their own thinking in response to environmental demands. This perspective does not subscribe to the notion of stages; rather, it presumes that thought processes are similar for people of all ages. The same thought processes in adults are found in children, but to a lesser degree. Development is seen as continuous.

Ethology theory stresses adaptation, survival, and the value of behavior in ensuring survival. This field has its origins in zoology and has become more influential in child development research in recent years. Observations of ethology scholars have led to the important concept of the *critical period,* which refers to a limited time span during which a child is prepared biologically to acquire certain adaptive behaviors but needs the support of appropriate environmental stimuli to do so. See Chapter 5 for further discussion of critical periods.

Finally, the contributions of the Russian psychologist Lev Semenovich Vygotsky have become increasingly important in child development theory. Vygotsky's perspective is sociocultural and focuses on how culture is transmitted intergenerationally. Vygotsky posited that children are active constructive beings. Unlike Piaget, he viewed cognitive development as being mediated socially and dependent upon support from adults. Rather than proceeding through stages, children acquire culturally relevant knowledge and skills gradually through cooperative dialogues with mature members of society. These dialogues become part of their thinking.

3.6 Emotional development

The emotional states of young infants can be observed from the time that they are newborns, primarily through facial expression and vocalization, and by the first few weeks their rhythms of contentment and distress can be monitored. These primary emotions continue to differentiate, and by 7–9 months of age children begin to understand that their subjective experiences and feelings can be understood by others. This leads to the possibility of caregiver capacity to harmonize or adjust their own affective responses and behaviors with that of the infant.

Social referencing is usually evident by 12 months of age, when infants turn to examine caregivers' facial expressions at times when they are confronted with potentially fearful situations or objects. In the second year of life infants become aware of their separateness from their primary attachment figure and the limitations of their control on her/his behavior. After attaining self-cognition, the child will exhibit more complex emotions of embarrassment and envy, which then evolve to feelings of shame, pride and guilt by the end of the second year.

During the preschool years, children begin to learn the nature of the relationship between emotions and behaviors and begin to understand the culturally defined rules associated with affect expression. As children move into the school years they experience the full range of adult emotions, although, in adolescence, emotions may be displayed more intensely. The most significant emotional issues in the lives of school-aged children concern personal worth, which is determined by a sense of competence and place (in family, peer group, and community). The drive to competence may be as important to the emotional and social development of the individual as libidinal drives.

3.7 Social development

The quality of the attachment relationship early in life has been shown to predict successful preschool social adaptation and a stronger sense of self-worth. Children are socially interactive from the first days of life. Between 7 and 9 months of age, infants develop separation protest and a negative reaction to the approach of a stranger. During the second half of the first year, the attachment of the infant to his or her parents evolves and it is within this context that "basic trust" is achieved.

By 18 months, play begins to be more directed toward peers, but this does not predominate until the third year of life. Along with the striving toward more personal autonomy, negative interactions emerge (the "terrible twos").

Gender differences emerge by two years of age. Boys are more aggressive and tend to play with toys that can be manipulated. Girls prefer doll play and artwork. By the end of the third year, gender preference in play has emerged, and the preference is to play with children of the same sex. This preference remains throughout childhood. Associative play, which refers to play that involves other children and the sharing of toys but does not include the adopting of roles or working toward a common goal, becomes more prominent during the preschool years. Cooperative play also emerges along with a strong tendency to include elements of pretend play into the cooperative sequences. The cultural context begins to shape the nature of social interaction even at these earliest stages of development.

During the school years, the role of peers in shaping social behavior becomes predominant. Small groups form, and the concept of clubs becomes important. Shared activities, including activities of collecting (dolls, athletic shoes etc.), are a common and important characteristic of this period. Sharing secrets and making shared rules also serve as organizing social parameters. Social humor develops, and appearance and clothing become an important social signaling system.

In adolescence and throughout the adult years, social and sexual relationships play a complex and powerful role in shaping experience. With the onset of strong sexual impulses and increasing academic and social demands in adolescence, the role of peer influences in shaping both prosocial and deviant behaviors becomes powerful.

The roles of adulthood are complex and focused on the most basic issues of marriage, parenting, working, and ultimately dealing with death.

3.8 Moral development

By the second year of life, the emergence of "moral emotions" such as embarrassment, shame, and guilt demonstrates that the beginning of a code of moral behavior, in the most primitive sense, is being established. By 36 months, most children demonstrate the internalization of parental standards even when their parents are not available to provide cues or reinforcement. The importance of emotions in the early evolution of moral behavior during the preschool years is particularly crucial and represents a distinct departure from the more traditional perspective that moral development does not occur until the establishment of concrete operation.

During the school years, the importance of rules and adhering to them become well defined. The moral code tends to be one of absolutes with strong consequences for transgressors.

The later evolution of moral principles is a complex process. With the development of abstract reasoning, adolescents progress through Kohlberg's stages of conventional morality, which entail meeting the expectations of others (stage 3) and subsequently accepting the maintenance of societal norms and rules as an appropriate standard (stage 4). These stages do not progress in a strictly sequential manner.

Stages 5 and 6, known as the principled or post-conventional stages, having to do with a view of justice superseding human-made laws, have not been easily codified and in his later years Kohlberg noted regression, inconsistency and suggested transition stages, as well as higher (stage 7) levels of moral development.

An alternative position to Kohlberg's has been posited by Carol Gilligan, who studied girls' and women's moral development. Gilligan posited that girls' moral development progressed differently from that of boys, and involved more emphasis on human relationships, as opposed to a masculine quasimathematical system for evaluating moral choices. There has been significant critical reanalysis of Gilligan's data and gender differences. For both boys and girls the development of morality reflects conventional thinking and measuring their evaluations with the rules of their society as they understand them. Although moral reasoning continues to evolve through and beyond adolescence, many of the standards that are developed for behavior during middle childhood are likely to remain internalized and used as self-evaluation measures into adulthood.

3.9 The importance of identity formation

A firm sense of personal identity is a critical achievement of adult development. This identity can change as the individual grows and develops, but a personal identity provides both an internal anchor and a stable way of relating to others in the world. Identity formation is both an internal process and a process achieved through interaction with others. It ends only when an individual develops new kinds of identification and long-term commitment to work and to others.

3.10 The emergence of mental illness

Within the developmental ecological model, the emergence of serious mental illness is seen as disrupting the resolution of a child's developmental tasks. This consideration is important, because many serious mental illnesses manifest themselves in childhood or adolescence. The individual's developmental stage and the particular tasks with which he or she is grappling determine the effects, and to some degree the trajectory, of the illness. Therefore, to understand the potential effects of any intervention, it is critical to assess and to understand the effects of proximal and distal influences in the person's environment and how those effects might be manifested in his or her behavior. This model stresses an appreciation of behavior as being developmentally based. It is also consistent with a stress–diathesis model of psychopathology that recognizes its multifactoral etiology. Biophysiologic characteristics interact and transact with environmental events. These important considerations allow clinicians across all disciplines to develop appropriate and individually crafted interventions. Multidimensionality of assessment and the importance of assessing multiple systems are discussed in Chapter 31.

3.10.1 Resilience

Resilience in humans is a phenomenon or process that reflects positive adaptation in the face of adversity or trauma. Although it is often reified, it is not something that can be directly measured; rather it is inferred on the basis of the idea of positive adaptation and risk or adversity. Risk or adversity constitutes conditions that carry high odds for maladaptation in certain domains of functioning. An example of this might be exposure to family violence. The idea of positive adaptation refers to a better than expected outcome than what might be expected with respect to exposure to the risk factor in question. Such outcomes have been identified in research studies as social competence or success at meeting stage-salient developmental tasks.

Teasing out actual operationally useful definitions of resilience is a thorny research issue. Most recently resilience researchers are more concerned with identifying vulnerability and protective factors that might mediate or modify the negative effects of adverse life circumstance, and identifying mechanisms or processes that could underlie associations that might be found.

3.10.2 Risk factors

Defining what constitutes a risk factor or condition is somewhat arbitrary, and many risk factors have been postulated. A complete discussion of risk and protective factors is beyond the scope of this chapter (see suggested readings). The four illustrative areas that are summarized in Table 3.1 have been studied extensively. Most studies document effects on broad outcomes of groups of children and families exposed to a given risk condition, and the results of these investigations provide only limited information. Moreover, an important caveat to bear in mind is that risk factors only rarely occur in isolation and their effects or sequelae may be interactive as well as cumulative.

3.10.3 Psychopathology across the lifespan

Research suggests that there is considerable stability that can be observed from childhood into adolescence for broad categories of mental disorders. Behavior disorders in childhood are associated with increased risk of a behavior disorder in adolescence; the more severe the disorder, the more likely it is to persist.

Psychopathology occurs throughout the life cycle. Certain forms of psychopathology are limited to specific stages in life, such as the autism spectrum disorders, but most can occur at any stage. Some disorders have a peak age at onset during the life cycle, which may be related to developmental themes of the stage in which they tend to develop. For example, disturbances in body image and eating behavior have peak ages of onset in adolescence and early adulthood.

From an early age, males and females differ in their susceptibility to certain disorders, the age at which they are at greatest risk, and prognosis. Boys are more susceptible to externalizing behavior disorders and girls to internalizing disorders.

Symptomatic expression of psychopathology may change in relationship to age. Disturbances in sexual functioning, for example, seem to manifest in early adulthood, while late-life risk for mood disturbances and memory or other impairments associated with the dementias are high.

KEY POINTS

- An integrative approach to patient care acknowledges the complexity and uniqueness of the whole person within his or her contexts, and makes use of many means of understanding them.

- A developmental ecological perspective (DEP) is useful for conceptualizing the influences of risk and protective factors on humans' development, simultaneously addressing individual and environmental characteristics.

- Understanding development is crucial for practitioners in that the life histories of patients demand developmental formulations to achieve a sense of understanding of the origins of the presenting symptoms and disturbing behaviors that bring the patients to psychiatric treatment.

- Within the developmental ecological model, the emergence of serious mental illness is seen as disrupting the resolution of a child's developmental tasks.

- Resilience in humans is a phenomenon or process that reflects positive adaptation in the face of adversity or trauma.

- Behavior disorders in childhood are associated with increased risk of behavior disorder in adolescence; the more severe the disorder, the more likely it is to persist.

Further Reading

Arnett, J.J. (2000) Emerging adulthood: a theory of development from the late teens through the twenties. *American Psychologist*, **55** (5), 469–480.

Arnett, J.J. (2006) The psychology of emerging adulthood: what is known, and what remains to be known, in *Emerging Adults in America: Coming of Age in the 21st Century* (eds J.J. Arnettand T.A. Tanner), American Psychological Association, Washington, DC, pp. 303–330.

Bronfenbrenner, U. ((1979) 2006) *The Ecology of Human Development: Experiments by Nature and Design*, Harvard University Press, Cambridge, MA.

Cicchetti, D.and Cohen, J.D. (eds) (2006) *Developmental Psychopathology: Risk, Disorder and Adaptation*, vol. **2**, Wiley, New York, NY.

Gilligan, C. (1993) *In a Different Voice: Psychological Theory and Women's Development*, Harvard University Press, Cambridge, MA.

Kohlberg, L. (1973) Continuities in childhood and adult moral development revisited, in: *Life Span Developmental Psychology: Personality and Socialization* (eds P.B. Baltesand K.W. Schaie), Academic Press, New York, USA.

Luthar, S.S., Burack, J.A., Cicchetti, D.,and Weisz, J.R. (eds) (1997) *Developmental Psychopathology: Perspectives on Adjustment, Risk, and Disorder*, Cambridge University Press, New York.

Luthar, S.S., Cicchetti, D., and Becker, B. (2000). The construct of resilience: a critical evaluation and guidelines for future work. *Child Development*, **71** (3), 543–562.

National Research Council (1993) *Understanding Child Abuse and Neglect*, National Academy Press, Washington, DC.

Roisman, G.I., Masten, A.S., Coatsworth, J.D. *et al.* (2004) Salient and emerging developmental tasks in the transition to adulthood. Child Development, **75** (1), 123–133.

Seanah, D.H., Boris, N.W.,and Larrieu, J.A. (1997) Infant development and developmental risk: a review of the past 10 years. *Journal of the American Academy of Child and Adolescent Psychiatry*, **36** (2), 165–178.

4

Psychiatric
Classifications

4.1 Introduction

The terminology used in the practice of psychiatry is very specific to psychiatric conditions and illnesses. Unlike other areas of medicine, psychiatric terminology is rarely used in the context of other medical disciplines. A working knowledge of psychiatric terminology and systematic medical classification of diseases is important because it serves as a communication tool for professionals.

This chapter examines the language of psychiatry. It traces the development of the American Psychiatric Association's *Diagnostic and Statistical Manual of Mental Disorders* briefly and describes the diagnostic process, the DSM's uses and shortcomings. In addition it will discuss the use and misuse of psychiatric "jargon."

4.2 Development of the diagnostic and statistical manual of mental disorders

Published by the American Psychiatric Association (APA), the DSM is the standard classification of mental disorders used by mental health professionals in the United States. There have been six editions of this collection of psychiatric nomenclature, each edition designated by a number. Historically the DSM has its genesis in the US War Department's *Technical Bulletin 203* of 1946, the *Standard Classified Nomenclature of Disease* of 1942, and the Veterans Administration Nomenclature. The *Medical 203* contained 47 mental illness diagnoses and it most heavily influenced what was to become DSM-I.

The fourth edition of the DSM (DSM-IV) was published in 1994. It contained 365 diagnoses and represented a leap forward in psychiatry in that it has eschewed the distinction between the mental and physical, considering it passé. It is unclear at this writing when a completely new DSM (DSM-V) will be ready for publication. However, because of new research information developed since the 1994 publication of DSM-IV, the APA revised its text in 2000. These text revisions (DSM-IV-TR) are minor and limited to criteria for "personality change due to a medical condition," several of the paraphilias (sexual disorders), and Tourette's disorder. In the latter two, it was no longer necessary that the person with the disorder suffer distress or impaired functioning.

4.3 Nosology, diagnoses, and the DSM

The DSM is intended to be applicable in a wide array of contexts and used by clinicians and researchers of many different orientations including biological, psychodynamic, cognitive, behavioral, interpersonal. The manual is designed to be used across settings that include inpatient,

Fundamentals of Psychiatry, First Edition. Allan Tasman and Wanda K. Mohr.
© 2011 John Wiley & Sons, Ltd. Published 2011 by John Wiley & Sons, Ltd.
This chapter is based on Chapter 40 (Michael B. First) of *Psychiatry, Third Edition*

outpatient, partial hospital, consultation-liaison, clinic, private practice, primary care, and with community populations. It is used by psychiatrists, psychologists, social workers, nurses, occupational and rehabilitation therapists, counselors, and other health and mental health professionals. It is a necessary tool for collecting and communicating among professionals.

The DSM consists of three major components: the diagnostic classification, the diagnostic criteria sets, and the descriptive text. The diagnostic classification is the list of the mental disorders that are officially part of the DSM system. Making a diagnosis consists of selecting those disorders from the classification that best reflect the signs and symptoms that are afflicting the individual being evaluated. Associated with each diagnostic label is a code, which is typically used by institutions and agencies for data collection and billing. These diagnostic codes are derived from the coding system used by all healthcare professionals in the US, known as the International Classification of Diseases (ICD-10) which will be discussed in a subsequent section of this chapter.

For each disorder included in the DSM, a set of diagnostic criteria indicates what symptoms must be present (and for how long) in order to qualify for a diagnosis, as well as the symptoms or conditions that must *not* be present. These are deemed "inclusion" and "exclusion" criteria.

The third component of the DSM is the descriptive text that accompanies each disorder. The text of the DSM systematically describes each disorder under the following headings: diagnostic features, subtypes and/or specifiers, recording procedures, associated features and disorders, specific culture, age and gender features, prevalence, course, familial pattern, and differential diagnosis.

The DSM uses a five-axis system to give a more comprehensive picture of the client's functioning. The five axes are as follows:

- Axis I – Clinical disorders consisting of all relevant major psychiatric disorders (e.g., schizophrenia, bipolar disorders, major depression).

- Axis II – Personality disorders and mental retardation (personality disorders as defined in the DSM-IV-TR are "deeply ingrained maladaptive, lifelong behavior patterns").

- Axis III – General medical conditions that are identified on the basis of a comprehensive history and physical examination, evaluation of symptoms, mental state examination, and supplementary assessment instruments. These include any medical condition (e.g., diabetes, hypertension, cystic fibrosis).

- Axis IV – Psychosocial and environmental problems (these can include stressors such a recent death of a loved one, being a victim of a crime, going through a divorce, losing one's job, among others).

- Axis V – Global assessment of functioning (GAF), written as numbers (0–100) meaning "current functioning"/"highest level of functioning in past year" with 100 being the highest optimization of functioning and 0 being the lowest.

Many patients have more than one diagnosis on the first three axes. This is known as *comorbidity* and is defined as two or more medical conditions that occur at the same time. From a psychiatric point of view, comorbidity means the coexistence of a psychiatric disorder – such as depression, anxiety, or a psychotic condition – with a chemical dependency disorder. These comorbid conditions are also referred to as "dual diagnosis." The term "comorbidity" tends to imply that the illnesses are equal, though they may not be. Disorders are listed in their order of importance for disposition and care. The multiaxial assessment helps to optimize reassessments of a patient's condition over time. It also affords a refinement of the validity of clinical diagnosis and can serve as an outcome measure of therapeutic intervention.

4.4 Validity, reliability, and limitations of the DSM

Although the DSM is universally used as a classification system, it has serious limitations. The categories are descriptions, not explanations. Clinicians must guard against the tendency to think that something has been explained when, in fact, it has only been named. In other words, giving a condition a label does not explain or confer any reality to it other than the name itself and the cluster of behaviors subsumed under it.

Also, as convenient as the DSM system is, its categories imply that sharp dividing lines exist between "normal" and "abnormal" behaviors and among different disorders. The reality, however, is that such categories are not so neat and some scholars argue that they are artificial. For example, three patients may suffer from the same disorder but the manifestations and the personal experience of that disorder will differ for each client. Also, while the DSM has criteria that specify that an individual must have, for example, six out of eight symptoms over the course of a month, it is not flexible enough to account for the individual who might have five of the eight over the course of three weeks and be in distress. Moreover, the DSM diagnostic categories differ somewhat from the taxonomies of other illnesses (e.g., hypertension, diabetes mellitus).

Although research is available to support most of the major psychiatric illnesses, many of these categories lack an empirical foundation. They were agreed upon by expert consensus and therefore are subject to question. Indeed, scholars both within and outside the psychiatric profession have criticized the DSM system. An example of such criticism and unanswered questions concerns the number of symptoms necessary for the diagnosis. If a person meets all but one of the criteria for the diagnosis, does he or she actually have the condition?

In particular, the diagnostic labels given to children have been found troublesome in that they were derived from adult categories. The most problematic issue related to this practice is that the diagnoses are not based on a comprehensive body of research on children; rather, they are derived from disorders that may have very different manifestations in adults. Depression is one such example. Moreover, making child categories downward extensions of adult categories is problematic because it assumes that children are little adults and that they can have the same adult illnesses. The reality is that some diagnoses are specific to children, while some are specific to adults.

Another caveat is that the DSM criteria may not be uniformly applicable to all cultures. Most studies on which the DSM criteria are based were conducted in the United States or Canada. The DSM lists a number of specific cultural syndromes, but that list is by no means comprehensive.

Other criticisms of the DSM among scholars include:

- It fails to clarify the exact relationship between Axis II and Axis I disorders and the way chronic childhood and developmental problems interact with personality disorders.

- Its differential diagnoses are vague and the disorders are insufficiently demarcated, resulting in excessive comorbidity especially on Axis II and in the area of childhood disorders.

- It contains little discussion of what distinguishes normal character from personality disorders.

- Numerous disorders contain a "not otherwise specified" addition. This is a catch-all addendum applied when all of the criteria for a certain disorder are not present.

- It does not speak to life circumstances, biological, and psychological processes, and lacks an overarching conceptual or explanatory framework.

- It is heavily influenced by fashion, prevailing social mores, and by the legal and business environment.

Other questions that arise about the DSM are in the area of its reliability. Diagnostic reliability concerns the likelihood that different users will assign the same diagnosis. High diagnostic reliability suggests that, if the DSM guidelines were followed, different clinicians would give the same label to a given person. A central claim about the DSM is that it is a highly reliable system. However, there is still not a major study available that shows that the DSM is used with high reliability by mental health clinicians in the practice setting.

Finally, the DSM system is not fixed. It is always a "work in progress" and should be thought of in that way. As knowledge expands, categories will appear and old ones may be revised, refined, or eliminated altogether. Because the manual omits a disorder, it does not mean that it does not exist.

Because of the space limitations of this book, complete diagnostic criteria are not listed comprehensively, rather reference is made generally to necessary signs, symptoms and other criteria. There are a number of searchable and comprehensive databases on the Internet that are freely available. The best are:

http://psyweb.com/Mdisord/DSM_IV/jsp/dsm_iv.jsp

http://www.behavenet.com/capsules/disorders/dsm4TRclassification.htm

http://allpsych.com/disorders/disorders_alpha.html.

4.5 The international classification of diseases

The International Classification of Diseases (ICD) is published by the World Health Organization and is the international standard classification for all diseases and health problems. It has been updated 12 times since its development. The tenth revision of the ICD was endorsed in 1990 and by 1994 was broadly used by the WHO member states. The ICD-10 is available in the six official languages of WHO (Arabic, Chinese, English, French, Russian, Spanish), as well as in 36 other languages.

In contrast to the DSM, the ICD provides two sets of diagnostic criteria for each disorder. One list is useful to the diagnostician and allows for some latitude and for the practitioner's exercise of judgment. The other set is far more precise and strict and intended to be used by scholars and researchers in their studies. Yet a third, simplified classification is applicable to primary care settings and contains only broad categories (dementia, eating disorder, psychotic disorder, and so on). The mental and behavioral disorders chapter, which includes all disorders of psychological development, can be accessed at http://apps.who.int/classifications/apps/icd/icd10online/.

With respect to clinical use in the United States, the DSM is the taxonomic system that is used almost exclusively. Also, with respect to diagnoses in academic psychiatry, the DSM criteria, rather than the ICD categories, are employed for the purpose of research.

4.6 Psychiatric terminology and accuracy in communication

The appendix of the DSM has a glossary of commonly employed psychiatric terms, and clinicians are encouraged to familiarize themselves with this terminology during their evaluation of cases. Psychiatric terminology is the specialized language of the mental health profession that functions as a kind of shorthand means of communication between members of the professional group.

Terminology can often be efficient and descriptive as a means of communication, but it can often be obfuscatory or pretentious, being employed to make the ordinary seem extraordinary or profound.

To the extent possible, clinicians are encouraged to use a data-based language and observations in their evaluations of patients. This is because psychiatric terminology, as opposed to data-based observations, is not theory-neutral because it is an interpretation of behavioral events.

Ideally, jargon terms should be followed by an objective observation that justifies using that term, in other words *data*. Thus, if a note in the chart indicates that a particular patient was secluded or restrained because he was were engaging in "aggressive behavior and was a threat to himself or others" it is incumbent on the professional who makes such a note to describe the aggressive behavior (e.g., was the patient kicking or choking someone or merely cursing loudly and making obscene or threatening gestures) and then to justify why these behaviors constituted a threat such that it became necessary to subject the patient to a potentially deadly intervention. The term "aggressive behavior" is subject to multiple interpretations, as is being a "threat to oneself or others" and they are often used as a shorthand way to justify restraining a patient. These terms should be operationally described and defined by the professional who is recording the events in the medical record. An operational definition of aggressive behavior would justify the use of the label as to what the person making the entry really means. It would break down the term to a series of discrete and objective descriptive observations.

Accuracy in communication is important in a legal–historical sense, because all that remains of a person's hospitalization is the medical record and the inaccurate and unreliable memories of all who are concerned with his care.

KEY POINTS

- Published by the American Psychiatric Association, the DSM is the standard classification of mental disorders used by mental health professionals in the United States.

- The DSM is intended to be applicable in a wide array of contexts and used by clinicians and researchers of many different orientations including biological, psychodynamic, cognitive, behavioral, and interpersonal.

- The DSM uses a five-axis system to give a more comprehensive picture of the client's functioning.

- In the DSM, each disorder has a set of diagnostic criteria indicating what symptoms must be present (and for how long) in order to qualify for a diagnosis, as well as those symptoms or conditions that must not be present.

- Although the DSM is a widely employed taxonomy, it has limitations, insofar as the diagnostic categories are descriptions, not explanations.

- Clinicians must guard against the tendency to think that something has been explained when, in fact, it has only been named.

- The ICD is published by the World Health Organization and is the international standard classification for all diseases and health problems.

- In order to ensure accuracy in communication, clinicians should strive for operational descriptions of behavior and not assume that all readers of assessments are conversant with psychiatric terminology.

Further Reading

American Psychiatric Association (2000) *Diagnostic and Statistical Manual of Mental Disorders Text Revision*, 4th edn, APA, Washington, DC.

Shorter, E. (1997) *A History of Psychiatry: From the Era of the Asylum to the Age of Prozac*, John Wiley & Sons, New York.

Wilson, M. (1993) DSM-III and the transformation of American psychiatry: a history. *American Journal of Psychiatry*, **150**, 399–410.

World Health Organization (2003) International Classification of Diseases, 10th revision, Clinical Modification (ICD-10-CM).

Psychiatry and the Neurosciences

5.1 Introduction

Research findings have made it abundantly clear that the brain is the organ of the mind. By the end of the twentieth century, equating a behavioral disorder with a dysfunctional brain had become a fundamental tenet in psychiatry. Just as the lungs exchange gases and the heart pumps blood, through a variety of mechanisms the brain influences and is responsible for behavior. Under the word "behavior" are subsumed all activities of the body, including respiration, fine and gross motor activity, sensory activity, as well as cognition or thought. More narrowly conceptualized, the brain is the major organ of the body that governs all forms of behavior which we observe in psychiatry and which our patients experience.

The goals of this chapter are to briefly summarize paradigms concerned with brain functions as they relate to psychiatric disorders. One operative word here is "brief," meaning that the neuroanatomical and basic neurophysiology content is *not* presented comprehensively. Moreover, knowledge in this area is vast and expanding so rapidly that to do it justice in a single chapter is impossible. Detailed information on such topics as gray and white matter, membranes, myelin sheaths, and so forth can be found in neuroanatomy textbooks. This chapter is limited to "need-to-know" rather than "nice-to-know" material. It is designed to give useful conceptual material. Clinicians can use this material to facilitate their understanding of the neuroscientific foundations of psychiatric illnesses, inform what they see in their clinical settings, and think about their interventions more creatively than generically.

The chapter explores evidence for the view that disorders that have normally been considered to be distinct entities frequently have shared or overlapping biologic underpinnings. The general relationship between brain and behavior and disorders of brain function and psychiatric disease are discussed, providing examples of evidence for biologic commonalities among different disorders. The chapter also discusses how an awareness of normal functions of different brain circuits can facilitate an understanding of the consequences of their disruption in psychiatric disease, and how dysregulation of the same brain circuits across different disorders can help clinicians understand aspects of their overlapping symptomatology. This discussion only scratches the surface of the rich neurobiology of these structures and the larger networks in which they are embedded.

Another operative word for this chapter is "relate." Because it is impossible to be exhaustive, the intention of this chapter is to relate (in a very broad sense) certain nervous system functioning to what clinicians might see in a clinical setting. For clinicians who want more in-depth information, the further reading list contains current textbooks and articles they may find especially useful.

Fundamentals of Psychiatry, First Edition. Allan Tasman and Wanda K. Mohr.
© 2011 John Wiley & Sons, Ltd. Published 2011 by John Wiley & Sons, Ltd.

5.2 Brain development

During infancy and childhood, the human brain develops rapidly, acquiring an entire set of capabilities. This process of development is sequential, from less complex to more complex capabilities, and is guided by experience. The brain modifies and changes itself in response to new experiences, with neurons and neuronal connections evolving in an "activity-dependent" manner. In other words, the activity to which the neurons are exposed drive their response. Thus, development of the brain is use-dependent. As certain neural systems are activated repeatedly, an internal representation of the experience corresponding to the neuronal activity is created in the brain. The use-dependent capacity of the brain to make such internal representations of the internal or external world suggests a basis for learning and memory.

The capacity and desire to form emotional relationships is related to the organization and functioning of specific parts of the human brain. The systems in the human brain that allow persons to form and maintain emotional relationships develop during the first years of life. Experiences during this vulnerable period are critical to shaping the capacity to form intimate and emotionally healthy relationships. This capacity is at its peak during childhood, making children far more malleable and receptive to environmental stimuli than adults. By the time children are three years old, the brain is 90% of its adult size, and the emotional, behavioral, cognitive, and social foundation is in place for the rest of life. A child's earlier repertoire of experiences provides an organizing framework or template through which subsequent experiences are filtered.

Human brains are most plastic (i.e., most receptive to environmental input) in early childhood. A child's brain organizes in a use-dependent fashion, mirroring the pattern, timing, nature, frequency, and quality of experiences. For brain development to take place, children must be exposed to appropriate sensory experiences. The consequences of sequential development are that as different regions are organizing, they require specific kinds of experiences targeting the region's specific function to develop properly. These developmental times are called *critical periods*.

The brain's ability to develop and alter in response to experience is known as *neuroplasticity*. The brain adapts to new conditions during its maturation and during its constant interaction with its environment. Stimuli that arise in the internal or external environment trigger neuroplastic mechanisms. In a sense this means that, to some degree, humans can create their own brains by exposing them to certain experiences or substances (see Chapter 18). The concept of neuroplasticity provides the foundation for learning, memory, and other complex mental processes. Neuroplasticity accounts for the brain's ability continue to grow connections, and exposure to new learning results in new brain changes, even into advanced old age.

5.3 Mind and brain in psychiatric illness

Psychiatric illnesses have been called "brain disorders," but that view masks enormous complexity. Clear, unitary, causes of symptoms are rare in psychiatry. More often, multiple causal factors, each with a small effect, act in concert to produce disease. The effects of causal factors for any one disorder include diverse genetic mechanisms, neurochemical systems, brain regions, and cellular abnormalities. The daunting complexity of psychiatric disorders poses a challenge to how one may meaningfully investigate biologic commonalities between disorders.

5.3.1 Endophenotypes

A way to come to terms with the complexity of the path from gene to mental illness is through the analysis of *endophenotypes*. These are important intermediaries along this path that assist in unraveling the contribution of genes. They are a measurable neurobiological or psychological parameter that meaningfully contributes to an aspect of a psychiatric disorder but is simpler, less heterogeneous, and more closely tied to measurable aspects of the underlying biology. Endophenotypes are inherited with, and closely linked to, the disease.

Endophenotypes may be shared across overtly distinct disorders, as can be seen by the presence of working memory impairments in schizophrenia, major depression, and attention-deficit hyperactivity disorder. Studies on endophenotypes may help bridge the explanatory gap between ultimate etiologic causes, such as genetic or environmental variables, and resulting psychiatric phenomenology.

There are two important classes of endophenotypes: biologic endophenotypes and symptom endophenotypes. Biologic endophenotypes are measurable biologic phenomena. There are many of these, ranging from the startle response to the neuroimaging response to information processing. Symptom endophenotypes are single symptoms associated with a mental illness and usually one of the DSM criteria for that illness. For example, guilt and insomnia are symptom endophenotypes that can be associated with major depressive disorder, and hallucinations and delusions are symptom endophenotypes that can be associated with schizophrenia.

One argument posits that certain discrete psychological functions are mediated through consistent, definable neural circuitry. Deficits in these psychological functions (i.e., endophenotypes) are therefore likely to be associated with abnormalities in the associated neural circuits. Furthermore, the presence of similar endophenotypes in otherwise disparate disorders predicts that related alterations may be observable in the same neural circuitry. The hypothetical path from gene to mental illness goes from the gene via molecules, circuits, and information processing (a biologic endophenotype), to symptom endophenotypes (a single symptom of a mental illness), to the full syndrome of symptoms of a mental illness.

The endophenotype approach to understanding different psychiatric disorders provides a powerful framework in which to conceptualize mental illness; namely, as a set of conditions that come about due to different combinations of endophenotypes.

5.3.2 Psychiatric genetics

After many years of study a new paradigm has emerged for genes and psychiatry. This paradigm conceptualizes genes not as direct causes of mental illness, but as direct causes of subtle molecular abnormalities that create risk for mental illness. Hence genes may act by biasing an individual's brain circuits toward inefficient information processing and possible breakdown into psychiatric symptoms under certain conditions.

Inherited, subtle molecular abnormalities in humans are not completely penetrant at the behavioral level. Some people with the same subtle molecular abnormalities and the same abnormal biologic endophenotypes in the same circuits can develop symptoms, while others do not. It is hypothesized that this may be due to the fact that genes exert variable effects throughout life and that it may depend on whether a person has a healthy compensatory back-up system for the abnormality or if there are additional genetic biases, molecular abnormalities, and additional independent causes of symptoms in the same circuitry.

5.3.3 The stress–diathesis model

The diathesis–stress model of psychiatric disorders hypothesizes that people are predisposed toward a particular mental or physiologic reaction and that the disorder will become manifest as a reaction to something other than genes. That "something other" is stress. Two major factors are postulated by the model: (1) individual response stereotype, consisting of a predisposition to respond physiologically to various situations and in a particular way; and (2) inadequate homeostatic restraints caused by stress-induced breakdown, toxins or trauma, or by genetic predisposition. Situational determinants play an important role, as does one's perception of the situation, which generates increased or decreased physiologic response.

A person experiencing multiple stressors and multiple genetic risks may not have sufficient back-up mechanisms to compensate for inefficient information processing within a "predisposed" circuit. The circuit may either be compensated unsuccessfully by overactivation, or it may break down and not activate at all. In either case, the abnormal biologic endophenotype would be associated with an abnormal behavioral phenotype, thereby producing a psychiatric symptom.

Although personality and individual coping styles are not postulates of this model, these can mitigate the effects of the stressor and the effects on the genome of the stressor may be negligible. Thus, good temperament, adaptability, and a healthy lifestyle can act as protective factors (see Chapter 32).

5.3.4 Neurotransmission

The basic cellular units of the nervous system are the neurons, whose function is to transmit messages and whose goal is to alter the biochemical activities of the postsynaptic target neuron in an enduring way. Neurotransmitters are chemicals that are synthesized and stored in the terminal region of the neuron. They are compounds that are released at a synapse and diffuse across the synaptic cleft to act on a receptor located on the membrane of a postsynaptic cell. The known neurotransmitters in the brain number several dozen (see Table 5.1), but there may be hundreds or thousands of these chemicals and these may ultimately prove to be important targets of pharmacotherapeutics as research emerges.

At this time a number of neurotransmitters are important clinically and clinicians should have a working knowledge of them because many of the medications used in psychiatry target them to increase or decrease their levels. Medications used in psychiatry often mimic the brain's natural neurotransmitters. The most commonly discussed neurotransmitters are sometimes referred to as the "classic" neurotransmitters. They include serotonin, dopamine, norepinephrine (noradrenaline), acetylcholine, glutamate, and gamma-aminobutyric acid. They are low-molecular-weight amines or amino acids. Other neurotransmitters, such as histamine, hormones, and various neuropeptides, are also important.

At one time it was believed that each neuron used only one neurotransmitter to send information and used that same neurotransmitter at all of its synapses. Research has shown that many neurons use more than one neurotransmitter at a single synapse. Input to each neuron at various sites also involves many neurotransmitters, and understanding these inputs is essential for combining certain medications to modify several neurotransmitters at the same time.

Neurotransmitters are referred to as "first messengers." These are molecules that communicate information or change *from one cell or cell group to another*. First messengers attach themselves to receptors outside of cell membranes and begin a cascade of events that activate receptors through second, third, fourth (and so on) messenger levels to produce an increasingly wider array of physiological effects.

Neurotransmitters can either inhibit the receptor cell or excite it. The inhibitory or excitatory nature of the neurotransmitter makes an axon discharge more or less likely. The nerve cell "decides" whether to send output as a result of the number of inhibitory or excitatory inputs it receives. Although the specific roles of neurotransmitters in the development of mental illness is not known, evidence suggests that no single neurotransmitter is responsible for any single disorder.

Table 5-1	Selected neurotransmitters
Type	**Transmitter**
Amines	Serotonin
	Dopamine
	Norepinephrine (noradrenaline)
	Epinephrine (adrenaline)
	Acetylcholine
	Tyramine
	Histamine
	Agmatine
	Octopamine
	Phenylethylamine
	Tryptamine
	Melatonin
Pituitary peptides	Corticotrophin
	Growth hormone
	Lipotrophin
	Alpha-MSH
	Oxytocin
	Vasopressin
	Thyroid stimulating hormone
	Prolactin
Hormones	Angiotensin
	Glucagon
	Insulin
	Leptin
	Estrogens
	Androgens
	Atrial natriuretic factor
	Progestins
	Thyroid hormones
	Cortisol
	Luteinizing hormone-releasing hormone
	Somoatostatin
	Thyrotropin-releasing hormone
	Growth releasing hormone
	Cholecystokinin
	Gastrin
	Motilin
	Pancreatic polypeptide
	Secretin
	Vasoactive intestinal peptide
Amino acids	GABA
	Aspartic acid (aspartate)
	d-serine
	Glycine
	Glutamate
Gases	Nitric oxide
	Carbon monoxide
Neurokinins	Substance P
	Neurokinin A
	Neurokinin B
Opiod Peptides	Dynorphin
	Beta-endorphin
	Met-enkephalin
	Leu-enkephalin
	Kyotorphin
	Nociceptin
Purines	ATP (adenosine triphosphate)
	ADP (adenosine diphosphate)
	AMP (adenosine monophosphate)
	Adenosine

5.3.5 Neurotransmission and gene expression

Chemical neurotransmission regulates the expression of genes. Neurotransmitters convert receptor occupancy by a neurotransmitter into the creation of third, fourth, and subsequent messengers, that eventually activate the transcription factors that "turn" genes on. The time that it takes from receptor occupancy by a neurotransmitter to gene expression is usually hours, but it takes longer for the gene activation to be fully implemented via the series of biochemical events that it triggers. These biochemical events can begin many hours to days after the neurotransmission occurred and can last days or weeks once they are put in motion. Understanding this process helps clinicians to appreciate the powerful effects of psychotropic drugs, as they induce prolonged alterations in brain function by influencing the brain's signal transduction pathways.

5.4 Other issues in neuroscience

5.4.1 Circadian rhythm

The word "circadian" means "about a day." Circadian rhythm can be compared to an internal clock that coordinates what happens in human bodies according to what approximates a 24-hour cycle. This cycle corresponds to the time that it takes for the Earth to spin on its axis, exposing all organisms to periods of dark, light, and temperature. The thinking on circadian rhythm is that, for the clock to function correctly, it must receive stimuli from its environment. The usual stimulus is thought to be sunlight, which seems to play a role in synchronizing body rhythms. Alterations in dark and light during the seasons are also thought to affect circadian rhythms. In some individuals, these dark–light cues can profoundly influence mood states.

5.4.2 Memory, repetition, and learning

Because of neuroplasticity, living organisms can change their behavior in response to environmental events (stimuli). This capacity underpins the ability of every life-form to learn and remember. Learning is a process that occurs when organisms take in and store information as a function of experience. Memory is the information that is stored as a result of learning. Learning results in neuronal changes at the level of existing synapses. It also results in the development of new synapses, thereby causing behavioral change. Structural changes are thought to result at the cellular level through changes in the effectiveness of existing synapses between cortical cells, through the formation of new synapses among existing cortical neurons, and through the creation of new neurons to support new memory.

Declarative or *explicit memory* storage, mediated by the medial temporal lobe of the brain and the hippocampus, constitutes a conscious memory for persons, places, and things. *Procedural* or *implicit memory* is unconscious, and those memories are evident only in performance rather than through conscious recall. Procedural memory is a collection of processes that involves several interrelated events, including cue recognition and various affective states associated with cues, to name just two. Both types of memory work in tandem; they overlap. Constant repetition (such as behavioral rehearsal) can transform declarative memory into procedural memory.

Whether conscious or not, memory is reflected in diffuse neuroanatomical changes. The plasticity capacity of the human brain is responsible for these changes and may be key to long-term change resulting from psychotherapeutic interventions.

KEY POINTS

- The brain is organized from the lower simpler regions to the more complex higher cortical areas. The lower parts mediate simple regulatory functions, whereas the cortical structures mediate more complex functions.

- Neurons are the basic unit of structure and function in the nervous system which transmit messages to other neurons with the help of neurotransmitters.

- Neurotransmitters either inhibit or excite cells and have been implicated in the development of psychiatric illnesses, but in what capacity remains unknown.

- Plasticity, a lifelong capacity, is a property of the nervous tissue, referring to its ability to shape or mold itself as a result of experience (exposure to environmental stimuli). Because of neuroplasticity, living organisms can change their behavior in response to environmental events (stimuli).

- Understanding the concept of plasticity is key to understanding why and how learning influences brain and behavior and why the repeated practice of new skills in the context of psychotherapy becomes part of a new behavioral repertoire.

- Genetics is playing an increasingly important role in understanding the basis and the expression of psychiatric illnesses.

- The diathesis–stress model of psychiatric disorders hypothesizes that people are predisposed toward a particular mental or physiologic reaction and that the disorder will become manifest as a reaction to stress in addition to genes.

- Circadian rhythm can be compared to an internal clock that coordinates what happens in human bodies according to what approximates a 24-hour cycle.

- Clear, unitary, causes of symptoms are rare in psychiatry. More often, multiple causal factors, each with a small effect, act in concert to produce disease.

Further Reading

Kandel, E.R. (2007) *Search of Memory: The Emergence of a New Science of Mind*, W.W. Norton, New York.
Kandel, E.R., Schwartz, J.H., and Jessell, T.M. (2000) *Principles of Neural Science*, 4th edn, McGraw-Hill, New York.
Snell, R.S. (2009) *Clinical Neuroanatomy*, 7th edn, Lippincott, Williams & Wilkins, Philadelphia, PA.

Unit 2
The Context of Care

6   Care Settings and the Continuum of Care

6.1 Introduction

Treatment settings for patients with psychiatric illnesses have undergone great upheaval since the 1960s, with inpatient psychiatric beds declining dramatically and the focus of care shifting from institutionalization to community-based management. In this chapter we describe the current role of inpatient settings and the continuum of care available to psychiatric patients and their families. Although effective services and pockets of excellence exist, care is uneven, and the situation described by the US Surgeon General over a decade ago, when he described the system as a "non-system," is too often the norm.

6.2 Background

The movement to bring mentally ill people out of institutions was made possible by the development of effective drugs, along with some change in attitude about the mentally ill. With the de-institutionalization movement, greater emphasis has been placed on viewing mentally ill people as members of families and communities. A significant catalyst of de-institutionalization was the Community Mental Health Act of 1963. It has been used by some governments and their agencies to attempt to save money by closing down, scaling back or merging psychiatric inpatient units. In 1999, the Supreme Court of the United States ruled in *L.C. & E.W.* v. *Olmstead* that states are required to provide community-based services for people with mental disabilities if treatment professionals determine that it is appropriate and the affected individuals do not object to such placement.

   People who must be hospitalized are less likely to be isolated and restrained than in the past, and they are often discharged early into day treatment centers. These settings are less expensive because fewer staff members are needed, the emphasis is on group rather than individual therapy, and people sleep at home or in halfway houses.

6.3 Inpatient facilities

In 2004, the Subcommittee on Acute Care of the New Freedom Commission (see Chapter 1) examined summary data regarding total inpatient bed capacity nationwide. They reported that from 1990 through 2000 the number of inpatient beds per capita declined by 44% in state and county mental hospitals, 43% in private psychiatric hospitals, and 32% in nonfederal general hospitals.

Fundamentals of Psychiatry, First Edition. Allan Tasman and Wanda K. Mohr.
© 2011 John Wiley & Sons, Ltd. Published 2011 by John Wiley & Sons, Ltd.

At this writing, for patients to receive inpatient care or hospital-based treatment, they must meet specific criteria which third-party payers (including private, state and federal insurance) have developed. Patients most likely to receive inpatient treatment are those who pose a risk of harm to themselves or others. Patients who qualify for admission may need short-term (acute) or long-term hospitalization depending on their unique circumstances.

Acute-care psychiatric hospitals provide highly structured settings in which staff can monitor patients. Patients who are experiencing suicidal or homicidal ideation, acute psychoses, disorientation, or confusion, or those in need of detoxification under close scrutiny, are candidates for these settings.

Some large general hospitals offer psychiatric services. These are used to stabilize patients who are triaged through the emergency department, or they serve as a safe environment in which patients can be evaluated and medicated until they can be sent to an acute psychiatric hospital.

Many facilities offer partial or day hospitalization programs (PHPs). These alternatives have been developed for patients who need some supervision but who are not appropriate candidates for long-term treatment. Partial hospitalization programs provide activities and therapy sessions for 6–8 hours per day. Patients then return to their homes or workplace. PHPs are a means of mainstreaming patients back to their communities.

Some patients are in need of longer term hospitalization due to the chronicity of their illnesses. If short-term stabilization cannot be achieved in an acute-care psychiatric hospital, patients may need longer term care. Most long-term facilities are state supervised.

Residential treatment facilities (RTFs) are institutions that provide intensive services, often focused at a specific population. They are often considered a "last resort" when other forms of treatment have been ineffective. Treatment is long-term and stays range from a few weeks to several months. Residential facilities have rules and regulations that facilitate the safety of patients, teach adaptive behaviors, and promote movement towards independence. They are not the optimal choice for patient care, especially when family involvement in therapy is crucial, as behaviors learned in RTFs tend not to generalize when patients return to their homes. Insurance coverage for this level of care varies and they are often expensive. Moreover, there have been a steady stream of abuses reported in some of these facilities. Hence clinicians should carefully investigate and evaluate the facility to which they may be referring patients and families. (See: Alliance for the Safe and Appropriate Use of Residential Treatment at http://astart.fmhi.usf.edu/.)

6.4 Community support programs

A community support system is a model of care that creates and delivers community-based care for a specific population who traditionally required long-term hospitalization. This system includes a range of supports: healthcare, mental healthcare, rehabilitation services, social networks, housing arrangements, and educational and employment opportunities. It offers these supports through several different program models. The goal is moving service approaches away from restrictive settings and into the community.

Community Support Programs (CSPs) are based on values implemented at three levels: the individual, the agency, and the community support system network. The patient is central to the system and she or he stays involved in decisions that affect the needed services. The central theme of community support is empowerment recognizing the following three tenets:

1. All people are valuable and should be afforded dignity, respect, and the opportunity to take full advantage of their human, legal, and social rights.

2. Every human being is capable of growth, development, and learning.

3. Services should be provided in a normative and socially valued way.

Key to this is a comprehensive understanding of each person as an individual with hope for a wide range of outcomes that includes improvement and recovery. The goal of the CSP is to enable those with severe mental illnesses to remain in the community and function as independently as possible. People having such challenges are a diverse group each having unique concerns, abilities, motivations, and problems. Hence, successful community support systems are based on services that provide for self-determination, individuation, normalization of settings and treatment offerings, least restrictive settings, and maximization of self-help.

6.5 Assertive community treatment

Assertive Community Treatment (ACT) is a service-delivery model that provides comprehensive, locally based treatment to people with serious and persistent mental illnesses. ACT provides highly individualized services directly to patients. ACT recipients receive the multidisciplinary, round-the-clock staffing of a psychiatric unit, but within their own home and community. To have the competencies and skills to meet a patient's multiple treatment, rehabilitation, and support needs, ACT team members include the disciplines of psychiatry, social work, nursing, substance abuse, and vocational rehabilitation (see Chapter 8). The ACT team provides these necessary services on a 24 hours a day basis.

The elements of ACT include psychopharmacologic treatment, individual supportive therapy, mobile crisis intervention, hospitalization if necessary, substance abuse treatment, including group therapy (for patients with a dual diagnosis of substance abuse and mental illness). It also includes elements of rehabilitation including behaviorally oriented skills teaching (supportive and cognitive–behavioral therapy), including structuring time and handling activities of daily living, supported employment, both paid and volunteer work, and support for resuming education. Finally, ACT includes support services such as education and skills teaching to family members, collaboration with families, and assistance to patients with children and direct support to help patients obtain legal and advocacy services, financial support, supported housing, money management services, and transportation.

ACT patients spend significantly less time in hospitals and more time in independent living situations, have less time unemployed, earn more income from competitive employment, experience more positive social relationships, express greater satisfaction with life, and are less symptomatic. In addition, the ACT model has shown a small economic advantage over institutional care. Despite the documented treatment success of ACT, only a few states in the US have statewide ACT programs.

6.6 Child and adolescent service system programs

Outcomes for children and youths with emotional and behavioral challenges have continued to be poor. Research findings demonstrate that children with these challenges, as a group, have the poorest long-term outcomes of any group with a disability. These children have serious problems in several domains, including social behavior, emotional and behavioral functioning, educational performance, and overall functioning.

In response to the multidimensional nature of emotional and behavioral challenges and the poor outcomes that children with such problems experience, reform efforts have focused on alternative ways of providing services. The guiding principles of programs providing services include: multidisciplinary and individualized community-based services in the least restrictive setting possible; a strengths-based approach; partnering with parents to design individual and culturally sensitive service plans for children; service coordination; a focus on natural and informal supports; and flexible funding streams. Service systems that adopt and use these principles are often referred to as systems of care (SOCs). All SOCs use some form of service coordination to connect the variety of systems, agencies, and individuals, including the family, that participate in the care of a child, and ensure effective, ongoing communication among parties so that services and interventions are consistent and directed toward common goals. A multiagency service coordination team is responsible for organizing and managing all the services received by the child and family. The SOC approach to service provision challenges teachers, clinicians, social workers, and other service providers to put aside professional biases and create partnerships both with one another and with families. All 50 states in the US have received federal grants to implement SOCs for troubled youths, but implementation across states is highly uneven.

6.7 Forensic settings

The care and management of the criminal offender with a psychiatric disorder challenges the collective wisdom of both the criminal justice system and the mental health system. Enduring contradictions about how to best meet the needs of the forensic population prevail. Forensic settings include those based in outpatient clinics within the community, secure units within general hospitals, state psychiatric hospitals, hospitals for the "criminally insane," and custodial-type settings such as young offender facilities, jails, and prisons.

Research findings suggest that, in any prison or jail population, up to 15% of those incarcerated will have a mental disorder, and up to 20% will require psychiatric intervention while incarcerated. As a rule, chronic severe schizophrenia, mood disorders, and organic syndromes with psychotic features are common. Psychotic presentations often are complicated by the coexistence of personality disorders, substance abuse, or both; many clients self-medicate with drugs and alcohol.

Increasing numbers of juvenile offenders are being detained in jails and prisons, and as a result are particularly vulnerable to adverse health outcomes. Although they require special services to meet their needs related to growth and development, education, and special health concerns, the behavioral problems associated with their criminal activity often draws attention away from their healthcare needs. The overcrowding in the prison system, along with the increased number of violent teen offenders, has resulted in the detainment of many young people in facilities designed for adults.

6.8 Court diversion schemes

In some jurisdictions, mentally disordered offenders, particularly those charged with minor offenses, are being diverted from the court process altogether and sent directly to treatment programs, mental health courts, or both. Although court diversion schemes have been in practice in the United Kingdom since the early 1990s, their existence in Canada and the United States varies, as does the type of diversion available (e.g., with the police, upon initial incarceration, upon arrival to court). Diversion schemes, although relatively new, are seen as a more humane form of treatment, are cost effective, and appear to contribute to reduced rates of recidivism among this population.

KEY POINTS

- Community support is crucial to quality of life for those with severe mental illness residing in the community. The goal of community support systems is to enable those with severe mental illnesses to remain in the community while functioning at optimal levels of independence.

- A community support system encourages participation from all people within it: clients, family members, government officials, and providers. The objective is to deliver a full range of life supportive care. Services are based on guiding principles that promote self-determination and individuation.

- Essential components of a community support system include active outreach efforts, help in ensuring access to services, psychosocial and vocational opportunities, rehabilitative and supportive housing options, crisis intervention services, case management, and family and community education programs.

- Reform efforts in children's social services have led to the establishment of systems of care, which create mechanisms for coordinating social services. They are designed to facilitate collaboration among parents, teachers, and other service providers so that they can gear services for students with multisystem needs toward common and agreed goals.

- Services must be developed with active participation from the consumer and family.

- Forensic settings include forensic psychiatric facilities, locked units of general hospitals, and state hospitals.

Further Reading

Allness, D. (2003) *The ACT Standards (revised). A Manual for ACT Start-Up: Based on the PACT Model of Community Treatment for Persons with Severe and Persistent Mental Illnesses*, National Alliance for the Mentally Ill, Washington, DC.

Human Rights Watch (2003) *Ill Equipped: US Prisons and Offenders with Mental Illness*, New York, HRW. Available at: http://www.hrw.org/reports/2003/usa1003/.

Stroul, B., Pires, S., Armstrong, M., and Zaro, S. (2002) The impact of managed care on systems of care that serve children with serious emotional disturbances and their families. *Children's Services: Social Policy, Research and Practice*, **5** (1), 21–36.

Systems of Care. Available at: http://systemsofcare.samhsa.gov/ and http://systemsofcare.samhsa.gov/2008ShortReport.pdf.

United States General Accounting Office (2007) *Residential Treatment Programs: Concerns Regarding Abuse and Death in Certain Programs for Troubled Youth*, USGAO, Washington, DC, GAO-08-147 T.

Cultural Context of Care

7.1 Introduction

Overall, international demographics indicate that the majority populations in most countries are composed of persons of color. Western (European) medicine, which is rooted in a high-technology, intervention-focused approach, however, continues to dominate the thinking of practitioners in many areas. Practitioners of Western medicine often disregard, supersede, or fail to recognize more traditional healing methods found in non-European cultures. A growing body of evidence shows that in addition to the mode of expressing psychological distress varying with cultural beliefs and practices, the causes, course and outcome of major psychiatric disorders are influenced by cultural factors as well. Lack of awareness of important differences between patient and practitioner can undermine the development of a therapeutic alliance and the negotiation and delivery of effective treatment (see Chapter 30).

A culturally competent healthcare system is one that acknowledges and incorporates, at all levels, the importance of culture. Such incorporation is evident through the system's assessment of cross-cultural relations, attention to the dynamics that result from cultural differences, growth of cultural knowledge, and adaptation of services to meet culturally unique needs. The system's behaviors, attitudes, and policies are congruent and help others to work effectively in cross-cultural situations. In this chapter we briefly summarize some of the concepts and factors that can inform culturally competent clinical practice.

7.2 Sociocultural aspects and influences

The ability to view patients through a cultural lens is becoming increasingly important as a consequence of the growing diversity found in the United States and Canada. Moreover, larger forces of globalization and migration have encouraged a fresh look at culture in every aspect of psychiatry, including psychosocial assessment, the boundaries of normality, and ethnopharmacotherapeutic issues (see Chapter 30).

Research has clearly demonstrated that the cause, course, and outcome of major psychiatric disorders are influenced by cultural factors. For example, international studies by the World Health Organization have provided compelling evidence that the prognosis for schizophrenia is better in some developing countries than it is in England or the US. Wide variations in the prevalence of many psychiatric disorders across geographic regions and ethnocultural groups have been documented with current standardized epidemiologic survey methods. In addition, social and cultural factors are major determinants of the use of healthcare services and alternative sources of help.

Fundamentals of Psychiatry, First Edition. Allan Tasman and Wanda K. Mohr.
© 2011 John Wiley & Sons, Ltd. Published 2011 by John Wiley & Sons, Ltd.
This chapter is based on Chapter 4 (Laurence J. Kirmayer, Cécile Rousseau, G. Eric Jarvis, Jaswant Guzder) and Chapter 39 (Juan E. Mezzich, Roberto Lewis-Fernández, Maria Angeles Ruiperez) of *Psychiatry, Third Edition*

7.3 Culture: the broad territory of a concept

Culture is the integration of human behaviors (which include thoughts, communications, actions, customs, beliefs, values, and institutions) of a racial, ethnic, religious, or social group. It represents the vast structure of ideas, attitudes, habits, languages, rituals, ceremonies, and practices peculiar to a particular group of people. Culture also provides people with a general design for living and with patterns by which to interpret reality.

Culture can greatly influence a person's perceptions of health and illness as well as how, when, and why he or she would seek treatment for a health problem. This factor becomes especially important in the area of mental health. Many aspects of psychiatric care involve self-perception, roles and relationships, family dynamics and interactions, attitudes toward medications, values, and community supports. Before mental healthcare providers can administer appropriate and effective treatment, they must understand the patient's cultural context and how it might influence his or her attitudes toward a particular health concern, its causes, and its treatment. Culturally relevant care is as diverse as the cultures represented. An understanding of the patient's cultural context also is necessary to appreciate the patient's attitude toward the clinician. This understanding is not a simple matter, as much has changed in anthropologists' views of culture, from one of finely balanced systems to a recognition of high levels of individual variability within even very small cultural groups and the active ways in which individuals and groups make use of a variety of forms of knowledge to fashion an identity and a way of life.

At the same time, anthropologists have come to recognize the high level of individual variability within even small cultural groups, and the active ways in which individuals and groups make use of a variety of forms of knowledge to fashion an identity and a viable way of living. In urban settings where many cultures meet, individuals have a wide range of options available, and can position themselves both within and against any given ethnocultural identity or way of life. This has led the anthropologists to rethink the notion of culture or even to suggest that it has outlived its usefulness.

Globalization and rapid technological developments have resulted in the intermixing of cultural worlds and the creation of new ethnocultural groups and individuals with multiple or hybrid identities. Many people now see themselves as transnational, with networks of affiliation and support that span great distances. The mental health implications of these new forms of identity and community have been little explored, and will be an increasingly important issue for psychiatry.

The notion of culture is broad and not easily described, and categories and characteristics of various cultural groups tend to stereotype and generalize. However, it is useful to distinguish notions of race, ethnicity and social class from culture, particularly in a society as diverse as that of North America.

"Race" is a term used to mark off groups within and between societies. Racial distinctions generally reflect a few superficial physical characteristics and hence have little correlation with clinically relevant genetic variation. The boundaries of any racial group are socially defined and have no biological reality. Race is usually ascribed by others and cannot be readily changed or discarded unless larger social criteria change. Race is significant as a social category that is employed in racist and discriminatory practices. Racism is clinically important because of its demonstrable effects on mental and physical health, individual and collective self-esteem, and health service use.

"Ethnicity" refers to the collective identity of a group based on common heritage, which may include language, religion, geographic origin, and specific cultural practices. Ethnic identity is often constructed *vis-à-vis* others and a dominant society. Hence, it is sometimes assumed that "foreigners" or minorities have ethnicity while the dominant group (e.g., Americans of British or Northern European extraction) does not. This obscures the fact that everyone may become aware of an ethnic identity in the right context.

Finally, "social class" reflects the fact that most societies are economically stratified and individuals' opportunities, mobility, lifestyle, and response to illness are heavily constrained by their economic position. Issues of poverty, unemployment, powerlessness, and marginalization may overshadow cultural factors as causes of illness and influences on identity and help-seeking behavior.

7.4 Gender

"Gender" refers to the ways in which cultures differentiate and define roles based on biological sex or reproductive functions. Hence there is a tendency to view gender differences as biologically given and determined. However, while some distinctions may be closely related to the physiological differences between males and females, most are assigned to the sexes on the basis of specific cultural beliefs. and social organization. There are also important gender differences in styles of emotional expression, symptom experience, and help-seeking. These vary cross nationally, although epidemiological surveys in the US have consistently shown that women tend to report more somatic symptoms and emotional distress, as well as to seek help for psychological or interpersonal problems.

7.5 Religion and spirituality

"Religion" or "spirituality" is a key marker of cultural identity and an important piece of an individual's "personhood." For many individuals and communities, it may structure the moral world more strongly than ethnic or national identity. Spirituality and religion are words often used interchangeably, but there are important differences.

Religion is the outward practice of a spiritual system of beliefs, values, codes of conduct, and rituals. It is an organized system of practices and beliefs in which people engage. Religion is a platform for the expression of spirituality, and is an important factor in the lives of most people in the US, and in many other parts of the world. Religion can be a source of cultural discrimination and prejudice as history has evidenced.

Spirituality has been described as a person's experience of, or a belief in, a power apart from his or her own existence. It also has been described as an individual search for meaning. Spirituality can be said to incorporate a sense of relationship with oneself, with others, or with a higher "power" – but not every person who professes to be spiritual is also religious or even believes in a deity. Spirituality is shaped by larger social circumstances and by the beliefs and values present in the wider culture. Cross-culturally, people express spirituality in many different ways.

Despite the ubiquity of religious and spiritual experience, it is frequently neglected during routine psychiatric evaluation. A thorough cultural formulation requires consideration of the patient's religion and spirituality. Areas to cover include religious identity, the role of religion in the family of origin, current religious practices (attendance at services, public and private rituals), motivation for religious behavior (i.e., religious orientation), and specific beliefs of the individual and of his family and community (see Chapter 30).

7.6 Cultural congruence

In a culturally competent healthcare system, care delivery should be culturally congruent, meaning that patients receive an overall message, conveyed both verbally and nonverbally, of personal and cultural validation. For mental health services to be culturally congruent, providers from all aspects of the delivery system must respond to diverse cultural values consistent with patients' and families specific contexts.

7.6.1 Culturally competent healthcare

Cultural competence means having the skills, both academic and interpersonal, that enable a person to understand and appreciate cultural differences and similarities within, between, and among groups. It is a process by which healthcare providers continuously strive to achieve the ability to effectively work within the cultural context of an individual or community from a diverse cultural or ethnic background. Skills in cultural competence are relevant for all variables to which differences may apply, including gender, race, ethnicity, language, country of origin, acculturation, age, religious and spiritual beliefs, sexual orientation, socioeconomic class, and disabilities. The culturally competent psychiatric professional is willing and able to draw on community-based values, traditions, and customs and to work with knowledgeable persons from the community to formulate appropriate interventions and supports for patients according to the different variables mentioned earlier. In culturally congruent mental healthcare, providers integrate the patient's value system, life experiences, and expectations about treatment into the therapeutic process; as a result, the full weight of the patient's cultural system can help support the healing process.

7.6.2 Transcultural assessment

To determine the influences on a patient's basic beliefs about illness and wellness, the practitioner must ensure that the assessment is transculturally focused (see Chapter 30).

Clinical Vignette

An ultra-orthodox Jewish family arrives for their consultation. The female psychiatrist, who is dressed in a short skirt, welcomes them by offering her hand to the father in greeting. He is confused and offended, avoids eye contact, and is reluctant to proceed with the session. The female doctor's style of dress and friendly handshake were viewed as disrespectful or as indicating her lack of familiarity with norms of conduct with observant orthodox families.

KEY POINTS

- Evidence suggests that the mode of expressing psychological distress varies with cultural beliefs and practices.

- Research also shows that the causes, course, and outcome of major psychiatric disorders are influenced by culture.

- A culturally competent healthcare system is one that acknowledges and incorporates, at all levels, the importance of culture. This includes a sensitivity to issues of race, ethnicity, sex or gender, socioeconomic status, religion and spirituality among other factors that are important to a person's identity and life.

- "Race" is a term used to mark off groups within and between societies.

- "Ethnicity" refers to the collective identity of a group based on common heritage, which may include language, religion, geographic origin, and specific cultural practices.

- "Gender" refers to the ways in which cultures differentiate and define roles based on biological sex or reproductive functions.

- "Religion" is a platform for the expression of spirituality, and is an important factor in the lives of most people in the US, and in many other parts of the world. Religion can be a source of cultural discrimination and prejudice.

- "Cultural competence" means having the skills, both academic and interpersonal, that enable a person to understand and appreciate cultural differences and similarities within, between, and among groups.

Further Reading

Boehnlein, J.K. (2000) *Psychiatry and Religion: The Convergence of Mind and Spirit*, American Psychiatric Press, Washington, DC.

Fulford, K.W.M. (1996) Religion and psychiatry: extending the limits of tolerance, in *Psychiatry and Religion: Context, Consensus and Controversies* (ed. D. Bhugra), Routledge, London, pp. 5–22.

Kleinman, A. (1996) How culture is important for DSM-IV, in *Culture and Psychiatric Diagnosis* (eds J. Mezzich *et al.*) American Psychiatric Press, Washington, DC.

CHAPTER

8

The Multidisciplinary Treatment Team and Working with Other Professionals

8.1 Introduction

Multidisciplinary teams are groups of professionals from diverse disciplines who come together to provide comprehensive assessments of patients, establish and carry out interventions for them, and engage in regular consultations about patients' progress. This chapter provides a brief outline of the roles and unique contributions of typical members of the treatment team. It also discusses professional relationships, and when to refer patients to other clinicians or specialists.

8.2 The multidisciplinary team

While the primary purpose of having a team of professionals caring for a person with a psychiatric illness is typically to bring the expertise of several disciplines to the plan of care, they have other roles. They can promote coordination between agencies. They also can identify gaps in service and breakdowns in coordination or communication between agencies or individuals. They also can enhance the professional skills and knowledge of individual team members by providing a forum for learning more about the strategies, resources, and approaches that different disciplines use.

Each discipline has its own perspective, jargon, mandates, and resources. When professionals fail to understand these differences, barriers, misunderstandings, or "turf" conflicts may develop. On the other hand, when professionals learn about the approaches, resources, and perspectives of colleagues from other disciplines, they can greatly expand their repertoire of skills, increase the resources they make available to patients, and enhance their understanding of various problems. Collaboration and interaction can facilitate interagency coordination, resulting in a more comprehensive range of services. As a result the likelihood decreases that patients will "fall between the cracks" of the service network, cutting down on wasteful overlap.

Professional disciplines typically represented in psychiatric–mental health settings include psychiatrists, psychologists, social workers, occupational therapists, professional dietitians, recreation therapists, substance abuse counselors, and nurses. Actual team compositions, however, are as diverse as the settings for patient care, and may include parole officers and other stakeholders from

Fundamentals of Psychiatry, First Edition. Allan Tasman and Wanda K. Mohr.
© 2011 John Wiley & Sons, Ltd. Published 2011 by John Wiley & Sons, Ltd.

the corrections system, as well as professionals from other local and state agencies. It can also include members of the advocacy communities.

Teams of professionals are generally found in an organized way in inpatient and residential treatment settings, in outpatient intensive case management settings, and in systems of care.

Table 8.1 illustrates modalities and aspects of patient care and staff members responsible for those modalities. The medical record should clearly indicate the fulfillment of the activities commensurate with the responsibility of each treatment team member.

8.3 Referrals

Most multidisciplinary teams operate in treatment programs that are tied to an institution, either inpatient or outpatient, system of care, or case management. But even in solo practice, no clinician can meet the needs of every patient, and there are times when referrals should take place. Below are situations in which we strongly recommend that clinicians seek referrals and/or supervision:

- The clinician feels incompetent in the required intervention or has not had education in, or experience with, the procedure under consideration.

- The clinician does not have interest in a particular condition, and/or feelings of counter-transference interfere with the patient's progress.

- The patient has experienced a failed attempt in achieving an acceptable outcome in treatment with a particular condition.

- Therapy is not moving forward.

- Patient or family are not engaged with the clinician and fail to adhere to treatment.

- The patient has a rare or relatively unknown condition that is best treated by a specialist who has seen and has treated these types of case.

8.4 Turf battles

Different clinicians stake out a scope of practice that gives them ownership rights to performing tasks within a specific clinical territory. In the arena of psychiatry, these scopes of practice sometimes overlap. Social workers, psychologists, licensed counselors, advanced practice nurses, as well as psychiatrists may have had training in certain psychotherapeutic techniques. Psychiatrists and advanced practice nurses can both perform physical assessments and prescribe medication.

In the past this overlap has sometimes resulted in turf battles over who "cares" for patients. In truth, all the above professionals care for patients and no one has a monopoly on caring. Turf battles do not solve any problems, but they certainly create many new ones. And they waste time. There is ample work and effort to keep everybody busy with our challenging and vulnerable psychiatric populations. Psychiatric clinicians and professionals are in service to patients and their families, and such battles are inappropriate.

8.5 Courtesies and professional relationships

Showing appreciation and acknowledgment for a referral or for a consultation is one of the best forms of motivation that exists. This can be accomplished by a formal letter thanking the referring professional, as well as a prompt telephone call and follow-up letter or note delineating findings that are pertinent.

Table 8-1   Professional/staff member modalities and responsibilities

Staff	Responsibilities
Psychiatrist	Admission evaluation/orders • Precautions • Diagnostic examination Relationship interventions • Individual meetings, daily rounds • Formal psychotherapy (individual and/or group) • Special therapies • Special procedures (e.g., orders seclusion and restraint) Therapeutic milieu • Team meetings • Patient staff meetings • Special inpatient meetings (e.g., eating-disorder groups) Somatic therapies • Pharmacotherapy • Other somatic therapies (e.g., ECT) Discharge planning and referrals
Generalist nursing care staff	Nursing assessment and care plan Relationship interventions • Individual meetings • Patient/staff group meetings • Social competency development Therapeutic milieu • Observe and reinforce impulse control • Patient government and unit meetings Activities of daily living • Personal hygiene, sleeping patterns, nutrition Somatic therapies • Administer medication • Medication education • Observe and record effects and adverse effects of all somatic therapies Health teaching (patient education) Discharge planning
Advanced practice nurse	• Limited prescriptive privileges within scope of practice in most states • Conducts physical assessments • Conducts formal psychiatric assessments • Conducts groups, counseling sessions, and medication checks • Conducts formal psychotherapy if has additional training and certification in the modality (e.g., CBT, IPT, DBT, etc.)
Activity therapist	Activity therapy evaluation • Evaluation of strengths and weaknesses and impairments • Occupational–vocational assessment Activity therapies (e.g., recreation and leisure skills, music, skills building) Discharge planning • Vocational rehabilitation
Clinical social worker	Social work assessment and plan • Family assessment • Contacts and working with family, friends, employers, teachers, and so on Relationship interventions Family therapy • Individual meeting with patients Discharge planning • Family casework • Contact with collateral resources
Psychologist	Diagnostic testing • Basic psychological assessment • Neuropsychological assessment Relationship interventions • Formal psychotherapy

(Continued)

Table 8-1 (*Continued*)	
Staff	**Responsibilities**
Pharmacist	• Evaluates the appropriateness of and fills medical prescriptions • Counsels patients on proper use and adverse effects of medications
Others	
Chaplain	• Religious counseling and spiritual guidance
Vocational counselor	• Vocational assessment, counseling, training
Dietician	• Nutritional planning and education
Teachers	• Education of children in pediatric settings
Substance abuse counselors	• Substance abuse assessments and counseling for specific dependency issues with licit or illicit substances

KEY POINTS

- The multidisciplinary teams consists of professionals representing diverse disciplines who work to provide comprehensive patient assessments, decide on interventions and treatment planning, and meet with patients and families to evaluate individual progress, revising the treatment plan as appropriate.

- Each discipline has its own perspective, jargon, and role in patient care.

- "Turf" conflicts may develop when individual professionals fail to understand differences in perspective and roles.

- A multidisciplinary approach is needed in the care of psychiatric patients, particularly when caring for the chronically mentally ill patient or with child populations since their problems are complex and different practitioners are needed to address their problems in the context of their community and families.

Further Reading

Baerlocher, M.O. and Detsky, A.S. (2009) Professional monopolies in medicine. *JAMA*, **301** (8), 858–360.
Fagin, L. and Garelick, A. (2004) The doctor–nurse relationship. *Advances in Psychiatric Treatment*, **10**, 277–286.
Housely, W. (2003) *Interaction in Multidisciplinary Teams*, Ashgate, Surrey, UK.
Nahata, M.C. (2002) Pharmacist's role in health care. *Annals of Pharmacotherapy*, **36** (3), 527–529.
Stein, L., Watts, D.T., and Howell, T. (1990) The doctor–nurse game revisited. *New England Journal of Medicine*, **322** (8), 546–549.
Stein, L. (1967) The doctor–nurse game. *Archives of General Psychiatry*, **16** (6), 699–703.

Ethical Practice

9.1 Introduction

Perhaps no other specialty area demands as great a need for knowledge of ethics as psychiatric medicine. The emotionally charged interpersonal process that often plays such a key role in psychiatric treatment necessitates a unique and generally more stringent ethical system than the basic principles of medical ethics. Psychiatric patients are especially vulnerable during treatment, to such an extent that the ethical character of the clinician has a unique and powerful potential to help or to harm our patients. The clinician must conduct accurate assessments, plan carefully, implement competent interventions, identify measurable outcomes, and work within the interdisciplinary process. While doing so, the clinician also must ensure that his or her practices meet professional standards, legal mandates, and ethical guidelines.

The goal of this chapter is to discuss ethical principles relevant to the practice of psychiatric medicine. It addresses basic and evolving rights of patients and addresses ethics as basic and obvious moral truths that guide deliberation and action when providing care to people with psychiatric disorders and discusses ethical considerations for the community psychiatric clinician. Finally, the chapter discusses the importance of professional boundaries when working in therapeutic relationships with patients. The discussion provided is by no means comprehensive and interested clinicians are encouraged to seek more in-depth material from the sources suggested at the end of this chapter.

9.2 Professional ethics

Ethics are principles that serve as codes of conduct about right and wrong behaviors to guide the actions of individuals. Although there are universal ethics, such as respect for others, ethics are often tailored for a specific professional culture. Psychiatric clinicians should understand ethical theories and use ethical principles to guide their decisions about patient care. They must clarify their own ethical beliefs and then combine their ideas with professional ethical principles to develop sound ethical decisions. By working to enhance their own positive character traits, psychiatric clinicians improve their potential to be able to be helpful. Positive character virtues that are likely to enhance the effectiveness of mental health professionals include respect for confidentiality, veracity, prudence, warmth, sensitivity, perseverance, patience, and generosity.

Ethical practice as a way of life focuses on interpersonal relationships and involves not only caring *for* but also caring *about* patients.

Responsibility and accountability are additional components of ethical practice. In addition to the universal principles of respect and responsibility, several other principles guide clinicians and other healthcare professionals in ethical decision making. They include autonomy, beneficence,

Fundamentals of Psychiatry, First Edition. Allan Tasman and Wanda K. Mohr.
© 2011 John Wiley & Sons, Ltd. Published 2011 by John Wiley & Sons, Ltd.
This chapter is based on Chapter 5 (Richard S. Epstein, Ahmed Okasha) of *Psychiatry, Third Edition*

Table 9-1	Six principles of medical ethics
Principle	**Description**
Autonomy	Respecting the patient's independence and right to make decisions
Beneficence	Applying one's professional abilities to patients' well-being
Confidentiality	Respecting patients' privacy
Justice	Equitableness in providing care regardless of patients' idiosyncrasies, background, or station in life
Non-maleficence	Avoiding doing harm to patients
Veracity	Exhibiting systematic behavior of honesty and truthfulness with oneself and with one's patients

paternalism, veracity, fidelity, and justice. As clinicians interact daily with patients, they make many ethical decisions and they must take full responsibility and accountability for his or her ethical decision-making. Such responsibility requires a code of ethics.

Most of the professional mental health workforce organizations have established codes of ethics that provide broad guidelines for mental health practitioners. The common factor in all codes is that the highest ethical priority is the well-being of the patient. The objectives of the mental health ethical codes include: (1) educating their associated workforce in sound ethical conduct; (2) providing a mechanism to ensure professional accountability, and (3) serving as a catalyst to improve practice. The primary purpose of the codes is to safeguard patient welfare. The six basic principles of medical ethics are summarized in Table 9.1.

9.3 Sources of ethics

Ethical codes and principles are derived from and embodied or articulated in three sources: law, religion, and professional associations. Ethics and law are related but not synonymous. Each nation has a legal system that attempts to embody ethical principles in the creation and interpretation of the law. But not every legal mandate is necessarily consistent with medical ethics and not every ethically supportable course of conduct is codified in law or legislation (see Chapter 10).

Many ethical decisions that confront practitioners have their roots in religion. Many contemporary issues including termination of pregnancy, refusal of treatment, and others are guided by patients' religious beliefs. Practitioners should be aware of these and the tensions that might inevitably arise when a patient's religious belief conflicts with ethical behavior on the part of the professional.

9.4 Ethical behavior of psychiatric physicians

Worldwide, the basic ideas of Hippocratic ethics are the cornerstone of professional behavior and the nucleus of subsequent ethical codes. Those are:

- **Declaration of Geneva**: (1948, amended in 1968) Adopted by the General Assembly of the World Medical Association (WMA), the Physician Oath seems to be a response to the atrocities committed by doctors in Nazi Germany. This oath requires the physician to "not use [his] medical knowledge contrary to the laws of humanity."

- **Nuremberg Code**: The judgment by the war crimes tribunal at Nuremberg laid down 10 standards to which physicians must conform when carrying out experiments on human subjects. The code articulated the requirement of voluntary informed consent of human subjects, recognized that risk must be weighed against expected benefits, and that unnecessary pain and suffering must be avoided. The principles of the Nuremberg Code have been incorporated into all codes of general medical ethics.

- **Declaration of Helsinki**: Developed by the World Medical Association as a statement of ethical principles for medical research involving human subjects, including research on identifiable human material and data.

- **Declaration of Madrid**: Specific declaration on standards for psychiatric practice developed by the World Psychiatric Association (WPA). The first of these was the Declaration of Hawaii in 1977. Currently all 130 societies of the WPA have adopted the Declaration of Madrid and abiding by the declaration is a prerequisite for joining the WPA. Elements of the Declaration of Madrid are summarized in Boxes 9.1 and 9.2.

Box 9.1 Summary of Declaration of Madrid

Physician must:

- Offer best treatment available
- Provide for least freedom-restrictive intervention
- Seek advice from experts when needed
- Advocate for equitable allocation of health resources
- Be familiar with scientific developments
- Assure that free and informed decisions are made
- Promote legal rights and human dignity
- Provide no treatment against a patient's will (unless there is a danger to life)
- Provide for informed consent for treatment based on findings of psychiatric assessment
- Maintain confidentiality (breach only when patient or third party is in danger)
- Research must be:
  - Approved by ethics committee
  - In keeping with scientific rules
  - Conducted by trained individuals
  - Respectful of patient's autonomy and integrity.

Box 9.2 Guidelines Regarding Special Situations

- Euthanasia
  - Duty is protection of life
  - Decisions of patient may be distorted by mental illness
- Torture
  - No participation under any circumstances
- Death penalty
  - No participation in assessment of competency for execution
- Selection of sex
  - No participation in decisions to terminate pregnancy for reasons of sex selection
- Organ transplantation
  - Ensure informed decisions and self-determination
- Psychiatrists addressing the media
  - No pronouncements on presumed psychopathology
  - Represent profession with dignity
  - Present research findings with awareness of their possible impact
- Ethnicity and culture
  - No discrimination
- Genetic research and counseling
  - Awareness of impact of genetic information
  - Genetic counseling respectful of patients' value system

- Protection of the rights of psychiatrists
  - Protection of the right of psychiatrists to live up to the obligations of their profession
  - Protection of the right of psychiatrists to practice at the highest level of excellence
  - Protection of the rights of psychiatrists to not be abused by
    - Totalitarian political regimes
    - Profit-driven economical systems
  - Protection of the right of psychiatrists not to become
    - Victims of discriminatory practices because of stigma
    - Outcast by the profession, ridiculed in the media or persecuted because of advocacy for the medical needs and the social and political rights of their patients
- Disclosing the diagnosis of Alzheimer's
  - Patient has the right to know or not to know
  - Patients and families should be told as early as possible
  - Exceptions to disclosure in cases of severe dementia, phobia, severe depression
- Dual responsibility
  - Obligation to disclose to the person being assessed the nature of the assessment (e.g., non-therapeutic and potentially damaging to the person's interests)
  - Need to advocate for limits to disclosure of information of informationother than what is absolutely essential

9.5 Selected ethical issues in psychiatric practice

The sections below discuss a few ethical issues specific to psychiatric practice, but a comprehensive discussion is beyond the scope of this chapter. The WPA standing committee on ethics has developed a teaching tool for students and practitioners entitled *Teaching Ethics in Psychiatry: Case Vignettes*. This resource contains 38 separate vignettes exploring various ethical dilemmas and their resolution and is available in its entirety on the Internet.

9.5.1 Boundaries and boundary violations

Despite the intensity of the therapeutic relationship that sometimes necessitates crossing into another's "space," clinicians must maintain certain boundaries in their interactions with patients. Patients with psychiatric disorders are highly vulnerable and interpersonal boundaries protect them from emotional harm that would impede their recovery. They must be initiated when the patient begins treatment and continue throughout treatment and, for the most part, continue even after the therapeutic relationship has ended. During treatment, providers must conduct interactions with patients within appropriate guidelines and focus on the patient's growth and movement toward wellness. Violations of boundaries are an infringement that interferes with the primary goal of providing care or causes harm to the patient, to the clinician, or to the fidelity of the treatment.

Boundary violations are usually insidious in their development. In the beginning, a healthcare provider may be unaware that the relationship is drifting from therapeutic interactions into a friendship or social relationship. As this relationship changes, the judgment of the healthcare provider becomes clouded, and the therapeutic needs of the patient slip from focus. Table 9.2 contains some indicators of potential boundary violations, with suggested remedial responses. Common boundary violations are more fully discussed below.

9.5.2 Violations of autonomy

Clinical actions that may interfere with the patient's autonomy include advice regarding non-urgent major life decisions; attempting to exert undue influence on issues unrelated to the patient's health; reluctance to allow patients to terminate treatment; seeking gratification by exerting power; and using power as a form of retaliation.

Table 9-2   Indicators of potential boundary violations with suggested remedial responses

Indicator	Suggested Remedial Responses
Clinician is frequently tardy starting sessions.	Avoid criticizing patient for complaining about lateness. Re-examine reasons for tardiness in light of patients' need for a stable treatment frame.
Clinician changes the treatment paradigm in "midstream," that is, switching from individual therapy with Mr A to couples therapy with Mr A and his wife.	Avoid dual relationships that may interfere with primary loyalty to the first patient. If dual relationships cannot be avoided, provide informed consent and explain risks to patient(s).
Clinician frequently advises patients on matters not related to treatment process.	Consider if this is a general pattern of need for control in one's non-clinical relationships. If so, consider ways to help patient to make his/her own decisions.
Clinician often relates to patient as if he/she were a personal friend.	Listen for signs that the patient feels burdened. Acknowledge pattern of role reversal and importance of clinician's fiduciary obligations to patient.
Clinician feels overly resentful about having to keep boundaries because they feel too constraining and spoil the "fun" and creativity of being a therapist.	Remember that therapy can often be difficult, burdensome, and frustrating work, and that boundaries are necessary for the patient's safety.
Clinician accepts gifts from patient.	Try to explore patient's motive for the gift. Consider refusing the gift by explaining that it might interfere with the effectiveness of treatment. Be prepared to work with patient's and one's own feelings of shame in this regard.
Clinician seeks contact with patient outside of therapy setting.	Avoid such contact, and explain the reason to patients. In settings where social contact is likely, discuss problems and options with the patient in advance.
Clinician is unable to confront patients who are late paying fees, remove items from the office, repeatedly try to prolong sessions, or torment therapist with insatiable demands.	Explore fear of one's own anger, the patient's anger, or of setting limits.
Clinician often tries to impress patients with personal information about him/herself.	Refrain from further disclosure and examine one's possible motives. Consider how such activity might relate to sexual feelings to patient or need to control patient.
Clinician becomes sexually preoccupied with patient.	Obtain supervision and/or personal psychotherapy if sexual preoccupations continue unabated.

9.5.3 Dual relationships

Clinicians should avoid treatment situations that place them in a conflict between therapeutic responsibility to patients and third parties. Examples of dual relationships in psychiatric practice include clinicians treating their own relatives and friends and the same therapist employing concurrent family and individual therapy paradigms with a given patient; and clinicians testifying as forensic witnesses for current psychotherapy patients.

Another source of dual relationship is associated with the expansion of prepaid care in the US and has provoked concern about a new source of role conflict for clinicians. Managed care generates serious concerns regarding potential conflicts of interest. Many managed care organizations (MCOs) have severely restricted the number of clinicians within a given community allowed to serve on their treatment panels. Patients' access to their regular treating practitioner may be limited For example, under the rules of some MCOs, physicians might be prevented from maintaining continuity of care for outpatients needing hospitalization. During their hospital stay, such patients must be attended by a preselected group of clinicians who conduct all hospital treatment for the plan. Since participation on a panel is often contingent on cost-efficiency profiles, clinicians who derive a significant portion of their income from a given MCO are discouraged from advocating for patients needing more expensive care. In addition, some managed care organizations refuse to pay for integrated treatment by clinicians for mentally ill patients enrolled in their panel. They may insist instead on a split treatment model in which the patient obtains psychotherapy from a social worker or psychologist, and is allowed only brief medication management visits with a physician or nurse practitioner. Practitioners attempting to do medication management under this model often have little contact with the psychotherapist, are very restricted in the frequency and duration of visits with the patient, and are thereby limited in making overall clinical decisions that might become necessary. Such a situation creates an ethical bind in which the medical responsibility is not accompanied by a commensurate degree of authority to direct the treatment process. A prudent course of action is for practitioners to be transparent and give informed consent regarding the risk to patients of their role conflicts and that payment under managed care may be stopped before patients feel ready to terminate.

9.5.4 Forensic roles

Questions as to dual relationship may exist regarding the ethical duties of forensic psychiatrists in settings where the sole function of the psychiatrist is to conduct an examination of an individual for the purpose of providing a report or testimony during legal proceedings. In US psychiatry the forensic examination is conducted as part of the legal process and is not considered a medical procedure. Prior to the forensic interview, the examinee is informed that the sole purpose of the examination is to report psychiatric findings to a third party, usually some type of legal or administrative forum. According to the latter position, no treatment relationship is ever established, and the sole ethical obligation of the forensic psychiatrist is to seek and report the truth in the interest of serving justice for the common good of the community.

9.5.5 Confidentiality

It is essential that clinicians treat their patients' communications as privileged. This means that patients alone retain the right to reveal information about themselves. The advent of managed care has raised even greater concern about the privacy of patients' personal communications because of the potential for an increasing number of persons connected with the MCOs to have access to material from patients' files. Clinicians should caution their patients about the potential limitations to confidentiality, and be prepared to explore the consequences of these exceptions. For example, if a patient is raising his or her mental health as an issue in litigation, some or all communications to a clinician could be legally discoverable.

Means of preserving confidentiality include obtaining proper authorization from patients before releasing information; explaining the need for confidentiality with parents of children and adolescents; and involving all participants in family and group psychotherapy in agreements about confidentiality. Problematic activities that may endanger confidentiality include stray communications with concerned relatives of patients in individual psychotherapy where there is not a prior expectation on the patient's part about discussions with relatives; discussion of privileged information with the clinician's own family members; releasing information about deceased patients; and failure to properly disguise case presentations.

9.5.6 Socialization and stepping out of the therapeutic role

Engaging in sexual behavior with current or former patients is absolutely contraindicated because it is almost invariably destructive, even though the damage may not be immediately manifested. In the therapeutic relationship, the patient's ability to consent to sexual activity with the psychiatric clinician is vitiated by the knowledge the latter possesses over the patient, and by the power differential or inequality that might lead to exploitation of the patient. Every professional group is unequivocal about sexual activity with current or former patients, stating that it is unethical in all circumstances.

Other risky forms of gratification include embracing or kissing patients; eating and drinking with patients; socializing with patients outside of the therapy setting; and failure to understand and resolve recurrent or obsessive sexual fantasies about a patient.

9.6 Rights of psychiatric patients

A patient bill of rights articulates the rights to which patients are entitled as recipients of healthcare services. It spells out the protections that healthcare providers should extend to patients. With respect to psychiatric patients, rights are particularly important insofar as their treatment tends to be more coercive, less voluntary and less open to public awareness or scrutiny. Legislation introduced in the US Senate in 2001 attempted to pass a patients' bill of rights for all Americans. The House of Representatives and the Senate passed differing versions, which remained unreconciled as of the spring of 2009. However, an alliance of mental health professional organizations have developed a bill of rights for patients in psychiatric settings. That document is summarized in Box 9.3. Subsequent sections under legal issues in psychiatric practice will more fully speak to the issues surrounding patients' rights and implications for professionals.

Box 9.3 Joint Initiative of Mental Health Professional Organizations:

Principles for the Provision of Mental Health and Substance Abuse Treatment Services

A Bill of Rights

Our commitment is to provide quality mental health and substance abuse services to all individuals without regard to race, color, religion, national origin, gender, age, sexual orientation, or disabilities.

Right to Know

- **Benefits**: Individuals have the right to be provided information from the purchasing entity (such as employer or union or public purchaser) and the insurance/third-party payer describing the nature and extent of their mental health and substance abuse treatment benefits. This information should include details on procedures to obtain access to services, on utilization management procedures, and on appeal rights. The information should be presented clearly in writing with language that the individual can understand.
- **Professional expertise**: Individuals have the right to receive full information from the potential treating professional about that professional's knowledge, skills, preparation, experience, and credentials. Individuals have the right to be informed about the options available for treatment interventions and the effectiveness of the recommended treatment.
- **Contractual limitations**: Individuals have the right to be informed by the treating professional of any arrangements, restrictions, and/or covenants established between third-party payer and the treating professional that could interfere with or influence treatment recommendations. Individuals have the right to be informed of the nature of information that may be disclosed for the purposes of paying benefits.
- **Appeals and grievances**: Individuals have the right to receive information about the methods they can use to submit complaints or grievances regarding provision of care by the treating professional to that profession's regulatory board and to the professional association. Individuals have the right to be provided information about the procedures they can use to appeal benefit utilization decisions to the third party payer systems, to the employer or purchasing entity, and to external regulatory entities.

- **Confidentiality**: Individuals have the right to be guaranteed the protection of the confidentiality of their relationship with their mental health and substance abuse professional, except when laws or ethics dictate otherwise. Any disclosure to another party will be time limited and made with the full written, informed consent of the individuals. Individuals shall not be required to disclose confidential, privileged or other information other than: diagnosis, prognosis, type of treatment, time and length of treatment, and cost. Entities receiving information for the purposes of benefits determination, public agencies receiving information for health care planning, or any other organization with legitimate right to information will maintain clinical information in confidence with the same rigor and be subject to the same penalties for violation as is the direct provider of care. Information technology will be used for transmission, storage, or data management only with methodologies that remove individual identifying information and assure the protection of the individual's privacy. Information should not be transferred, sold or otherwise utilized.
- **Choice**: Individuals have the right to choose any duly licensed/certified professional for mental health and substance abuse services. Individuals have the right to receive full information regarding the education and training of professionals, treatment options (including risks and benefits), and cost implications to make an informed choice regarding the selection of care deemed appropriate by individual and professional.
- **Determination of treatment**: Recommendations regarding mental health and substance abuse treatment shall be made only by a duly licensed/certified professional in conjunction with the individual and his or her family as appropriate. Treatment decisions should not be made by third party payers. The individual has the right to make final decisions regarding treatment.
- **Parity**: Individuals have the right to receive benefits for mental health and substance abuse treatment on the same basis as they do for any other illnesses, with the same provisions, co-payments, lifetime benefits, and catastrophic coverage in both insurance and self-funded/self-insured health plans.
- **Discrimination**: Individuals who use mental health and substance abuse benefits shall not be penalized when seeking other health insurance or disability, life or any other insurance benefit.
- **Benefit usage**: The individual is entitled to the entire scope of the benefits within the benefit plan that will address his or her clinical needs.
- **Benefit design**: Whenever both federal and state law and/or regulations are applicable, the professional and all payers shall use whichever affords the individual the greatest level of protection and access.
- **Treatment review**: To assure that treatment review processes are fair and valid, individuals have the right to be guaranteed that any review of their mental health and substance abuse treatment shall involve a professional having the training, credentials and licensure required to provide the treatment in the jurisdiction in which it will be provided. The reviewer should have no financial interest in the decision and is subject to the section on confidentiality.
- **Accountability**: Treating professionals may be held accountable and liable to individuals for any injury caused by gross incompetence or negligence on the part of the professional. The treating professional has the obligation to advocate for and document necessity of care and to advise the individual of options if payment authorization is denied. Payers and other third parties may be held accountable and liable to individuals for any injury caused by gross incompetence or negligence or by their clinically unjustified decisions.

KEY POINTS

- Psychiatric patients are especially vulnerable during treatment, so that the ethical character of the clinician has a unique and powerful potential to help or to harm patients.

- Autonomy, beneficence, non-maleficence, confidentiality, veracity, and justice are the six ethical principles of medical ethics and are common to all clinicians' codes of ethics.

- Boundaries are essential in the therapeutic relationship; violations of boundaries are an infringement that interferes with the primary goal of providing care or causes harm to the patient, to the clinician, or to the fidelity of the treatment.

- Stepping outside the boundaries of the professional role can compromise a patient's movement toward recovery.

- Clinicians must treat their patients' communications as privileged.

- Clinicians should avoid treatment situations that place them in a conflict between therapeutic responsibility to patients and third parties.

Further Reading

American Nurses Association (2001) *Code of Ethics for Nurses with Interpretive Statements*, ANA, Silver Springs, MD.

American Psychiatric Association (1993) *Principles of Medical Ethics with Annotations Especially Applicable to Psychiatry*, APA, Washington, DC.

Beauchamp, T.L. and Childress, J.F. (2001) *Principles of Biomedical Ethics*, 5th edn, Oxford University Press, New York.

Carmi, A., Moussaoui, D., and Arboleda-Florez, J. (2005) *Teaching Ethics in Psychiatry: Case Vignettes*, International Center for Health Law & Ethics, University of Haifa, Haifa, Israel. Available at: http:// medlaw.haifa.ac.il/index/main/4/teaching%20ethics%20in%20psych%20new.pdf.

Corey, G., Corey, M.S., and Callanan, P. (2003) *Issues and Ethics in the Helping Professions*, Brooks/Cole, Pacific Grove, CA.

Declaration of Geneva (1948) Adopted by the General Assembly of World Medical Association at Geneva, Switzerland, September 1948.

1982 President's Commission for the Study of Ethical Problems in Medicine and Biomedical and Behavioral Research (1982) *Making Health Care Decisions: The Ethical and Legal Implications of Informed Consent in the Patient–Practitioner Relationship*, vol. 1, US Government Printing Office, Washington, DC.

World Medical Organization (1996) Declaration of Helsinki. British Medical Journal, **313** (7070), 1448–1449.

World Psychiatric Association (1996) Madrid Declaration on Ethical Standards for Psychiatric Practice. WPA General Assembly, Madrid.

10 • Legal Context of Psychiatric Practice

10.1 Introduction

Psychiatric professionals practice within the context of a legal system that impacts the way they provide care on a daily basis. While clinicians are not expected to be experts in legal matters, this context is one that requires a clear understanding of how clinical work intersects with the law and how law affects and constrains their decision-making.

Clinicians should value, respect, and be aware of laws, legislation, and the legal processes that regulate, impede, and facilitate professional practice. By being aware of such standards, staying informed about new and changing legislation that affects clinical practice, and understanding proposed and past legislation affecting mental healthcare, they can provide quality care that safeguards the rights and safety of clients. The goal of this chapter is to discuss legal principles relevant to the practice of psychiatric medicine. It addresses different types of commitment and other significant legal issues that apply to special patient populations. The following sections discuss relevant legal issues to practice divided broadly into civil issues and criminal issues.

10.2 Hospitalization

When patients with psychiatric disorders are hospitalized, the type of admission determines the treatment plan. *Civil commitment admissions* include the following:

- Voluntary admissions

- Emergency admissions

- Involuntary commitments (indefinite duration).

Each state has specific statutory regulations pertaining to each admission status that mandate procedures for admission, discharge, and commitment for treatment.

10.2.1 Voluntary hospitalization

Patients who present themselves at psychiatric facilities and request hospitalization are considered voluntary admissions. Likewise, patients evaluated as being a danger to themselves or others or are so seriously mentally ill that they cannot adequately meet their own needs in the community but are willing to submit to treatment and are competent to do so have voluntary admission status.

Fundamentals of Psychiatry, First Edition. Allan Tasman and Wanda K. Mohr.
© 2011 John Wiley & Sons, Ltd. Published 2011 by John Wiley & Sons, Ltd.
This chapter is based on Chapter 6 (David M. Benedek, Thomas A. Grieger) of *Psychiatry, Third Edition*

Voluntary patients have certain rights that differ from the rights of other hospitalized patients. Specifically, they are considered competent (unless otherwise adjudicated) and therefore have the absolute right to refuse treatment, including psychotropic medications, unless they are dangerous to themselves or others, as in a violent destructive episode within the treatment unit (*Rennie* v. *Klein*, 1981).

Voluntary patients do not have an absolute right to discharge at any time but may be required to request discharge. This time delay gives the healthcare team an opportunity to initiate a procedure to change a patient's admission status to involuntary if the patient meets the necessary statutory requirements. Many people with mental illness can be voluntarily treated; however, the state cannot require that a patient receive treatment in any setting if he or she refuses. Therefore, many people with psychiatric disorders whose behavior causes family, community, and social problems do not and cannot receive psychiatric care if they are unwilling to be voluntary patients.

10.2.2 Emergency admissions

Patients are considered to have emergency admission status when they act in a way that indicates that they are mentally ill and, due to the illness, are likely to harm themselves or others. State statutes define the exact procedure for the initial evaluation, the possible length of detainment, and attendant treatment available.

All patients who enter the hospital as emergency admissions enter healthcare facilities for the purposes of diagnosis, evaluation, and emergency treatment. At the end of the statutorily limited admission period, the facility must discharge the patient, change his or her status to voluntary admission, or send representatives to a civil hearing to determine the need for continuing treatment on an involuntary basis.

During the emergency admission, the patient's right to come and go is restricted, but the right to consult with an attorney to prepare for a hearing must be protected. Patients may be forced to take psychotropic medications, especially if they continue to be dangerous to self or others. However, more invasive procedures, such as electroconvulsive therapy or psychosurgery, are not permitted unless they are ordered by the court or consented to by the patient or legal guardian. No treatment should impair the patient's ability to consult with an attorney at the time of a hearing.

10.2.3 Involuntary hospitalization

In the US, a person who refuses psychiatric hospitalization or treatment but poses a danger to self or others and is mentally ill and for whom less drastic treatment means are unsuitable may be adjudicated to involuntary admission status for a period of time. The exact legal procedure may differ in each state, but the standards for commitment are similar. Although the statutory language for involuntary hospitalization (civil commitment) varies from state to state, three principles serve as the basis for all commitment laws. The individual must be:

- mentally ill, and

- dangerous to self or others, or

- unable to provide for his or her own basic needs (i.e., "gravely disabled").

Involuntary hospitalization, even when accomplished entirely in the patient's best interests, represents an extreme curtailment of civil liberty. To deprive a person of liberty by involuntary commitment is a serious matter, and the legal protections are strict. The statutes of each state concerning commitment procedures must reflect the Supreme Court's standard of the protection of the right to liberty. In most statutes, the term "mentally ill" is not clearly defined but requires the petitioner (e.g., the psychiatrist) to state the psychiatric problem necessitating hospitalization and in some states that proof must be "clear and convincing" (*Addington* v. *Texas*, 1979). In some states, additional criteria such as an overt act of violence toward self or others or damage to property within a specified period of time, or the absence of available less restrictive treatment alternatives, must also be established before people can be hospitalized against their expressed desires. Most states allow for a period ranging from 1 to 20 days of emergency hospitalization for the purposes of providing immediate crisis intervention and completing a more detailed evaluation. All states require periodic reassessment of the need for continued involuntary hospitalization. Most states require that a clinician other than the primary treatment provider must certify mental illness, dangerousness, and/or grave disability under these circumstances.

When persons are involuntarily hospitalized, they generally maintain their rights to manage their own financial matters, to communicate with others via phone or mail, and to receive personal visitors. They also have rights to privacy including space to secure valuables, private bathing and toilet facilities, and personal space. These rights are typically statutorily quantified. In most states, the right of psychiatric inpatients (including those involuntarily committed) to refuse therapy and/or medication is also preserved. Involuntarily hospitalized patients require a separate judicial proceeding to establish incompetence to manage finances before a guardian can be appointed or to establish incompetence to make medical decisions before involuntary medications may be ordered. Patients' rights in hospital settings may be restricted by the clinical judgment of treating professionals in consideration of both the patient's interests and the rights and safety of other persons within the hospital. Disputes over violations of patient's rights in such situations are inevitable. In many jurisdictions, a civil rights officer or ombudsman is mandated to assist in resolving these disputes.

10.2.4 Minors and hospitalization

A special population of psychiatric patients is minors or juveniles. Until recently in the US, parents or guardians had an almost absolute privilege to admit their minor children younger than 18 years for mental health treatment. State recognition of some rights of more mature children (12–18 years old) to protest such treatment, however, has eroded this absolute right.

In 1979, the US Supreme Court, in *Parham* v. *J.R.*, gave a more definite standard for juvenile admissions, to which state statutes and hospital policy should conform. The Court held that parents can authorize the admission of juveniles, but accompanying the admission, some neutral fact-finder should determine whether statutory requirements for admission are satisfied. Furthermore, an adversarial hearing for admission is not required, nor does due process require that the fact-finder be legally trained or be a hearing officer. By ruling in this way, the court balanced the competing interests of the rights of parents and guardians to control the lives of their children with the right of children to due process before their liberty is limited.

Psychiatric clinicians need to be mindful of these procedural protections for the benefit of their juvenile patients. Limiting hospitalization to statutory requirements is an important advocacy activity for pediatric patients with mental illness.

10.3 Informed consent

In situations where patients must be involuntary hospitalized, it is impossible to obtain informed consent, but in all other instances practitioners are obliged to obtain consent for treatment.

The requirement that a physician obtain an individual's informed consent to medical treatment (*Canterbury* v. *Spence*, 1972; Natanson v. Kline, 1960) is based on a consensus that individuals have the right to control access to their own bodies and to make informed decisions about their own health and well-being decisions. Informed consent means consent that a recipient of healthcare gives to treating providers in an interaction (or series of interactions) that enables him or her to understand a proposed treatment or procedure, including the following:

- The way the treatment or procedure will be administered
- The prognosis if the treatment or procedure is given
- Side-effects
- Risks
- Possible consequences of refusing the treatment or procedure
- Other alternatives.

In the US, the landmark *Canterbury* v. *Spence* (1972) decision ruled that patients could truly be informed only if their provider shared with them all things that the patient "would find significant" in deciding whether to permit or participate in a particular treatment regimen. Informed consent requires that healthcare professionals give patients adequate and accurate knowledge and information. It mandates that the patient have the legal capacity to give consent and give it voluntarily.

All patients have the right to give informed consent before any healthcare professionals perform interventions. The administration of healthcare treatments or procedures without a patient's informed consent can result in legal action on the patient's part against the primary provider and the healthcare agency. The patient will prevail in such a lawsuit, alleging battery (touching another without permission), if it can be proven that he or she did not consent to the procedure. Consent is an absolute defense against battery, which is why informed consent is so necessary in healthcare situations.

As a broad mandate for informed consent, the US Congress passed the Patient Self-Determination Act (PSDA), which went into effect on 1 December 1991. The PSDA requires healthcare facilities to provide clear written information for every patient concerning his or her legal rights to make healthcare decisions, including the right to accept or refuse treatment.

Informed consent also protects patients from being subjected to experimental treatments and research projects without their knowledge and agreement. Because of the complexity of informed consent issues with patients who have psychiatric disorders, institutions with programs involving research or experimental treatment approaches must have institutional review boards to evaluate such projects and programs and to approve or disapprove them based on strict patient protection criteria.

There are several exceptions to the requirement of informed consent. In emergency situations where the patient experiences an acute threat to life requiring immediate medical attention, consent is implied when the patient is unable to communicate a choice (e.g., is unconscious). Circumstances and options when the patient is incompetent are addressed elsewhere in this chapter. A competent patient may also decline being informed of all facts relating to a medical decision (*waiver*) and a physician may choose to withhold full disclosure if disclosure would seriously worsen a patient's condition or impede rational decision-making (*therapeutic privilege*). In situations where a psychiatrist asserts an exception to informed consent, his or her reasoning should be clearly documented in the medical record.

10.4 Consent to the treatment of minors

Competent individuals have the right to consent to or to refuse treatment, but the same rights are rarely extended to minors. The legal rights of children in the context of healthcare in the US are a patchwork of competing opinions, laws, and attitudes and there are a number of court decisions affecting children's rights that are not necessarily coherent. In fact these decisions may range from a paternalistic or progressive approach, which focuses on nurturance and protection, to an individual rights approach, which emphasizes the child's age-appropriate right to personal autonomy. Nevertheless, it is crucial to engage children in their treatment to the extent that the clinician can make this happen, because consent, assent and transparency go to the heart of the therapeutic alliance, and effective treatment as patient choice appears to be an important determinant of treatment success.

Effective residential treatment of children often depends on the facility's relationship with both the child *and* the family. One of the major components of positive child outcomes in residential treatment for children is a family's involvement in their child's treatment planning. Family involvement in residential care is also a major component in some successful restraint reduction programs.

Although family involvement may be essential to successful treatment outcomes, this tripartite relationship among the child, parent or guardian, and care provider increases the complexity of the informed consent process since the roles of each often are more difficult to define. Each party may have conflicting obligations, interests, needs, desires and wishes that are further compounded by medical, ethical and legal standards, case law, and parental rights. When these events occur, the duty of the pediatric healthcare professional to a youth exists independent of parental desires, and the professional may be forced into an adversarial relationship requiring court intervention.

Another issue adding to the complexity of informed consent for children is a child's assent or dissent to treatment. Assent, is a lesser standard than informed consent; however, like informed consent, it indicates that children have been told about the treatment and agree to it. Obtaining assent or dissent to treatment for children and young people recognizes developmental maturation and that, as they mature, they become the "primary guardians of their personal health and the primary partners in medical decision-making" (American Academy of Pediatrics Committee on Bioethics, 1995). Quality treatment acknowledges children's rights and encourages them to play a major part in their treatment planning. Although parental authority still overrides children's assent or dissent, whether a youth assents or dissents may play a powerful role in treatment success.

Although there is no current and generally accepted framework for gaining informed consent from parents for children and adolescents in the mental health field, there is agreement in the pediatric community that parents and practitioners should not exclude children and adolescents from decision-making without persuasive reasons such as age, compromised developmental capabilities, limited intellectual and emotional competency, comprehension or rationality. Most medical standards differentiate the informed consent processes according to age categories such as infants and preschool children, primary school-aged children, adolescents, and emancipated minors. These are summarized below.

10.4.1 Primary-school children (ages 7–12)

Although primary-school children may not have full decision-making capabilities, at age seven they should be given information appropriate to their level of comprehension so that they may participate in their medical and treatment decisions.

10.4.2 Adolescents (ages 13–18)

Many adolescents have the capability to make treatment decisions based on their best interests. They may have ability to understand and communicate relevant information about themselves and their circumstances, the ability to choose and to think, and their ability to assess the potential benefits, risks, harm, or consequences. Informed consent with these youths involves gaining parental permission and adolescents' assent.

10.4.3 Emancipated and mature minors

Minors under the age of 18 can give sole consent to treatment if they are deemed "emancipated" or free from parental authority, if they are self-supporting or living independently with court permission, in the military, pregnant, or married. In the case of emancipated minors with appropriate awareness and understanding, informed consent can be obtained directly from them.

10.4.4 Special problems with families and children

The problem faced by children's psychiatric facilities is that children who present for treatment often are compromised medically, have histories of multiple placements and severe trauma, and may be adjudicated. These conditions may lead to distrust and impaired decision-making. Coercion, either real or perceived, is a danger where these dynamics are present. In these cases an advocate such as the child's law guardian or guardian *ad litem* may be an essential partner in the informed consent process, especially if the advocate defines his or her role as addressing the child's wishes, desires, and needs.

10.5 Substituted consent

When a patient cannot give informed consent, healthcare providers must obtain substituted consent for necessary treatments or procedures. Substituted consent is authorization that another person gives on behalf of a patient who needs a procedure or treatment but cannot provide such consent independently. The appointment of a healthcare proxy is one example of the concept of substituted consent.

Substituted consent can come from a court-appointed guardian or in some instances from the patient's next of kin. If the patient has not previously been adjudicated incompetent and if the law so permits and no next of kin are available to give substituted consent, the healthcare agency may initiate a court proceeding to appoint a guardian so that treatment professionals can carry out the procedure or treatment. In an emergency, the patient who is in danger of harming self or others can be given medication or be restrained or secluded without consent

10.6 Refusal of treatment and competence

The doctrine of informed consent implies that patients have the right to choose or refuse medical and health treatment. Clinicians are obliged, through interpersonal relationships and client education, to convince patients about the need for certain treatments; however, only in rare or life-threatening instances will courts intervene in treatment decisions.

Psychiatric consultation tends to be requested only when questions arise surrounding a patient's decision-making, such as when a patient refuses an important diagnostic or therapeutic procedure, or refuses physician-recommended treatment. In these situations, it may be necessary to determine whether the patient is competent to make treatment decisions. As with involuntary hospitalization, "competency" is a legal determination. All persons are presumed competent unless they have been explicitly declared legally incompetent by the appropriate court. This rule holds for even the most severely psychotic or demented patients. While a determination of incompetence is a legal one, in practice the judicial system relies heavily on medical expert testimony in making such determinations. Therefore, psychiatrists should be comfortable with processes used to assess the extent to which a patient's *capacity* to make a particular decision may be impaired. Capacity – or functional impairment – is a clinical rather than legal determination.

Decision-making capacity and competence are task specific. Patients may be competent (e.g., demonstrate the capacity) to make some medical decisions but not others depending on the complexity and consequences of the medical decision and the complexity of the medical information the patient must understand. Since there is no single legal standard for competency, appropriate criteria for assessing decision-making capacity may vary from jurisdiction to jurisdiction. Beyond clinical judgment about the complexity of the medical decision and relevant clinical information, basic principles underlying legal determinations of medical competency are summarized in Box 10.1.

Box 10.1 Elements of competency to make medical decisions.

- Ability of patient to communicate a choice
- Ability of patient to understand the relevant facts
- Ability of patient to appreciate his/her own particular circumstances and apply the facts to his/her particular case
- Ability of patient to rationally manipulate data in reaching a decision

All courts have accepted the notion that patients who are unable to communicate a choice are not competent to make medical decisions. Therefore, a comatose patient, or a psychotically paranoid patient refusing to speak to all clinicians, would be declared incompetent to make treatment decisions. More than merely communicating a decision, most courts have determined that a patient's stated decision must be sufficiently stable to be considered evidence of competence. A patient may change his mind upon further consideration.

Thus for all patients, including those hospitalized involuntarily, the right to refuse treatment is preserved unless they are declared legally incompetent to make medical treatment decisions. While most courts recognize understanding of the relevant facts and ability to communicate a choice as sufficient standards for competence, in their assessments of decision-making capacity, professionals should comment on the patient's abilities to apply the relevant facts to his or her particular case and the ability to rationally manipulate data. The clinician should focus on signs that demonstrate that the patient is (or is not) applying the facts to his or her own situation (e.g., weighing the expected side-effects of a treatment in association with his or her own social and occupational priorities), considering and balancing alternatives, and prioritizing. The clinician may not base determination on the extent the patient's ultimate decision corresponds to clinical recommendations. Except in emergencies, patients lacking medical decision-making capacity need an authorized representative or court-appointed guardian to make treatment decisions.

The time and cost of formal legal proceedings for an adjudication of incompetence may be daunting for many families, and may delay appropriate treatment. Some states allow for legally authorized proxy consent of the next of kin when a patient is *thought to be* incompetent. All states allow for the establishment of a durable power of attorney, which allows for patients' next of kin to consent when a patient becomes incompetent. Some states have passed healthcare proxy laws creating documents similar to durable power of attorneys but limited to healthcare decisions. Since consent options vary from state to state, psychiatrists should be aware of the options available to patients and their families in the jurisdictions they reside.

10.7 Confidentiality

It is a professional and an ethical duty to use knowledge gained about patients only for the enhancement of their care and not for other purposes. Psychiatric professionals must maintain the confidentiality of verbal and written information.

Preserving confidentiality is especially important in the care of patients with mental illness. Despite some advances, society still attaches a tremendous stigma to anyone with a diagnosis of psychiatric illness. Any breach of confidentiality of data about patients, their diagnoses, symptoms, behaviors, and the outcomes of treatment can certainly affect the rest of their lives in terms of employment, promotions, marriage, insurance benefits, and so forth. The practitioner, however, must maintain a delicate balance. With managed care companies (MCOs) being the payers for behavioral health services in many cases, providers (hospitals, nurses, social workers, physicians) must provide clinical information to the managed care company case manager to justify admission and continued treatment of patients. Thus, healthcare providers must obtain "fiscal informed consent" from the patient or family. It is the provider's responsibility to know the legal requirements regarding clinical confidentiality and the requirements of managed care companies to be informed of the patient's clinical condition for reimbursement.

10.7.1 The health insurance portability and accountability act

The Health Insurance Portability and Accountability Act (HIPAA) of 1996 outlines appropriate use and disclosure of the health information of patients, identifies patients' privacy rights, requires certain privacy practices of healthcare providers, and requires the development and implementation of administrative, technical, and physical safeguards to ensure the security of patients' health information.

HIPAA's Final Rule (45 C.F.R. Parts 160 and 164), which became effective on 15 October 2002, provides standards for the privacy of individually identifiable health information. Under this privacy rule, healthcare providers and others must guard against the misuse of any patient's identifiable health information. The rule also limits sharing such information and affords significant new rights to enable patients to understand and to control the use and disclosure of their health information. Protected health information under HIPAA is broadly defined as any individually identifiable health information, and includes demographic data that either identifies or could reasonably be used to identify the individual. The Privacy Rule covers healthcare providers who transmit health information electronically. Providers may use and disclose protected health information without consent, authorization, or both when they are conducting treatment, payment, and healthcare operations. Information may be disclosed without consent or authorization if so required by state or federal reporting requirements such as those related to public health, abuse, neglect, and domestic violence. Providers may disclose protected information to law enforcement officials under various specific circumstances. Providers also may disclose protected information without authorization to comply with laws related to workers' compensation, to a party responsible for paying the benefits, and to any agency responsible for handling the workers' compensation claim. Special provisions for authorization apply to psychotherapy notes.

10.7.2 Privileged communication

Privileged communication is provided by statute in each state in the US. These statutes delineate which categories of professionals are given the legal privilege to withhold conversations and communications. Although statutes differ among states, they customarily provide this privilege to physicians, attorneys, clergymen, and in some states, psychologists, nurses, and other healthcare providers. Psychiatric practitioners should be aware of statutorily privileged communication, and if the privilege is limited or nonexistent, they should know what boundaries to set in therapeutic interviews. In the absence of statutory privileges for a certain class of practitioner, he or she may be subpoenaed and required to repeat professional communications. It is a prudent practice to not encourage the patient to share sensitive or incriminating data that is not necessary for treatment planning.

In the US, some cases have involved the issue of the identification of the appropriate circumstances that warrant breach of the confidential relationship with a patient. A leading case in this area is *Tarasoff* v. *Board of Regents of University of California* (1974), which held that therapists might have a duty to protect a person who is threatened by a patient. Subsequent decisions discuss the issues of foreseeable violence and the amount of control that the therapist could reasonably use to prevent the harm. In these types of cases, courts have said that the mandate on therapists to hold patients' verbalizations in confidence is cut off when those confidences include threats against the lives of others.

Courts have held that, although the duty of confidentiality between patient and therapist should be recognized, a higher duty to protect the public safety intervenes and supersedes the duty of confidentiality. Other types of situation in which a breach of confidentiality may be required by law include allegations of child abuse, threats of suicide, and allegations of sexual misconduct made against a therapist. Box 10.2 summarizes the exceptions to the professional and legal responsibility to confidentiality.

Box 10.2 Exceptions to confidentiality.

- Patient requests release of records to third party
- Duty to protect (e.g., warn police or potential victim)
- Emergencies
- Mandatory reporting statutes (e.g., child abuse)
- Court-ordered evaluations
- Patient initiates litigation (e.g., defense of malpractice).

10.8 Responsible record-keeping

According to *A Patient's Bill of Rights* of the American Hospital Association, each patient has a right to a written record that enhances care. Accrediting agencies such as JCAHO also require each patient to have a medical record. Records may be kept manually or electronically. Records are legal documents that can be used in court; therefore, all notes and progress records should reflect descriptive, nonjudgmental, and objective statements. Examples of significant data include here-and-now observations of the patient through the use of the clinician's critical assessment, an accurate report of verbal exchanges with patients, and a description of the patient outcomes of the care provided. The medical record is the best source of legal protection in a malpractice suit.

10.9 Lawsuits and legal redress

Professional negligence, commonly referred to as "malpractice," is a particular kind of tort action that a patient plaintiff brings against a defendant professional when the plaintiff feels that an injury has been sustained within the professional relationship. For a plaintiff to receive monetary damages in a malpractice suit, he or she must prove the following elements of professional negligence:

1. The professional had a duty of due care toward the plaintiff.

2. The professional's performance breached the duty owed to the plaintiff by falling below the accepted standard of care.

3. As a result of the failure to meet the standard of care, the plaintiff was injured, and the professional's action was the proximate *cause* of the injury and that it was forseeable that the action would cause an injury.

4. The plaintiff sustained injury or harm.

To decrease their chances of liability for malpractice, professionals must ensure that their professional practice is within the bounds of statutory and professional standards. In a malpractice action against a nurse, proof of the "standard of care" becomes essential. Both sides usually present expert witness testimony to give the jury perspectives about what are considered professional practices and standards. The appropriate expert witness for psychiatric practice is another psychiatric practitioner who knows about the standard of care in the same or similar situations. Both sides include such expert testimony and submit it with all other testimony and evidence to the jury for a decision. The issue of negligence refers to a peer standard for reasonableness of action, not a standard for excellence of action. Thus, when making legal decisions, the court asks the jury to apply the "reasonable person" test to the facts of the case at hand. The "reasonable person" test, as applied to the psychiatric professional, is what a reasonably prudent professional of the same discipline would have done under similar circumstances if that clinician came from the same or a similar community.

Although it is estimated that 50–65% of all physicians will experience at least one malpractice lawsuit during their career, psychiatrists and other mental health clinicians tend to be sued less often than other practitioners. One reason is that their treatments are less likely to kill or maim. Also, the focus that mental health practitioners have on the importance of the therapeutic relationship may be a mitigating factor in preventing litigation. Both patients and families view such relationships positively. Lawsuits tend to occur when a bad outcome is associated with bad feelings about the professional on the part of the plaintiff.

Patient suicide is one of the most frequent outcomes associated with lawsuits in psychiatry. Suicides occurring in hospitalized patients often result in litigation, since one purpose of hospitalization is to provide close monitoring and safety for potentially suicidal patients. In a hospital environment, psychiatrists and staff are assumed to have greater control of their patients' actions. In such situations malpractice is more likely to be established when medical staff members fail to adhere to hospital or Joint Commission policies and regulations regarding the monitoring of suicidal patients.

"No-suicide contracts" have been used by clinicians under the mistaken belief that these will protect them from liability. These contracts have never been shown to reduce suicide, litigation, or adverse legal outcomes. Indeed they may be harmful in that they can create a barrier to patient communication and they may reduce or diminish vigilance for suicidal potential.

The courts have recognized that current medical knowledge does not fully allow for the prediction of suicidal behavior – particularly in less restrictive (e.g., outpatient) settings. Consequently, outpatient psychiatrists are somewhat less likely to be sued when patients commit suicide. However, routinely assessing for risk of suicide, monitoring changes in risk, and providing treatment informed by ongoing risk assessment are considered part of the standard of psychiatric care in both inpatient and outpatient settings The courts have generally held that suicide should be prevented if it is *reasonably foreseeable*, suggesting that a psychiatric risk assessment should be reasonable (e.g., include an examination for known risk factors such as history of suicide attempts, depression, anxiety, psychosis, recent socioeconomic or interpersonal loss, possession of firearms, and substance abuse). Treatment plans should also be altered to reflect changing risk factors. Psychiatrists should carefully document and periodically update suicide risk assessment in their patients as well as interventions aimed at mitigating the risk.

10.10 Liability for supervising other professionals

When a professional supervises another practitioner, the supervisor gives active guidance and professional direction and retains responsibility for patient care. The legal doctrine of *respondeat superior* – "let the master answer for the deeds of his servant" – provides the basis for the assumption of liability by the supervising psychiatrist in malpractice cases involving the care provided by those whom he supervises.

When a clinician provides consultation, guidance provided may be accepted or declined by the professional seeking consultation. Therefore, the consulting professional is not considered to have assumed responsibility for the patient's care.

Frequently, the relationship between a psychiatrist and non-physician therapist takes the form of collaboration. Here, the responsibility for patient care is shared between the two clinicians in accordance with the professional qualifications and limitations of their respective professions.

10.11 Criminal issues

In contrast to the civil issues outlined above, practicing psychiatrists interact much less frequently with the criminal law system. But there are circumstances in which mental health professionals become involved with patients who are charged with criminal acts:

1. For the evaluation of a defendant's competency to stand trial and administration of concomitant pretrial treatment, if needed

2. For the evaluation of a defendant's mental condition at the time of an alleged crime and administration of concomitant treatment if the defendant pleads and is acquitted on an insanity defense.

This specialized area is called *forensic psychiatry*. Ideally, the mental health team responsible for providing forensic evaluations and services is composed of a psychiatrist; clinical psychologist; social worker; psychiatric nurse practitioner; and/or other personnel who are active in the patient's evaluation and treatment.

10.11.1 Competency to stand trial

Competency to stand trial refers to a defendant's mental condition at the time of the trial. Mental health professionals determine whether the defendant is competent by assessing the following in the defendant:

* Ability to assist the attorney with defense

* Understanding of the nature and consequences of the charge against him or her

* Understanding of courtroom procedures.

A decision handed down by the US Supreme Court in *Jackson* v. *Indiana* (1972) resulted in state statutes designed to protect the rights of criminal defendants who continue to be incompetent to stand trial by virtue of their mental illnesses. These defendants can no longer be detained for an indefinite time without the benefit of the same type of commitment hearing to which all civilly committed patients have a right. In other words, these pretrial defendants should be returned to court as soon as they are competent to stand trial, which should be the primary goal of pretrial treatment.

10.11.2 *Pleas of insanity or mental illness*

If the defendant chooses to plead an insanity defense, mental health professionals are involved in evaluating the defendant's mental condition at the time of the alleged crime. A person found not guilty by reason of insanity is involuntarily admitted to a psychiatric facility for a statutorily defined evaluation period. During this time, mental health professionals evaluate the need for hospitalization and any other appropriate disposition. On completion of the evaluation, the professionals notify the court of their recommendations, at which time a hearing may be scheduled to determine the court's order for release or for continuation of mandatory commitment for treatment. As soon as patients are considered not committable, they must be released into the community, possibly with some mandatory requirements for aftercare.

A great deal of controversy surrounds the verdict of "not guilty by reason of insanity," particularly as a consequence of the acquittal of John Hinckley following his attempt to assassinate President Ronald Reagan in 1981. As a result of this controversy, some states have passed a "guilty but mentally ill" plea, meant to mandate psychiatric treatment of criminals with mental illness in correctional facilities.

Clinical Vignette

A businessman referred his 23-year-old stepdaughter Sara to a psychiatrist, explaining: "I told her she could only come to work in my office if she got her act together, stopped partying so much, stopped acting so down and out every time things didn't go her way, and acted more responsibly."

At the initial evaluation, Sara relates a lengthy history of low self-esteem, intermittent episodes of depression accompanied by neurovegetative symptoms, a history of deliberate self-injurious cutting behaviors when particularly feeling "overwhelmed by my life," and of suicide attempts (via combinations of medication and alcohol overdoses) and related psychiatric hospitalizations. She notes that she has neither attempted suicide nor been hospitalized since her mother remarried 8 months ago.

At the time of the evaluation Sara denies depressed mood or neurovegetative symptoms of depression. "The only good thing my last doctor did was start me on paroxetine and I think that's helped," but she reports "increasing anxiety since starting work for my stepdad, since he expects me to work on odd hours and my boyfriend doesn't seem to like it when I can't be at his beck and call." Her affect is labile during the interview, but she does not appear anxious and she denies significant anxiety except surrounding her boyfriend "who means everything to me." She denies current suicidal ideation, but reports increased urges to cut herself when her boyfriend (of four weeks) threatens to terminate the relationship. He has done this twice in the last two weeks, but they have reconciled on each occasion. Sara also reports weekly binge alcohol use with her boyfriend, but denies alcohol-related legal or occupational difficulties. She notes: "I drink a lot less then my real father, and unlike him, I don't abuse anyone when I'm loaded."

The psychiatrist obtains Sara's informed consent to begin individual psychotherapy and group dialectical behavior therapy, and to continue the paroxetine started by her family physician. He recommends that she consider specific treatment aimed at reducing her alcohol use and provides information on Alcoholics Anonymous and phone numbers for local AA meetings. Sara declines participation: "I've got enough on my plate with my appointments with you, this DBT group thing, work, and my boyfriend."

Two weeks later Sara is killed in a single-vehicle alcohol-related motor vehicle accident. The police investigation reveals that, on the night of her death, after her boyfriend broke up with her at a local bar, she fled in tears. Her boyfriend notes that her last words to him were: "If this is goodbye it is my last goodbye. Life isn't worth it." The police determine the accident to have been a suicide. The businessman sues the psychiatrist for failure to sufficiently treat the patient's depression.

At the trial, the psychiatrist produces medical record documentation of his thorough diagnostic evaluation, his diagnostic assessment (including a risk assessment for suicide) and his efforts to target modifiable risk factors for self-injury. These included continued treatment and monitoring for depressive symptoms, addressing anxiety-provoking situations and behaviors in therapy, and continued efforts to enroll the patient in alcohol-specific treatments. The psychiatrist had addressed the issues of the potential for acute mood and behavioral changes precipitated by workplace or social stressors with the patient; the medical records indicated that he had provided the patient with his emergency phone number as well as the number for 24-hour emergency coverage associated with his practice. The records indicate that the patient had agreed to utilize these numbers if she believed she needed help between appointments.

The psychiatrist's lawyer obtains expert testimony acknowledging the standard of care for comorbid depression, borderline personality disorder, and alcohol abuse, and the effort the psychiatrist had taken to anticipate the potential for self-harm. The expert also identifies the intervening variable (the boyfriend's decision to break off the relationship) as one over which the psychiatrist had no control. The psychiatrist's lawyer argues that no deviation from the standard of care occurred, that the relationship break-up precipitated the suicide, so there was neither "deviation" nor "direct causation." The defense was successful, and the jury determined that no malpractice occurred.

KEY POINTS

- A failure to meet the standard of care that results in an injury to a patient makes the clinician liable for negligence or malpractice.

- To provide legally acceptable psychiatric care, clinicians should be informed about a variety of legal issues, including patient rights, and take responsibility to see that patient rights are protected.

- All patients have the right to give informed consent before any healthcare professionals perform interventions.

- When questions arise surrounding a patient's decision-making, such as when a patient refuses an important diagnostic or therapeutic procedure, or refuses physician-recom-mended treatment, it may be necessary to determine whether the patient is competent to make treatment decisions.

- Psychiatric professionals must maintain the confidentiality of verbal and written information.

- It is a prudent practice to not encourage the patient to share sensitive or incriminating data that is not necessary for treatment planning.

- Patient suicide is one of the most frequent outcomes associated with lawsuits in psychiatry.

- The medical record is the best source of legal protection in a malpractice suit.

Legal Citations

Addington v. *Texas*, 99 S. Ct. 1813, 441 U.S. 418 (1979).
Canterbury v. *Spence*, 464, F2nd 772, 786, (D.C. Cir. 1972).
HIPAA Final Rule, 45 C.F.R. Parts 160 & 164 (2002).
Jackson v. *Indiana*, 46 U.S. 715 (1972).
Nathanson v. *Kline*, 350 P2nd 1093, 1106 (Kan, 1960).
Parham, Commissioner, Department of Human, Resources of Georgia et al. v. *J.R. et al.*, 442 U.S. 584 (1979).
Rennie v. *Klein*, 653 F.2d 836 (1981).
Tarasoff v. *Board of Regents of University of California*, 592 P.S. 553 (1974).

Further Reading

American Academy of Pediatrics Committee on Bioethics (1995) Informed consent, parental permission, and assent in pediatric practice. *Pediatrics*, **95**, 314–317 (Reaffirmed October 2006).
Bioethics Committee Canadian Paediatric Society (2004) Making treatment decisions for babies, children, and teens. *Paediatrics & Child Health*, **9**, 99–103.
Bursztajn, H.J. and Brodsky, A. (1994) Authenticity and autonomy in the managed-care era: forensic psychiatric perspectives. *Journal of Clinical Ethics*, **5**, 237–242.
Felthous, A. (1999) The clinician's duty to protect third parties. *Psychiatric Clinics of North America*, **22** (1), 49.
LeFrancois, B.A. (2008) "It's like mental torture": participation and mental health services. *International Journal of Children's Rights*, **16**, 211–227.
Mulvey, E.P. and Peoples, F.L. (1996). Are disturbed and normal adolescents equally competent to make decisions about mental health treatments? *Law and Human Behavior*, **20**, 273–287.
President's Commission for the Study of Ethical Problems in Medicine and Biomedical and Behavioral Research (1982) *Making Health Care Decisions: The Ethical and Legal Implications of Informed Consent in the Patient-Practitioner Relationship*, vol. **1**, US Government Printing Office, Washington, DC.

Unit 3
Clinical Disorders

Pediatric Disorders

11.1 Introduction

This chapter presents an overview of mental health issues in children and adolescents with brief discussions of common psychiatric disorders, pervasive developmental disorders, and mental retardation. It is beyond the scope of this book to include a discussion of in-depth care of each individual disorder. Depression, attention deficit hyperactivity disorder, and other commonly diagnosed conditions in children and adolescents that clinicians will encounter in practice receive special focus within this chapter. For more in-depth material, readers are referred to the sources listed at the end of this chapter. Issues concerning child abuse and neglect and reactive attachment disorders, substance abuse, and eating disorders are discussed in other chapters.

11.2 Risk factors

No single cause can explain child and adolescent psychopathology. Risk factors that may cause a child to be more susceptible include: family history of a mental illness; immature development of the brain; brain abnormality; family problems and dysfunction; poverty; mentally ill or substance-abusing parents; teen parents; abuse; discrimination based on race, creed, or color; chronic parental conflict or divorced parents; and chronic illness or disability. The developmental ecological model of psychopathology and a discussion of risk and protective factors is more fully explained in Chapter 3 of this book.

11.3 Importance of the family context

The importance of the family environment and its influence in the life of children cannot be over-stated. Children cannot be understood in the absence of understanding their family context, and families are integral to successful treatment. Parent–child transactions are two-way, reciprocal relationships. Children largely acquire the coordination of affect, cognition, and behavior, which they need to relate successfully to others within the socializing context of the parent–child relationship.

Families do not operate in a vacuum – the behavior of each family member affects the others, and each member is affected by other contexts to which he or she is exposed. Therefore, many situations affect family dynamics, and those dynamics may change from more to less adaptive depending on the nature of contextual factors. For example, a family may function adaptively given one set of circumstances (e.g., death of a grandparent) but maladaptively given another (e.g., sudden unemployment).

Because they function within a family that helps to buffer the effects of social change, children are less susceptible to sociocultural influences than are adults. As they grow and mature, however,

Fundamentals of Psychiatry, First Edition. Allan Tasman and Wanda K. Mohr.
© 2011 John Wiley & Sons, Ltd. Published 2011 by John Wiley & Sons, Ltd.

children increasingly come into contact with the larger society. Stable, nurturing forces in the child's home protect him or her from noxious exogenous influences. If children do not have stable nurturing forces in the home, they may be at risk for maladjustment.

Parents' fears, anxiety, depression, and aggression, as well as their love, nurturance, and concern, shape the youth's developing sense of self and the world. What parents believe about their world is often reflected in their child's skills or deficits.

11.4 General interventions

Increasing recognition of the complexities of the etiologies of psychopathology have moved the field of child and adolescent psychiatry beyond a disease model and simple social explanations. Research into genetic, neurophysiologic, and environmental variables and their effects on behavior have provided understanding of adaptation and maladaptation (see Chapter 3). Although the knowledge base for child and developmental psychopathology has grown exponentially in the last decade, it has been and continues to be compromised by the atheoretical, unsystematic, and somewhat fragmented fashion in which research findings have accrued. That is changing to some degree, but change comes slowly to the practice arena, and clinicians may find interventions in place in service provision to children and their families that are not based in the current science.

11.4.1 Coordination of care

Many mental health professionals participate in the care of a mentally ill child or adolescent. They include psychiatrists, advanced practice clinicians, social workers, psychologists, recreational therapists, and occupational therapists among others. Although some disciplines overlap in the care they provide, each discipline contributes a unique service. For example, reviewing psychological testing results helps the clinician develop a comprehensive picture of a patient's diagnosis and condition.

11.4.2 Treatment settings and continuum of care

Treatment for mentally ill children is provided in many different settings, from the most restrictive levels of care for a seriously disturbed youth to the least restrictive level. Treatment services within these levels include preventive services, early intervention, crisis stabilization, inpatient hospitalization, crisis in-home services, residential treatment, partial hospitalization, day treatment, therapeutic foster care, case management, family support services, outpatient counseling, and medication management. Discharge planning, a collaborative process involving the youth, family, and mental health team, begins with admission to the inpatient unit or other treatment service.

Current structures of service provision, known as systems of care (SOCs), are slowly replacing the former wrap-around services models. These SOCs are a comprehensive spectrum of mental health and other necessary services organized into a coordinated network. This network is dynamic and changes as the needs of the children and families change.

11.4.3 Early identification

Early identification and treatment are the keys to reducing the harm caused by psychiatric disorders in children and adolescents. Clinicians play integral roles in detecting early symptoms, such as depression, and referring children and families to appropriate psychiatric care providers. Screening for, and prevention of, psychiatric disorders needs to start during infancy. In addition, early intervention with children and teens at risk can prevent more serious maladjustment and emotional turmoil later in life.

11.4.4 Types of interventions and therapies

Several different forms of therapy are available to treat the child or adolescent with a psychiatric disorder. Whichever type of therapy is used, it is important to consider the child's and family's culture (see Chapter 7).

Individual therapy focuses on the needs and problems of the child or adolescent. Individual therapy is often of the cognitive and behavioral types, as these have the greatest empirical support in terms of efficacy. Behavioral and cognitive therapy is based on the concept that psychiatric disorders represent learned behavior. Thus, learning principles are applied to modifying these behaviors. Behavioral techniques include the use of token economies, time-out (from positive reinforcement), and rewards for – and reinforcements of – desired behaviors (see Chapter 32). Participation in devising a written behavioral contract helps increase a youth's adherence to the treatment plan. Cognitive therapy, which assists with problem-solving and stopping negative self-perceptions, is likely to work well with older adolescents who may view a behavioral management system as a type of adult control. Other forms of empirically validated individual therapies are cognitive problem skills training and multisystem therapy.

Brief psychotherapy addresses a central issue in a specified time. The provider and child do not discuss extraneous issues. The provider openly explores the central problem with the child and family.

Play therapy is a vehicle that offers children an opportunity to express their fears, anxieties, frustrations, and aggression. Play is the child's work and natural medium for expression. Play therapy is, however, a misnomer. The play is the means for the therapy to take place. In play therapy, the assumption is that the child expresses and works out conflicts and problems through play. There is no support, however, for the supposition that play therapy can be used as a way to establish the truth of past events. Moreover, despite its ubiquity in many child settings, empirical evidence is not available to verify its effectiveness. Most research on play therapy consists of case reports and trials comparing play with other forms of therapy, but does not account for the effects of the intense attention that the child receives.

Family therapy is based on the premise that the behavior of one person in the family affects everyone else in the family. No behavior of an individual can be understood without understanding the behavior of other family members. Interventions are directed at the family as a whole and their behavior patterns, not at one member. The idea in family therapies is that treating a child or adolescent successfully necessitates modifying how the home environment is reinforcing his or her behavior.

Parent management training (PMT) refers to procedures in which parents are trained to alter their child's behavior in the home on the premise that the child's maladaptive behavior is inadvertently developed and sustained by maladaptive parent–child interactions. Altering those interactions is hypothesized to reduce these problem behaviors. PMT involves educating and coaching parents to change their child's problem behaviors using principles of learning theory and behavior modification. The aim of PMT is to decrease or eliminate a child's disruptive or inappropriate behaviors at home or school and to replace problematic ways of acting with positive interactions with peers, parents, and such authority figures as teachers. In order to accomplish this goal, PMT focuses on enhancing parenting skills. The goal is to replace coercive behavior with prosocial behavior between parent and child interchanges. This training has been extensively studied and is a promising treatment for children with a conduct disorder.

Group therapy is especially helpful for adolescents for whom the influence of peers is strong; adolescents are more likely to accept feedback and suggestions from their peers than from adults. The exception to this is with conduct-disordered children, in which negative behaviors may actually be reinforced by the group. Group therapy is less threatening than individual therapy and allows the adolescent to identify with others who have similar problems. Groups provide opportunities to learn to identify and dismiss defeating cognitions and practice new behaviors.

A *therapeutic milieu* is a planned treatment environment that should be flexible and normalizing, as well as geared toward helping children develop self-responsibility and healthy interdependence with others. Ideally, the milieu should be planned to support and guide children toward greater responsibility and a more robust locus of control within their individual capacities. In a therapeutic milieu, interactions become opportunities for therapeutic intervention, and open, clear communication is modeled. Through the day-to-day normalizing experiences the child or teen can learn how to manage activities, deal with feelings, and get along with others. Milieu staff members work to model supportive and respectful behavior. Inpatient or residential milieu settings must offer safety, security, clear and reasonable limits, behavioral consequences, age-appropriate activities, and 24-hour availability of mature, caring adults.

The *collaborative problem-solving* (CPS) model is an approach to communicating and interacting with children who are inflexible and often explosive. It is posited on the idea that a child's capacity for complying with a caregiver's directives or expectations is unique to each child, and if the caregiver's demands exceed that capacity the child's responses deviate from those expected. These deviations may increase frustration levels for both parties, and may result in response biases on the part of both. The CPS model assumes that children "do well if they can." It aims at helping challenging children and their adult caregivers to learn to resolve conflicts, disputes, and disagreements in a collaborative, mutually satisfactory way. The approach consists of three steps. The first is to identify and understand a child's concern about a given issue and to reassure the child that the issue will not be resolved through coercion. The second is identifying the adult caregiver's perspective on the same issue or problem. The third is to invite the child to brainstorm possible solutions with the goal being to mutually agree upon a realistic course of action.

Special education describes an educational alternative that focuses on teaching students with academic, behavioral, health, or physical needs beyond those met by traditional educational programs or techniques. Ideally, this process involves the individually planned and systematically monitored arrangement of teaching procedures, adapted equipment and materials, accessible settings, and other interventions designed to help students with special needs achieve success in school and community than would be available if the student were only given access to a typical classroom education.

The goals of special education are as follows:

- Decrease the child's disturbing behavior.

- Increase the child's rate of learning to enable him or her to remediate and progress.

- Reintegrate the child into regular classes as soon as possible.

Coordination and collaboration between school and other care systems is critical.

Pharmacologic therapy is an important part of any treatment program. Medication does not solve all the child's or teen's problems. If it is combined with therapies, family education, parent guidance, and special education, medication improves the likelihood that the child's symptoms will decrease and his or her functioning will improve. Psychotropic medication must be given cautiously to children and adolescents because of the idiosyncratic reactions they can have, and because their rates of metabolism may be quite different from that of adults (see Chapter 33).

11.5 Common psychiatric disorders

Many psychiatric illnesses affect children and adolescents. Some of these illnesses are usually first diagnosed during infancy, childhood, or adolescence. Alternatively, some disorders develop in childhood or adulthood, but the manifestations, treatment, or both in children and adolescents may differ from that of the adult. The disorders discussed in this section include the most common child and adolescent mental disorders from each category.

11.5.1 *Mental retardation*

In the DSM-IV-TR taxonomy, mental retardation is defined on the basis of three features:

- Intellectual functioning with an IQ of approximately 70 or below

- Concurrent deficits or impairments in present adaptive functioning in at least two of the following areas: communication, self-care, home living, social/interpersonal skills

- Onset before 18 years of age.

Mental retardation (MR) affects 2–3% of the general population, although some experts argue that only about 1% should receive the diagnosis. The large majority of retarded persons fall in the mild range of retardation (intelligence quotient, IQ = 50–70), and smaller numbers are moderately (IQ = 35–49), severely (IQ = 20–34), or profoundly (IQ < 20) retarded. Children with severe and profound MR come to attention earlier than those with borderline or mild MR. More males than females are affected, and retardation can coexist with psychological disorders and physical disabilities.

ICD-10 characterizes mental retardation as a condition resulting from a failure of the mind to develop completely. There are several hundred disorders associated with mental retardation. The most common factor associated with severe mental retardation (including the moderate, severe, and profound levels of mental retardation) has been chromosomal abnormality, particularly Down syndrome. In approximately 20–30% of the individuals identified with severe mental retardation the cause has been attributed to prenatal factors, such as chromosomal abnormality. Perinatal factors such as perinatal hypoxia account for about 11%, and postnatal factors such as brain trauma account for 3–12% of severe mental retardation. In 30–40% of cases, the cause is reported to be unknown.

Knowledge of the sequence of development traversed by normal children has proved useful in early behavioral interventions with mentally retarded children. Studies of programs serving retarded children aged below 5 years have shown that particular types of cognitive and social stimulation can increase levels of functioning.

Research on older retarded children has shown that motivational factors play the major role in determining how productive and independent the children ultimately become. As retarded children face increased failure experiences compared to normal children, however, they may develop traits that work against their becoming independent. They often become overly wary of adults and develop a lower expectancy of success (i.e., they do not expect to succeed at challenging tasks). At the same time, children with MR are more likely to become dependent on adult approval and to accept adult (as opposed to their own) solutions to difficult problems. The net effect is that these children frequently perform below the level of their intellectual abilities on a variety of experimental and real-life tasks.

The range of psychiatric disorders in people with MR is similar to that of "normal" populations. Appropriate assessment of psychopathology in patients with dual diagnosis is important because: (a) it can suggest the form of treatment; (b) it may ensure access to and funding for special services; and (c) it can be used to evaluate subsequent interventions. Brain damage, epilepsy and language disorders are risk factors for psychiatric disorders and are often associated with mental retardation. Social isolation, stigmatization, and poor social skills put individuals with mental retardation at further risk for affective disorders.

Because children with mental retardation often have other problems, it is necessary to involve a team of practitioners from different disciplines (e.g., child psychiatrist, social worker, child psychologist, special education teacher, speech and language specialist, and community agencies), in the comprehensive diagnosis and care. The involvement of the family in the decision-making processes is crucial. In the United States, Public Law 99–457 and Public Law 102–119 *require* the involvement of parents and professionals in early intervention services. A family-centered inter-disciplinary approach involves an assessment of the child (including school history, obtained from parents and school records), family (family marital and parenting history), and community resources. Medical, developmental and psychiatric histories are obtained. Behavioral analysis, psycho-educational, speech and language testing are completed. Medical and neurological assessments are performed. The team presents these results to the parents who are actively involved in evaluating and implementing treatment recommendations.

11.5.2 *Autism spectrum disorders*

Autism spectrum disorders, also called *pervasive developmental disorders,* have as their core features impairments in socialization, impairments in communication, and restricted repertoire of behaviors.

In 2007, the Centers for Disease Control and Prevention (CDC) in Atlanta reported that across the US autism rates were in the range of 6.7 per 1000, with approximately 1 in 150 eight-year-old children affected by an autism spectrum disorder.

11.5.2.1 Autism

Autism is a genetic disorder of neuronal organization occurring more in boys than girls. Chromosomal abnormalities are present in 5–6% of children with autism, and the role of genetic mechanisms is suggested by the observation that siblings of affected people are at a 22-fold or greater risk of autism than the general population. Autims is not caused by vaccinations.

Children with autism develop language slowly or not at all. They may use words without attaching meaning to them or communicate with gestures or noises instead of words. They spend time alone and show little interest in making friends. Approximately 50–80% of people with autism also are classified as mentally retarded. Their most distinctive feature, however, is that they seem isolated from the world around them. This detachment and aloofness helps distinguish people with autism from those who are solely mentally retarded. Children with autism are less responsive to social cues such as smiles or eye contact. They often have some degree of sensory impairment, including sensitivity in the areas of sight, taste, hearing, touch, or smell.

Children with autism do not play spontaneously or imaginatively. They act socially aloof and indifferent. They do not imitate others' actions or participate in pretend games. They may act aggressively and throw tantrums for no obvious reason. In addition, they may *perseverate*; that is, show an obsessive interest in some item or activity and engage in ritualistic behavior. They often adhere to routines and do not tolerate changes in routine well. These characteristics are evident in children with autism before the age of 3 years.

11.5.2.2 Asperger syndrome

Asperger syndrome, a condition occurring more frequently in boys, is a severe developmental disorder characterized by major difficulties in social interaction and restricted and unusual interests and behavior. Although there is not a significant general delay in language, people with Asperger syndrome use monotone speech and rigid language. They tend to be concrete and naive. Despite not grasping nonverbal communication cues and an inability to show empathy to others, they want to meet people and make friends. Mental retardation usually is not observed with Asperger syndrome, although occasional cases of accompanying mild mental retardation have been noted.

People with Asperger syndrome have an obsession with facts about circumscribed and odd topics. For example, they may have a tremendous interest in, and talk incessantly about, a topic that would not have interest or appeal to others. They are often rigid and perfectionistic.

11.5.2.3 Childhood disintegrative disorder

Childhood disintegrative disorder is a rare condition that is characterized by the development of an "autistic-like" picture and a marked regression following a period of normal development. It is often mistaken for autism. In this condition, onset of skill deterioration begins between ages 3 and 4 years. Skills lost are usually those of communication and motor development. Males are more likely to be affected. Prevalence rates are approximately 1 in 100 000 children. The outcome for children with childhood disintegrative disorder is usually very poor, worse than for children with autism. The loss of language, cognitive, social and self-care skills tends to be severe and permanently disabling. As a result, children with the disorder may eventually need residential care in a group home or long-term care facility.

11.5.2.4 Treatments

Improved outcomes are achieved with early detection. An easy screening tool for 18-month-olds is the Checklist for Autism in Toddlers (CHAT), which is used to evaluate the child's ability to pretend, enjoyment in peekaboo games, attempts to engage the parent, and eye contact.

Treatment for patients with autism, Asperger syndrome, and related disorders centers on behavioral interventions, particularly cognitive and behavior therapy, special education, social skills training in groups, language therapies, occupational therapy, and sometimes pharmacotherapy. Behavior modification techniques include those used to enhance and reduce certain behaviors.

Medication may be needed to manage the symptoms of hyperactivity, irritability, aggression, self-injury, ritualistic behavior, and obsessive–compulsive behavior. These can span a wide range of psychoactive medications, including the SGAs, anticonvulsants, and mood stabilizers.

Treatment needs change according to the age of the developing child. Speech and language therapy and assistance to parents are critical when the child is very young. An older child or adolescent may need cognitive–behavioral therapy and medication to deal with obsessive–compulsive symptoms. The child's prognosis is more positive when language development and social interaction are less impaired.

Children with an autism spectrum disorder need a structured environment and social–emotional training. The goal may be to learn to imitate social behavior that other children learn intuitively. In addition, special education placement in public school settings with measurable goals and objectives for the child is necessary.

Parents require accurate information, training in becoming advocates for their child, respite programs, and inclusion in individualized, collaborative treatment planning to understand and help their child. Future needs of the child with autism spectrum disorder might include vocational training and placement, use of sheltered workshops, supported employment, and community-based programs such as group home or supervised apartment living.

11.5.3 Learning disorders

A comprehensive discussion of learning disorders is beyond the scope of this chapter and book. Readers are directed to references contained at the end of this chapter for more in-depth information.

The generic term "learning disabilities," used when children are classified for education purposes, encompasses seven categories. Under the guidelines for special education, these categories are listening, speaking, basic reading skills, reading comprehension, written expression, mathematics calculation, and mathematic reasoning. School guidelines do not include other learning problems, but such problems certainly affect academic functioning. These would include problems of concentration, attention, memory, and executive function. In the US, when a learning disability is suspected, a complete multidisciplinary evaluation can be requested at the child's local public school (even if the child attends a private school or is home-schooled), or the child can be referred to the appropriate psychology, speech and language, or education professionals for discipline-specific evaluation.

11.5.4 Disruptive behavior disorders

Three disruptive behavior disorders are commonly seen in children and adolescents: ADHD, oppositional–defiant disorder, and conduct disorder.

11.5.4.1 Attention-deficit hyperactivity disorder

Attention-deficit hyperactivity disorder (ADHD) is a psychiatric disorder characterized by inattention, impulsivity, and hyperactivity. ADHD is diagnosed by means of comprehensive clinical evaluation, as well as parents' and teachers' ratings of inattention, hyperactivity, and impulsivity. Approximately 5% of the population has ADHD. ADHD occurs in families. If a child has ADHD, the chance of a sibling having ADHD is 30%; if a parent has ADHD, the risk for a child may be as high as 25–50%. The exact etiology is unclear, but it seems to be a heterogeneous disorder involving neurologic and genetic factors. Recent studies done through magnetic resonance imaging have identified differences in brain function in patients with ADHD.

The primary symptoms of ADHD are inattention and hyperactivity or impulsivity. In children and adolescents, these symptoms often take the following forms:

- Forgetting to do or to turn in homework

- Failing to hear or follow directions

- Daydreaming during school and at times when attention is required

- Talking excessively and inappropriately

- Constantly moving and climbing

- Not remaining seated during class or meals

- Taking extraordinary risks

- Losing objects, particularly those needed for schoolwork, such as books, pencils, and paper.

These symptoms eventually lead to poor performance or failure in school. Adolescents tend to have more inattentive and impulsive symptoms than hyperactivity and, therefore, may be ignored, under-diagnosed, and under-treated. Children with ADHD also grow up with stigma and negative feedback from others about their behavior. As a result, they may view themselves as stupid, frustrated, "messing up," helpless, and worthless.

ADHD continues into adulthood for at least 50% of youths who are diagnosed and causes impairment in 11% of them. Teens and adults who seem to no longer have the same level of problems they had when younger most likely learned a variety of coping skills to compensate for their symptoms. These skills would include various ways to increase focus and maintain attention during tasks.

Adults with ADHD may have a history of poor performance in work and school settings, inattention, distractibility, restlessness, procrastination, disorganization, impulsive behavior, and driving problems. They have a higher-than-average risk for drug and alcohol abuse and accompanying legal problems.

Comorbid psychiatric conditions often accompany ADHD, especially untreated ADHD, in both children and adults. These include oppositional–defiant disorder (see below), conduct disorder, depressive disorders, early-onset substance abuse disorders, and learning disorders. These comorbid disorders may require additional pharmacologic treatment.

Treating ADHD involves psychopharmacologic as well as psychosocial interventions. Medication used in conjunction with other treatments is more effective than medication used alone. The goals of treatment are to improve self-regulation and social functioning.

Stimulant medication is the primary pharmacologic treatment for ADHD. About 70–75% of youths and adults with ADHD respond favorably to these medications. Stimulants increase concentration or focus, decrease hyperactivity, impulsivity, and aggression. The most commonly used stimulant medications are methylphenidate, dextroamphetamine, and a combination of mixed amphetamine salts. A newer medication, atomoxetine (a selective norepinephrine re-uptake inhibitor), is not a part of the stimulant class and has also been found useful in treatment of ADHD. Pemoline is a less-useful stimulant medication because of the risk of serious or lethal liver toxicity. Pemoline has been removed from the market in Canada (see Chapter 33).

Other medications that have been used to treat ADHD, particularly for patients who cannot tolerate stimulants, include bupropion, clonidine, and first-generation cyclic antidepressants. But none of these has been shown to be as effective as the stimulant class of medication. The American Academy of Pediatrics has issued a practice guideline for the treatment of school-aged children with ADHD (available at: http://aappolicy.aappublications.org/cgi/content/full/pediatrics;108/4/1033).

Psychosocial, or non-pharmacologic, treatment interventions include education for patient and family, organizational coaching, supports provided at school and home, and behavior therapy. One school system uses specially trained, paraprofessional classroom aides who design and implement a behavioral program for the struggling student. Adolescents may benefit from behavior management and cognitive therapy to manage their trouble in controlling impulses, focusing attention, and following rules. Educational and support groups and organizations can provide important information and help for families.

11.5.4.2 Oppositional–defiant disorder

Oppositional–defiant disorder (ODD) is marked by negativistic, defiant behaviors such as stubbornness, resistance to directions, and unwillingness to negotiate with adults or peers. Children or adolescents with ODD persistently test limits, usually by ignoring directions, arguing, or failing to accept responsibility for behavior. They direct their hostility at adults or peers through verbal aggression or deliberately annoying actions. They do not see themselves as defiant but justify their behavior as a response to unreasonable demands. Symptoms may be present at home but not seen at school.

ODD is one of the more common disorders seen in adolescents, although children also have the disorder. Prevalence rates range from 2% to 16%. ODD is more common in boys before puberty but equally prevalent in both sexes after puberty. Symptoms are generally more confrontational and persistent in boys. There may be comorbid ADHD, depression, or learning problems. The etiology of ODD is unknown.

School-age children with ODD are likely to exhibit low self-esteem, mood lability, low frustration tolerance, swearing, precocious use of alcohol, tobacco, and other drugs, and interpersonal conflicts. Parents and their children or adolescents often bring out the worst in one another. Youths with ODD may be at risk for conduct disorder. Although adolescents are typically oppositional, those with ODD show more severe behaviors with more serious consequences and impairment in home, school, and social functioning.

Appropriate pharmacotherapy is used to treat comorbid conditions such as ADHD and depression. Psychosocial treatments include: parent management training programs to help parents and others manage the child's behavior; individual psychotherapy to develop more effective anger management; family psychotherapy to improve communication and mutual understanding; cognitive problem-solving skills training and therapies to assist with problem-solving and decrease negativity; and social skills training to increase flexibility and improve social skills and frustration tolerance with peers.

11.5.4.3 Conduct disorder

Adolescents with conduct disorder are often unmanageable at home and disruptive in the community. They have little empathy or concern for the feelings and well-being of others. They may be callous and lack appropriate feelings of guilt and remorse, although they may express remorse superficially to avoid punishment for their behavior. They often blame others for their actions. Risk-taking behaviors such as drinking, smoking, using illegal substances, experimenting with sex, and participating in criminal actions are common. Cruelty to animals or people, destruction of property, theft, and serious violation of rules are diagnostic criteria of conduct disorder.

The onset of conduct disorder is usually late childhood or early adolescence. Conduct disorder in adolescents is seen frequently in mental health treatment centers. Prevalence rates range from 6% to 16% in boys and from 2% to 9% in girls younger than 18 years. A youth with conduct disorder may have comorbid ADHD, ODD, a learning disorder, depression, an anxiety disorder, or substance abuse. Risk factors for conduct disorder include physical and sexual abuse, inconsistent parenting with harsh discipline, lack of supervision, early institutional living or out-of-home placement, association with a delinquent peer group, maternal depression, and parental substance abuse.

Behavioral techniques may reduce some of the symptoms of conduct disorder, but their application requires a great deal of consistency. Specifically these are the ones mentioned in the section on ODD. Aggression and impulsivity can be treated with several medications, including the atypical antipsychotics, lithium, and other mood stabilizers such as valproic acid. Comorbid disorders must be treated with appropriate psychosocial and pharmacologic means.

11.5.5 Anxiety disorders

Children and adolescents experience several anxiety disorders, including obsessive–compulsive disorder, phobias, social anxiety disorder, generalized anxiety disorder, separation anxiety disorder, and post-traumatic stress disorder. Children with these types of disorder often have symptoms of fear, anxiety, physical complaints, and sleep disturbances, including nightmares and night terrors. In all age groups, sleep problems are associated with mental illness.

11.5.5.1 Obsessive–compulsive disorder

Obsessive–compulsive disorder (OCD) is characterized by recurrent intrusive thoughts (*obsessions*) and repetitive behaviors that the person realizes are senseless but feels he or she must perform (*compulsions*). Obsessions and compulsions consume hours of the day and cause the child or teen great distress. OCD occurs in families; if a parent has OCD, the child has an increased likelihood to also have OCD.

Treatment of OCD in children and adolescents involves behavioral and psychopharmacologic intervention. Behavioral techniques include *exposure* (deliberately confronting the patient with stimuli that trigger obsessions and provoke the urge to perform rituals) and *response prevention* (either instructing the patient to delay the ritual or blocking the child from performing the ritual). These two techniques allow the child to experience the rise and fall of anxiety. Effective medications for treating OCD symptoms are fluvoxamine, clomipramine, fluoxetine, and paroxetine.

11.5.5.2 Phobias

A phobia is a morbid, irrational, and persistent fear of certain situations, activities, things, or people. The main symptom of this disorder that makes it so disabling is the excessive and unreasonable desire to avoid the feared subject. Phobias should be distinguished from normal fears, which are so common in childhood that mild passing fears are considered part of normal development. Children may express the anxiety of a specific phobia by crying, clinging, or having tantrums. Phobias can be incapacitating.

Treatment of specific phobias includes pharmacotherapy with a selective serotonin-reuptake inhibitor; preparation of the child for traumatic experiences; behavioral training such as relaxation, desensitization, and modeling; and psychotherapy for the child who has experienced a traumatic event.

11.5.5.3 Social anxiety disorder

Children and adolescents with social anxiety disorder ("social phobia") avoid contact with unfamiliar people and performing or speaking in front of others. This behavior interferes with typical day-to-day functioning, such as with peers or at school. These children may appear socially withdrawn, embarrassed, shy, self-conscious, and anxious if asked to interact with strangers. The avoidance and anxious anticipation cause marked distress in new or forced social situations.

Treating social anxiety disorder requires both pharmacologic and psychosocial interventions. Selective serotonin-reuptake inhibitors are the pharmacotherapeutic agents of choice. Exposure, relaxation, and cognitive behavior therapy are the psychotherapeutic interventions with the greatest efficacy. In addition, affected children need support in learning and using social skills by means of role-playing and other forms of practice.

11.5.5.4 Generalized anxiety disorder

Children with generalized anxiety disorder (GAD) have excessive or unrealistic anxiety. They worry about past and future events, the weather, their own school performance or health, the family's finances, and the welfare of others. Physical symptoms of anxiety such as stomach ache, headache, nausea, shortness of breath, and dizziness often accompany GAD.

The anxiolytic buspirone or a selective serotonin-reuptake inhibitor may help reduce anxiety and promote a sense of well-being. In addition, relaxation techniques, and cognitive behavior therapy are psychotherapeutic interventions of choice.

11.5.5.5 Separation anxiety disorder

Children with separation anxiety disorder experience severe anxiety to the point of panic when separated from a parent or attachment figure. When apart or threatened with separation from his or her parent, the child may be very fearful of accidents or injuries befalling the parent, may be extremely homesick, may cling to or shadow the parent, may have nightmares about separation, and may refuse to attend school or spend the night away from home. The child may complain of headaches and stomach aches and may vomit when separated from the parent. Children with separation anxiety often have sleep disturbances. Adolescents usually complain of physical ailments and refuse to attend school. The prevalence of separation anxiety drops as the young person moves into adolescence.

The anxieties of children and adolescents with separation anxiety usually respond well to a selective serotonin-reuptake inhibitor. Behavioral therapy includes imagery, self-talk, and cognitive techniques.

11.5.5.6 Post-traumatic stress disorder

Post-traumatic stress disorder (PTSD) can result in children who are exposed to the pervasive trauma of inner-city life, suffer physical or sexual abuse, are exposed to community or family violence, or witness the wounding or death of a close family member. Whether a child or adolescent develops PTSD in response to a traumatic event depends on several factors, including the risk and protective factors in the child's environment, as well as individual vulnerabilities and strengths.

Interventions for PTSD include psychotherapy with a skilled therapist and medications to treat symptoms. For example, a child or adolescent with PTSD may need an antipsychotic medication for auditory hallucinations, an antidepressant for depressive symptoms and thoughts of self-harm, or both types of medication.

11.5.6 Tic disorders

Tics are sudden repetitive movements, gestures, or utterances. Tics are brief and may occur in bouts. They tend to increase during periods of stress and lessen during absorbing activities. Tics can be motor or vocal, simple or complex.

11.5.6.1 Tourette syndrome

Tourette syndrome is the most severe tic disorder. It is characterized by multiple motor tics and one or more vocal tics many times throughout the day for one year or more. The disorder impairs functioning at home, in school, and with peers. Obsessions, compulsions, hyperactivity, disinhibited speech or behavior, and impulsivity may be associated features. The child may also have depression and school and behavioral problems.

Tic disorders are treated with supportive counseling, school modifications, parent guidance, and individual therapy, as needed. Pharmacotherapy with haloperidol, pimozide, clonidine, clomipramine, desipramine, fluoxetine, and sertraline is useful to diminish tics.

11.5.6.2 Trichotillomania

Children with trichotillomania have an irresistible urge to pull out their hair; they feel tension before pulling out the hair and relief or pleasure during and after pulling. They may then examine, chew on, or eat the hair. The hair loss is noticeable. Trichotillomania is a chronic impulse control condition, and it impairs the child's or adolescent's social or school life. Typically, people with trichotillomania try to deny or hide their behavior, so the hair pulling is done privately. This results in social withdrawal because the person fears that he or she may have a strong urge to pull hair while with others. Feelings of shame and humiliation, poor self-image, and problems with mood, anxiety, or addictions are common.

At least 2.5 million people in the US have trichotillomania. It occurs with the same frequency in boys and girls. The average age of onset is 12–13 years, although many younger children have the disorder. Children and adults most commonly pull out their scalp hair, then eyelashes, eyebrows, and pubic hair. They may pull hair in certain circumstances, such as while watching television, reading or studying, or lying in bed waiting to fall asleep. Causes for the disorder seem to be biological (links have been seen between trichotillomania and Tourette syndrome) and behavioral (e.g., the patient relies on hair pulling as a tension-reducing action, and it becomes a habit).

Treatment for trichotillomania includes both behavior therapy and pharmacotherapy with clomipramine, fluvoxamine, fluoxetine, or another serotonin-reuptake inhibitor. Habit reversal therapy (HRT) is the method used to increase awareness of the hair pulling. HRT is a set of behavioral procedures that involves awareness training, teaching a competing response, contingency management, relaxation training, and generalization training. In addition, teaching alternative coping activities and maintaining motivation through social support are methods useful for treatment.

11.5.7 Childhood psychosis

Childhood-onset schizophrenia is a rare but severe form of psychotic disorder that occurs at age 12 years or younger (as early as age 6) and is often chronic and persistently debilitating. Prevalence of the disorder is thought to be about 1 in 10 000. The younger the onset of the condition, the poorer the prognosis.

Although there is a vast literature on psychosis in adults, there is correspondingly very little literature on psychosis in children. Some symptoms include social withdrawal, incoherent speech, decrease in ability to practice self-care, illogical thinking, agitation, inappropriate or severely attenuated emotions, delusions, hallucinations, violent or destructive behavior, and withdrawal from social activities. The onset is insidious and gradual, becoming slowly more serious and noticeable to the child's family. Psychotic children may attempt suicide, exhibit an absence of emotion, and indulge in uncharacteristic behaviors, such as stealing or sexual promiscuity.

Early identification and treatment is essential to preserve as much functioning as possible. Pharmacotherapy is essential with antipsychotics. Occasionally children may need a benzodiazepine for sedation. The child with schizophrenia requires multimodal care. This should include social skills training, a supportive environment, and a structured individualized special education program. Supportive psychotherapy is used to encourage reality testing and to help the child monitor for warning symptoms of impending relapse. Electroconvulsive therapy has also been used adjunctively in rare cases.

Family education is an essential component of a multifaceted treatment approach for these children. Family members need to know the warning signs of impending relapse.

11.5.8 Mood disorders

Mood disorders, including unipolar depression and bipolar disorder, occur in children as well as adults. The most prominent signs and symptoms are specific to the age and developmental level of the child. Some of the signs and symptoms of mood disorders in children and adolescents are similar to the normal mood swings that all people go through, so mood disorders in children and adolescents are often unrecognized by families and clinicians. Mood disorders in young people often co-occur with other mental disorders, such as anxiety, disruptive behavior, or substance abuse, as well as with physical illnesses.

Several factors contribute to the failure to recognize depressive disorders in children and adolescents. The way that young people express symptoms is a function of their developmental stage and the attendant tasks of that stage. Substance abuse also may contribute to a missed diagnosis of depression. In addition, a major problem is that children and adolescents sometimes have difficulty expressing their internal mood states and emotions. Sometimes, the only way they can express these emotions is through acting out and behaving inappropriately. Parents, teachers, and other adults, however, may misinterpret such clues as disobedience or insolent behavior.

Early diagnosis and treatment of mood disorders is essential for the continued healthy emotional, social, and behavioral development of children and adolescents. Identifying and treating mood disorders early reduces their duration, severity, and resulting functional impairment.

11.5.8.1 Depression

Mental health organizations and the US Public Health Service estimate that at least 5% of children and adolescents are depressed at any point in time. Incidence of adolescent major depression is about 4.7%, although about one-third to one-half of adolescents report symptoms of depression. Early identification and treatment are essential to prevent depression, especially long-term depression later in life. As with adult depression, depression in children involves some combination of genetic vulnerability and psychosocial or environmental factors.

Dysthymia is a mild form of depression that lasts a year or more in a child or teen. Because the symptoms are less debilitating than with major depression, nurses in school and clinic settings may see youths with dysthymia. They are at risk for developing major depression.

Depression affects children and teens in all areas of physical, emotional, and cognitive development. The duration and intensity of symptoms differentiate depression from sadness. Depressive behavior differs significantly from the child's usual behavior and interferes with his or her life in relation to family, schoolwork, and friends.

Depression in children and adolescents is easily confused with other childhood disorders, such as ADHD. Because children often cannot tell adults what they are feeling, they communicate their feelings by acting out. A prepubertal child with depression often exhibits irritability and separation anxiety, whereas an adolescent may be negativistic, antisocial, defiant, socially withdrawn, and failing at school. Signs of depression in children and adolescents are listed in Box 11.1.

Half of children and adolescents with depression have another psychiatric illness, such as GAD, OCD, ADHD, or conduct disorder. In addition, adolescents with depression may abuse drugs or alcohol.

The recovery rate from a single episode of major depression in children and adolescents is relatively high; 70–80% can be treated effectively. Episodes of depression, however, have a high rate

---

Box 11.1 Childhood Major Depression Signs and Symptoms

- Depressed or irritable mood, low frustration level, overreaction to simple requests, loss of joy, moodiness
- Psychomotor agitation or retardation; the child may talk slowly and pause before responding
- Changes in appetite and sleep; the child may eat everything or very little, not sleep restfully, have trouble falling or staying asleep, or awaken very early
- Physical complaints such as headache, stomach ache, fatigue, and loss of energy
- Depressive themes expressed in play, dreams, or verbalizations; themes may include feeling worthless or guilty, minimizing one's own strengths and maximizing failures, and blaming self as the cause of problems in the family
- Social withdrawal
- Intense anger or rage
- Anhedonia (loss of pleasure in hobbies or activities of interest)
- Acting-out behaviors, such as abusing drugs and alcohol, playing truant, dropping out of school, running away, exhibiting antisocial behavior, inflicting self-injury, practicing sexual promiscuity
- Decreased ability to think, concentrate, or make decisions; this often results in falling academic performance
- Thoughts of, and verbalizations about, death or wishing he or she had never been born; teens may express their thoughts through music, films, or writing with morbid themes
- Stressors, such as a breakup with a boyfriend or girlfriend, which may trigger suicidal thoughts

of recurrence and 40% of children with one depressive episode will experience another within 2 years.

Cognitive–behavioral therapy for younger children, parent and family consultation, and medication constitute the necessary treatment for children and adolescents with depression. Neither therapy alone nor medication alone has been found to be as effective as the combination treatment. Cognitive–behavioral therapy can decrease errors in thinking and improve developmental skills. Family consultation helps family members understand mood disorders, support their child or adolescent with depression, and develop more effective parenting skills. Parents also learn to identify risk factors that will worsen depression, such as alcohol and nicotine use.

The most commonly used antidepressant medications for children and adolescents are the selective serotonin-reuptake inhibitors. Antidepressants are given for 6 months to 2 years to treat the depression fully and decrease its likelihood of recurrence. Several years ago, the US Food and Drug Administration issued a black-box warning (see Chapter 33) cautioning that the use of SSRI antidepressants was associated with a higher rate of suicidal ideation in children and in August of 2009 confirmed their concerns over increase in suicidal ideation in young people under the age of 25 taking SSRIs (see: http://www.reuters.com/article/idUSN11535486). Clearly, the SSRIs or any psycopharmacotherapeutic agent should be prescribed only by a clinician with a solid knowledge of psychopharmacology and pediatrics, and patients should be closely monitored. Families should also be educated as to the proper use of antidepressants and for the signs of increased suicidal thoughts.

For children with depression who also experience aggression, severe agitation, or the psychotic symptoms of delusions and hallucinations, antipsychotic medications, particularly the atypical antipsychotics, are most often used. Traditional antipsychotic medications are used less frequently in children.

11.5.8.2 Bipolar disorder

Juvenile-onset bipolar disorder is marked by rapid, wide swings of emotion, arousal, excitability, and movement. Other symptoms include severe irritability, dysphoria, and "affective (or emotional) storms" or rages (i.e., prolonged, aggressive temper outbursts). These children may be prone to violence, show poor school performance, have sleep disturbances, and experience rapid mood swings that may occur in rapid cycles. Children do not show the classic manic picture of elated mood seen in adults with bipolar disorder. Sometimes it is difficult to identify episodes of cycling (i.e., switching from one mood to another) because the symptoms seem to be chronic. A child also may exhibit delusions, hypersexuality, pressured speech, or flight of ideas.

Adolescents may demonstrate hallucinations, delusions, labile mood, or idiosyncratic thinking. Although adolescents may have symptoms that resemble those of adults, it is still difficult to determine cycling of moods. Incidence of substance abuse is high in adolescents with bipolar disorder, making the diagnosis difficult. Childhood-onset bipolar disorder may have comorbidity with ADHD, ODD, and conduct disorder, or it may have features of those conditions.

Children or adolescents with bipolar disorder and their families need several types of treatment including education, family therapy, special education or school modifications, support groups, individual or play therapy, and mood-stabilizing medication. The goals of treatment for the child with bipolar disorder are to alleviate symptoms and improve day-to-day functioning.

Studies suggest that patients who have had prior episodes of bipolar disorder may have a poorer response to lithium and that a person's past history in terms of episodes and mood instability will affect treatment response. If bipolar disorder remains unrecognized and unchecked in the child, future episodes of illness may occur with greater frequency and the child may become resistant to treatment. Therefore, early identification of bipolar disorder in the child is urgent.

Although early treatment is essential, it is also crucial that clinicians are certain of a diagnosis prior to prescribing medications. It is essential that the child undergo a detailed, thorough, longitudinal history before medications are prescribed because rushing to judgment can have unintended consequences. For example, medications that are completely appropriate for the treatment of ADHD may worsen the course and prognosis of bipolar disorder.

Mood-stabilizing medications, including lithium, divalproex, and carbamazepine, have calming and anti-aggressive effects and help to prevent depressive and manic symptoms. Lithium is particularly effective in patients whose behavior is manic or elated rather than depressed. Moreover, lithium has strong suicide preventive properties and generally is recommended as a first-line treatment for bipolar disorder. The anticonvulsant mood stabilizers divalproex and carbamazepine are more effective in treating rapid cycling, angry, or depressed states. Other medications for mood stabilization and augmentation are discussed in Chapters 33 and 34. Children with bipolar disorder who also have psychosis may be given an antipsychotic medication, most likely an atypical antipsychotic.

11.5.9 Enuresis

There are two main types of enuresis in children. *Primary enuresis* occurs when a child has never established bladder control. *Secondary enuresis* occurs when a person has established bladder control for a period of 6 months, then relapses and begins wetting. To be diagnosed with enuresis, a person must be at least 5 years old or have reached a developmental age of 5 years. Below this age, problems with bladder control are considered normal.

Most children achieve some degree of bladder control by 4 years of age. Daytime control is usually achieved first while nighttime control comes later. The age at which bladder control is expected varies considerably and is dependent on many variables. Enuresis is a problem of the young and is more common in boys than girls. At age five, about 7% of boys and 3% of girls have enuresis. This number declines steadily in older children. By age 18, only about 1% of adolescents experience enuresis.

Although there is no good evidence that the condition is primarily psychogenic, it is often associated with a psychiatric disorder, and enuretic children are frequently referred to mental health services for treatment.

Biological factors described in the literature on enuresis include a structural pathological condition or infection of the urinary tract (or both), low functional bladder capacity, abnormal antidiuretic hormone (ADH) secretion, abnormal depth of sleep, genetic predisposition, and developmental delay. Evidence has also been found for sympathetic hyperactivity and delayed organ maturation as seen by delay in ossification. Scholars have also demonstrated an association between enuresis and developmental delay with impaired acquisition of gross motor (sitting/crawling) and language milestones in future bed-wetters.

Obstructive lesions of the urinary outflow tract, which can cause a urinary tract infection (UTI) as well as enuresis, have been thought to be important, with a high prevalence of such abnormalities seen in enuretic children referred to urologic clinics. UTIs has been found to occur frequently in children, especially girls, and a large proportion (85%) of them have been shown to have nocturnal enuresis. Also, in 10% of bed-wetting girls, urinalysis results show evidence of bacterial infection. The consensus is that, as treating the infection rarely stops the bed-wetting, a UTI is probably a result rather than a cause of enuresis.

Research exploring the notion that children who are bed-wetters sleep more deeply than others has been inconclusive, with studies both upholding and not upholding this hypothesis. The evidence for some genetic predisposition is strong. Approximately 70% of children with nocturnal enuresis have a first-degree relative who also has or has had nocturnal enuresis.

Psychiatric disorder occurs more frequently in enuretic children than in other children. The relative frequency of disorder ranges from two to six times that in the general population but there have been no specific types of psychiatric disorder identified in children with enuresis. There is little evidence that enuresis is a symptom of underlying disorder because psychotherapy is ineffective in reducing enuresis.

A final possibility is that enuresis and psychiatric disorder are both the result of joint etiologic factors such as low socioeconomic status, institutional care, parental delinquency, and early and repeated disruptions of maternal care. Shared biological factors may also be important in that delayed motor, speech, and pubertal development, already shown to be associated with enuresis, have proven to be more frequent in disturbed enuretic children than in those without psychiatric disorder.

The presence or absence of conditions often seen in association with enuresis, such as developmental delay, UTI, constipation, and comorbid psychiatric disorder, should be assessed and ruled out as appropriate. Other causes of nocturnal incontinence should be excluded, for example, those leading to polyuria (diabetes mellitus, renal disease, diabetes insipidus) and, rarely, nocturnal epilepsy.

Information on the frequency, periodicity, and duration of symptoms is needed to make the diagnosis and distinguish functional enuresis from sporadic seizure-associated enuresis. If there is diurnal enuresis, an additional treatment plan is required. A family history of enuresis increases the likelihood of a diagnosis of functional enuresis and may explain a later age at which children are presented for treatment.

For patients with secondary enuresis, precipitating factors should be elicited, although such efforts often represent an attempt to assign meaning after the event. It is important to inquire about previous management strategies used at home, such as fluid restriction, nightlifting (getting the child out of bed to take him to the toilet in an often semi-asleep state), and rewards and punishments.

All children should have a routine physical examination, with particular emphasis placed on detection of congenital malformations, which are possibly indicative of urogenital abnormalities. A midstream specimen of urine should be examined for the presence of infection. Radiological or further medical investigation is indicated only in the presence of infected urine, enuresis with symptoms suggestive of recurrent UTI (frequency, urgency, and dysuria), or polyuria.

Treatment for enuresis is not always necessary. About 15% of children who have enuresis outgrow it each year after age 6. Behavior modification is the treatment of choice. A night alarm is the most effective. The child's bedding includes a special pad with a sensor that rings a bell when the pad becomes wet. The bell wakes the child, who then gets up and goes to the bathroom to finish emptying his bladder. Over time, the child becomes conditioned to waking up when the bladder feels full.

Another behavioral technique involves setting an alarm clock to wake the child every night after a few hours of sleep, until the child learns to wake up spontaneously. In trials, this method was as effective as the pad-and-alarm system. Waking children during the night to use the bathroom and restricting liquids starting several hours before bedtime have not been shown to be effective.

A miniature ultrasound bladder volume measurement instrument during sleep seems to be a promising treatment for nocturnal enuresis in that it prevents the enuretic event, appears to facilitate a permanent cure, and is noninvasive.

There are two main drugs for treating enuresis. Imipramine reduces the frequency of enuresis in about 85% of bed-wetters and eliminates enuresis in about 30% of these individuals. Nighttime doses of 1–2.5 mg/kg are usually effective and a therapeutic effect is usually evident in the first week of treatment. It is not clear why this antidepressant is effective in treating enuresis when other antidepressants are not.

Desmopressin acetate (DDAVP), a synthetic ADH, has been widely used to treat enuresis since the 1990s. It is available as a nasal spray or tablet. Both imipramine and DDAVP are very effective in preventing bed-wetting, but have high relapse rates if medication is stopped.

11.5.10 Encopresis

Encopresis is defined as the intentional or involuntary passage of stool into inappropriate places in the absence of any identified physical abnormality in children older than 4 years. Encopresis that is present from birth is called *primary encopresis*. *Secondary encopresis* occurs when a child has an established period of fecal continence that is then interrupted by incontinence.

The overall prevalence of encopresis in 7- and 8-year-old children has been shown to be 1.5%, with boys (2.3%) affected more commonly than girls (0.7%).

Encopresis may occur after an acute episode of constipation following illness or a change in diet. In addition to the pain and discomfort caused by attempts to pass an extremely hard stool, a number of specific painful perianal conditions such as anal fissure can lead to stool withholding (retentive type) and later fecal soiling. Stressful events such as the birth of a sibling or attending a new school have been associated with up to 25% of cases of secondary encopresis.

In non-retentive encopresis, the main theories center on faulty toilet training. Stress during the training period, coercive toileting leading to anxiety and "pot phobia," and failure to learn or to have been taught the appropriate behavior have all been implicated.

Having identified the presence of encopretic behavior and formed some idea of the type of encopresis (primary, secondary, or retentive, or a combination), the remaining task is to discover the presence and extent of any associated conditions, both medical and psychological. The comprehensive assessment process should include a medical evaluation, psychiatric and family interviews, and a systematic behavioral recording.

The medical evaluation should include a history, review of systems, physical examination, and appropriate hematological and radiological tests. Although the vast majority of patients with encopresis are medically normal, a small proportion may have pathological features of etiological significance which should be referred to an appropriate specialist.

Behavioral therapy is the mainstay of treatment for encopresis. In the younger child who has been toilet trained, this focuses on practical elimination skills, for example, visiting the toilet after each meal, staying there for a maximum of 15 minutes, using muscles to increase intra-abdominal pressure, and cleaning oneself adequately afterward. Parents or caretakers, or both, should be educated in making the toilet a pleasant place to visit and should stay with the younger child, giving encouragement and praise for appropriate effort. Small children whose legs may dangle above the floor should be provided with a step against which to brace when straining. Systematic recording of positive toileting behavior, not necessarily being clean (depending on the level of baseline behavior), should be performed with a personal star chart. For the child with severe anxiety about sitting on the toilet, a graded exposure scheme may be desirable.

In patients with retention leading to constipation and overflow, medical management is nearly always required, although it is usually with oral laxatives or microenemas alone. The use of more intrusive and invasive colonic and rectal washout or surgical disimpaction procedures is nearly always the result of the clinician's impatience rather than true clinical need.

Clinical Vignette 1

Adam was the third of three children born to a social worker and an office manager. No medical problems were reported during pregnancy or birth, and his medical and family history was unremarkable. His pediatrician expressed mild concern during the first 24 months of his life because his motor milestones (e. g., sitting up, walking) consistently fell at the late end of normal limits. His language development was precocious; he had amassed a formidable vocabulary by 12 months and, by 24 months, was using four- to five-word sentences. He displayed great interest in trains and dinosaurs, and he spent large amounts of time as a young child examining books about these topics.

Adam's parents viewed his facility with language and extensive knowledge favorably and perceived him to be intellectually gifted. They noted that Adam had great difficulty putting aside these activities; he also became extremely flustered with unexpected changes in his schedule. They worked around this rigidity by providing Adam with extensive notice before any activity or change in schedule was initiated.

First concerns emerged at age 4, when Adam was expelled from nursery school for physical aggression. His preschool teachers reported that he was extremely possessive of his favorite toys and would strike children who attempted to play with them. This behavior pattern continued into grade school, and Adam was considered a "behavior problem" by many of his teachers. Adam displayed minimal interest in developing friendships, preferring to focus on a newfound interest, American history.

In third grade, Adam was referred for a psycho-educational evaluation because of difficulties with math. Results of testing indicated a significant discrepancy between his strong verbal skills and his weak visual–spatial abilities and poor fine motor control. The evaluator noted his strong preoccupation with a particular topic and its intrusive effects on adaptive functioning in the social and academic realms. Despite his strong language skills, the evaluator described poor conversation skills, a tendency to speak in a pedantic tone, and poor modulation of the volume and inflection of his voice. The evaluator diagnosed Adam with Asperger's disorder.

Adam began participation in social skills groups at school and enrolled in individual therapy to work on his understanding of social mores and for explicit instruction in social behavior. He developed several social relationships based around his area of interest (with a local historical society).

As Adam approached adolescence he became increasingly interested in social interaction and romantic relationships. At this time, Adam became acutely aware of his social difficulties and experienced depression, which was successfully addressed through pharmacotherapy. Adam graduated from high school, enrolled in a junior college transition program for individuals with developmental disabilities, and eventually obtained a bachelor's and obtained employment as a library employee.

Clinical Vignette 2

Tim was a 6-year-old boy brought to clinic for an initial visit. On entering the examination room, the evaluator observed Tim spinning in circles on the stool while his mother cried: "If I have to tell you one more time to sit down!" Tim was not permitted to begin first grade until his immunizations were updated. His mother explained that Tim had visited several physicians for immunization but was so disruptive that the physicians and nurses always gave up. She hoped that with "counseling" Tim's behavior might improve such that he would comply with his immunizations and be allowed to progress to the first grade.

The mother described a several-year history of aggressive and destructive behavior, as well as four school suspensions during kindergarten. Tim had recently been suspended from school for the fourth time for violent behavior towards other children, often resulting in injuries. He had been attending his current school for only nine months.

Tim often became "uncontrollable" at home and had broken dishes and furniture. Last year, Tim was playing with the gas stove and started a small fire. Tim frequently pulled the family dog around by its tail. Tim's older sisters watched him in the past but refused to do so after he threw a can of soup at one of them.

(Continued)

Tim's father was a long-haul truck driver who saw him every 3–4 weeks. The family history indicated that Tim's father was incarcerated for auto theft and assault when Tim was 6 months old. Tim's mother frequently left Tim unsupervised overnight as she was a night nurse. Her job required her to be away from home often for 12-hour shifts. For the most part, childcare arrangements were poorly planned and ad hoc when he was "suspended" from day care owing to uncontrollable rages during which he hit other children and staff and destroyed day-care property.

Tim lived at home with his mother. His father had a history of antisocial behavior, with a number of juvenile offenses, and there was a family history of alcohol abuse. Tim had been in child (day) care since he was one. His mother reported a "very normal" childhood. No records of his previous behavior or development were available, as his family had moved from state to state and the mother did not know where his records were.

Tim's mother did not initially see Tim's behavior as problematic for her and blamed the school for his behavioral problems. In fact, she was quite hostile to the school as a report had been made to Child Protective Services with concerns about his care. The Services investigated and found that Tim and his brother were at no significant risk.

When asked what modes of discipline she used with Tim, his mother informed the evaluator that the primary means of control were whipping across his buttocks and thighs with a belt when he misbehaved, and making him swallow Tobasco sauce. When asked if this "worked," she became defensive and answered that this was the way her mother had disciplined her and "I turned out just fine."

Early in his kindergarten career, his school urgently referred Tim to the Department of Education psychologist, who found it very difficult to gain a complete assessment as he did not cooperate during the interview. Tim was then referred to a psychiatrist who specialized in high-risk cases. After assessment a discrete number of problem areas were identified that were most urgently in need of attention:

- Rages that included violence toward others
- Hitting, kicking and bullying behavior at school
- Lack of remorse about his behavior
- Lack of empathy.

Risk factors for Tim included:

- Poor family network/support
- Inadequate supervision at home
- Exposure to TV violence (no supervision during leisure hours)
- Harsh and inconsistent parenting.

On evaluation, Tim's IQ tested at 102 (average). Tim was sullen in his attitude and frequently got up from his chair. When redirected, he became verbally abusive. It took several visits to fully evaluate him. He was unwilling to focus and twitched and paced around the office when he was asked to perform for more than 15 minutes. He would fly into rages spontaneously and seemingly without provocation. He was oriented and manifested no evidence of a thought disorder. The psychiatrist determined that Tim had childhood-onset *conduct disorder*. He and his parents were referred to a parent management training program and multisystemic therapy.

KEY POINTS

- The effects of child and adolescent mental illness include the increased likelihood of the disorder continuing into later life, feelings of guilt and blame, unmet needs of siblings and other family members, marital stress and conflict, diminished productivity of lives, and direct and indirect costs.

- Factors placing the child or adolescent at risk for development of mental health disorders include biological ones, such as a family history of a mental illness, immature development of the brain, or a brain abnormality; psychological ones, including family problems and dysfunction; and stressors, including poverty, mentally ill or substance-abusing parents among others.

- Early intervention with children and adolescents at risk can prevent more serious mental disturbance later in life.

- Child and adolescent mental illness is treated by biologic interventions such as psychotropic medication, psychosocial interventions such as therapies, therapeutic approaches designed for each client, school modifications, and community-based services.

- Children and adolescents are affected by many psychiatric illnesses, including ones that are usually first diagnosed during infancy, childhood, or adolescence and ones that, although common in adults, have different manifestations and require different treatment in children and adolescents.

- The most common from each category include ADHD, conduct disorder, ODD, adjustment disorder, OCD, phobias, social anxiety disorder, GAD, separation anxiety disorder, PTSD, depression, bipolar disorder, autism spectrum disorders, substance abuse, trichotillomania, and tic disorders.

- Treatment of children focuses on the family as a whole and involves educating them about treatment and behavioral strategies, helping the family cope, managing developmental and academic issues, teaching social skills, and improving self-esteem.

This chapter contains material from the following chapters in *Psychiatry, Third Edition*: Chapter 45 (James McPartland, Ami Klin, Alexander Westphal, Fred R. Volkmar); Chapter 46 (Jeffrey H. Newcorn, Iliyan Ivanov, Vanshdeep Sharma, Kurt Schulz, Jeffrey M. Halperin); Chapter 48 (Matt W. Specht, Courtney Pierce Keeton, John T. Walkup); and Chapter 49 (Christopher P. Lucas, David Shaffer).

Further Reading

Findling, R.L. (2007) *Clinical Manual of Child and Adolescent Psychopharmacology*, American Psychiatric Press, Washington, DC.

Goodman, R. and Scott, S. (2005) *Child Psychiatry*, John Wiley & Sons, New York.

Greene, R.W. (2001) *The Explosive Child: A New Approach for Understanding and Parenting Easily Frustrated, Chronically Inflexible Children*, 2nd edn, Harper Collins, New York.

Heffernan, K. (2002) *Child Psychopathology*, 2nd edn, Guilford, New York.

Kazdin, A.E. (2008) *Parent Management Training: Treatment for Oppositional, Aggressive, and Antisocial Behavior in Children and Adolescents*, Oxford University Press, New York.

Mikkelsen, E.J. (2001) Enuresis and encopresis: ten years of progress. *Journal of American Academy of Child and Adolescent Psychiatry*, **40**, 1146–1159.

Paul, R. (2006) *Language Disorders from Infancy Through Adolescence: Assessment and Intervention*, Elsevier, New York.

12 ● Sleep Disorders

12.1 Introduction

Nearly a half of all people in the United States report a sleep-related disorder and more than 50% of them are untreated. A sleep disorder can cause emotional disturbance, concentration and memory problems, impaired motor skills, and decreased work efficiency. It can even contribute to cardiovascular disorders and morbidity. Sleep disturbances are a major feature of several psychiatric conditions as well as being primary disorders in and of themselves. Given the importance of sleep for well-being, clinicians should have a working knowledge of sleep disorders and include sleep assessment as part of their patient assessments. This chapter reviews the normal physiology of sleep and discusses sleep disorders, their evaluation and treatment.

12.2 The physiology of sleep

The function of sleep remains unknown. Although experience suggests that sleep is a restorative process that results in the person feeling rested, researchers have not yet been able to establish the physiological reasons for this, despite many years of investigation. Various theories about the purpose of sleep have been proposed, but none has been proven conclusively.

Sleep involves many complex physiological processes in virtually all body systems. Although sleep is considered a time of inactivity and rest, many physiological events occur throughout the sleep cycles, such as changes in heart rate, blood pressure, and respiration. Growth hormone and prolactin levels increase, and cortisol and thyrotropin (TSH) levels decrease. These normal events may be altered markedly in conditions of disturbed sleep, such as sleep deprivation.

12.2.1 Stages of sleep

There are two types of sleep: non-rapid eye movement (NREM) and rapid eye movement (REM). Both are marked by characteristic physiologic changes. Each stage is associated with characteristic patterns of EEG activity.

NREM sleep includes stages 1, 2, 3, and 4. During stage 1, the person is roused most easily, and as the sleep stages progress it becomes more difficult to awaken the person. Stages 3 and 4 are referred to as "deep sleep" and people perceive these stages as high-quality sleep. NREM has been described as a relatively inactive yet actively regulated brain in a movable body. During NREM sleep, heart rate, blood pressure, and respiratory rate generally decrease.

Rapid eye movements and vivid dreams characterize REM sleep, which is also associated with great electrical brain activation and loss of muscle tension, or *atonia*. In contrast to NREM, heart rate and blood pressure are more variable and may increase.

Fundamentals of Psychiatry, First Edition. Allan Tasman and Wanda K. Mohr.
© 2011 John Wiley & Sons, Ltd. Published 2011 by John Wiley & Sons, Ltd.
This chapter is based on Chapter 79 (Milton Erman, Sonia Ancoli-Israel) of *Psychiatry, Third Edition*

12.2.2 *Sleep regulating processes*

The two primary physiologic processes that regulate sleep cycles are the circadian rhythm and the homeostatic process. The *circadian rhythm* is a pacemaker or biological clock that regulates the daily patterning of sleep. Circadian characteristics result in sleep and wake occurring during predictable times of the day and night. The circadian pacemaker stimulates changes in the daily patterns of sleep and wakefulness that are endogenous to the organism. The changes occur in an approximately 24-hour rhythm, but exogenous factors also influence the timing of these changes. An example is environmental changes in light and dark. Sleep disturbances may result from changes in exogenous factors, such as night work or changes in time zones associated with air travel.

Homeostasis describes the coordinated physiological processes that maintain most steady states in an organism. In humans, the need for sleep increases as the time awake increases. Prolonged periods of wakefulness result in decreased alertness, increased sleepiness, and greater amounts of slow-wave (NREM stage 4) sleep. Once sleep occurs, homeostasis, or the steady state, is accomplished and the accumulated "sleep debt" is replenished and patients awake feeling rested.

12.2.3 *Normal age-related changes in sleep and wakefulness*

Newborns spend nearly 50% of total sleep time in REM sleep. Because infants may sleep up to 16 hour a day, they may spend 8 hours in REM sleep. Children display a polyphasic sleep–wake pattern, with short bouts of sleep and wakefulness throughout the 24-hour day, until several months of age when they eventually sleep through the night. Daytime napping, however, often persists until the age of 4–6 years.

Maximal "depth" of sleep may occur during the prepubertal period, when children are often difficult to awaken at night. Adolescents often still need at least 10 hours of sleep. Yet, during adolescence, stages 3 and 4 sleep decline and daytime sleepiness increases, partially in association with the normal Tanner stages of pubertal development. Teenagers are also phase-delayed, which means that they may not get sleepy until the early morning hours (e.g., 2–3 a.m.) and do not naturally wake up until the later morning hours. Early school start times and social pressures may produce mild sleep deprivation during weekdays, with some "catch-up" occurring on weekends.

As adults enter middle age and old age, sleep often becomes more shallow, fragmented, and variable in duration and circadian timing compared with that of young adults. Stages 1 and 2 and the amount of time spent awake during the night tend to increase; REM latency and slow-wave sleep decline. Most age-related sleep changes occur in early and mid-years of the human lifespan, and in healthy older adults sleep remains fairly constant between the ages of 60 and 90 years.

Daytime sleepiness and napping usually increase with age, often as a function of disturbed nocturnal sleep. Adults in the sixth decade and older may experience advanced sleep phase syndrome, which involves falling asleep early in the evening and awakening very early in the morning. Although many sleep experts believe this finding to be a normal developmental pattern, advanced sleep phase syndrome may interfere with preferred work and leisure activities. Many clinicians believe that it is normal for older adults to report more sleep disturbances than young and middle adults. The belief that sleep disturbance is a normal part of aging is particularly common among older adults and may prevent them from seeking help with genuine sleep problems. Studies suggest that observed higher rates of sleep disturbance among older adults are associated with medical or psychiatric illness. For this reason, clinicians should be especially cognizant of performing sleep assessments with older adult patients and assisting them with interventions to improve sleep.

12.3 Sleep hygiene

Sleep hygiene includes strategies to manipulate environmental conditions and personal behaviors to support effective sleep. Just as human beings need a balanced diet to promote and maintain health, they need habits and a structure to promote effective sleep. The general principles of sleep hygiene include maintaining a regular sleep–wake schedule, environmental modifications, and reductions in sources of arousals.

Although numerous strategies have been recommended, no universal consensus has been reached about the best strategies to use, and more research is needed. Most sleep specialists teach patients to maintain a regular sleep schedule on weekdays and weekends, to modify the sleeping environment to reduce noise and light, to maintain a comfortable environmental temperature, and to sleep in a comfortable bed. Clinicians should discourage patients from eating a large meal or spicy foods near bedtime; conversely, they instruct patients to avoid going to bed on an empty stomach. Many sleep specialists recommend that patients consume a light snack of carbohydrate-containing foods or warm milk prior to bedtime and avoid caffeine within 6 hours of bedtime.

12.4 Sleep disorders

Sleep disorders include dyssomnias and parasomnias. Dysomnias are abnormalities in the amount, quality, or timing of sleep and include narcolepsy, breathing-related sleep disorders, periodic limb movement disorder, and insomnia. Parasomnias are abnormal behavioral or physiologic events associated with sleep. Parasomnias include problems such as sleepwalking and tooth grinding and are not discussed in this chapter.

12.4.1 Insomnia

Insomnia, a perception of insufficient sleep or not feeling rested after a habitual sleep episode, is the most prevalent sleep disorder. People with insomnia report difficulty falling asleep, staying asleep, or both, or not feeling rested on awakening. Insomnia can range in duration from a few days to many months or years. Patients with insomnia often report distress in social, occupational, or other areas of functioning.

Primary (idiopathic) insomnia occurs when no cause of a sleep disturbance (e.g., a mental health or medical diagnosis) can be identified. The etiology is unclear. It often begins in young or middle-aged adults and tends to be more common in women. Patients with idiopathic insomnia have had difficulty sleeping since childhood.

Psychophysiologic insomnia is chronic insomnia in which patients worry about sleep, are cognitively and physiologically over-aroused at bedtime, and have poor daytime functioning. This leads to further worry about sleep. This, in turn, may lead to a vicious cycle in which insomnia leads to more insomnia.

The development of insomnia is multifactorial. Influences include the person's predisposition, developmental factors, environmental/situational characteristics, medical disorders, psychiatric disorders, drugs, and other ingested substances. Predisposing characteristics may include genetics, personality, and coping style. Normal developmental events, such as pregnancy, the postpartum period, and menopause, also may contribute.

Environmental changes and stressful situations are very common causes of acute insomnia. Acute illness, bereavement, and significant life changes are also stressors that may influence the development of insomnia. Many patients have difficulty initiating and maintaining sleep in an environment to which they are unaccustomed, such as the hospital or a hotel.

Treatment of insomnia is multidimensional, requiring behavioral and pharmacologic approaches. Behavioral techniques include sleep hygiene (promoting habits that help sleep), sleep restriction, cognitive–behavioral therapy, and relaxation techniques. (For expanded explanations of these, see the National Sleep Foundation website: http://www.sleepfoundation.org/.)

The only US Food and Drug Administration approved medications for insomnia are the benzodiazepine receptor agonists (the older benzodiazepines and the newer non-benzodiazepines) and one MT receptor agonist (see Chapter 33). The older benzodiazepines are non-selective agonists of BZD benzodiazepine receptors whose advantages are decreased sleep latency and increased total sleep time, but whose risks include daytime sedation, cognitive impairment, motor incoordination, dependence and abuse, tolerance development, and rebound insomnia after withdrawal. The newer, non-benzodiazepine receptor agonists have fewer side-effects as they act on selected alpha subunits of the GABA receptors. Ramelteon is a selective agonist of MT (MT1 and MT2) receptors, and is the only FDA-approved hypnotic that is not a controlled substance owing to its lack of significant or clinically relevant residual effects such as abuse potential, dependence, development of tolerance, or withdrawal syndrome/rebound insomnia in clinical trials. In reviewing the benzodiazepine receptor agonists, the US National Institutes of Health concluded that short-, intermediate-, and long-acting benzodiazepines are all efficacious. Patients should be educated about the anticipated benefits and limitations of sleeping pills, side-effects, and appropriate use, and should be followed up by office visits or phone calls regularly if prescriptions are renewed. Treatment of these patients should focus on the lowest possible effective dose for the treatment of insomnia.

12.4.2 Insomnia comorbid with a psychiatric disorder

Subjective and objective disturbances of sleep are common features of many psychiatric disorders. Complaints may be of insomnia or hypersomnia, parasomnias (such as nightmares, night terrors, and nocturnal panic attacks), and circadian rhythm disturbances (early morning awakening). Before assuming that a significant sleep complaint invariably signals a psychiatric diagnosis, clinicians should go through a careful differential diagnostic procedure to rule out medical, pharmacologic, or other causes. Even if the sleep complaint is primarily related to an underlying psychiatric disorder, sleep disorders in the mentally ill may be exacerbated by many other factors, such as: increasing age; comorbid psychiatric, sleep, and medical diagnoses; alcohol and substance abuse; effects of psychotropic or other medications; use of caffeinated beverages, nicotine, or other substances; lifestyle; past episodes of psychiatric illness; and cognitive, conditioned, and coping characteristics such as anticipatory anxiety about sleep as bedtime nears. Some features of these sleep disorders may persist during periods of clinical remission of the psychiatric disorder and may be influenced by genetic factors. Finally, even if the sleep complaint is precipitated by a non-psychiatric factor, psychiatric and psychosocial skills may be useful in ferreting out predisposing and perpetuating factors involved in chronic sleep complaints.

Although signs and symptoms of sleep disturbance are common in most psychiatric disorders, an additional diagnosis of insomnia or hypersomnia related to another mental disorder is made according to DSM-IV-TR criteria only when the sleep disturbance is a predominant complaint and is sufficiently severe to warrant independent clinical attention. Many of the patients with this type of sleep disorder diagnosis focus on the sleep complaints to the exclusion of other symptoms related to the primary psychiatric disorder. For example, they may seek professional help with complaints of insomnia or oversleeping when they should be at work, excessive fatigue, or desire for sleeping pills, but initially they minimize or strongly deny signs and symptoms related to poor mood, anxiety, obsessive rumination, alcohol abuse, or a personality disorder.

12.4.3 Narcolepsy

Narcolepsy is a disorder of unknown etiology characterized by excessive daytime sleepiness and associated with cataplexy (sudden bilateral loss of postural muscle tone) and other REM sleep phenomena. It often begins in adolescence and seems to have a genetic component.

In addition to excessive daytime sleepiness and cataplexy, patients also may have sleep paralysis, hypnagogic hallucinations (dream-like images, sounds, or sometimes smells before falling asleep or waking up), automatic behaviors, or disruptions of nocturnal sleep episodes. Narcolepsy can negatively impact virtually every domain of a patient's life (e.g., professional performance, ability to drive and operate machinery, social interactions) and depressed mood can accompany this disorder.

Treatment for narcolepsy focuses on managing the symptoms of excessive daytime sleepiness and cataplexy. Stimulants such as methylphenidate (Ritalin) and, more recently, modafinil (Provigil) are used to decrease daytime sleepiness. Tricyclic antidepressants are used to treat the distressing symptom of cataplexy. Scheduled naps appear useful in assisting patients with severe sleepiness not addressed by the use of stimulant medication.

12.4.4 Breathing-related sleep disturbance

Breathing related sleep disturbance (BRSD) is sleep disruption resulting from sleep apnea or alveolar hypoventilation, leading to complaints of insomnia or, more commonly, excessive sleepiness. Many individuals with BRSD cannot sleep and breathe at the same time and therefore spend most of the night not breathing or not sleeping.

Obstructive sleep apnea (OSA) is characterized by repetitive episodes of upper airway obstruction that occur during sleep, resulting in numerous interruptions of sleep continuity, hypoxemia, hypercapnia, bradytachycardia, and pulmonary and systemic hypertension. It may be associated with snoring, morning headaches, dry mouth on awakening, excessive movements during the night, falling out of bed, enuresis, cognitive decline and personality changes, and complaints of either insomnia or, more frequently, hypersomnia. Patients with OSA may be unaware that they have apnea or hypopnea or that they snore during sleep and reports of others who witness these events are helpful in establishing the diagnosis. The disorder is most common in middle-aged men; however, its prevalence appears to increase in women in the menopausal years. Risk factors for both men and women include obesity and large neck size.

Patients with OSA are at risk for lapses in memory, slowed reaction time, and falling asleep while working, operating machinery, or driving a motor vehicle. Patients should be discouraged from operating machinery or driving motor vehicles until their OSA is treated.

Effective treatments include weight loss, nightly nasal nocturnal continuous airway pressure (CPAP), and oral appliances designed to maintain patency of the upper airway during sleep. Surgical procedures on the soft palate and pharyngeal tissue also may be helpful.

12.4.5 Periodic limb movement disorder and restless leg syndrome

Periodic limb movement disorder (PLMD) is a condition in which the legs move repetitively during the night. These movements occur in approximately 90-second repetitive patterns. They result from contractions of the leg muscles during sleep. This condition causes frequent nighttime arousals and results in non-restorative sleep and excessive daytime sleepiness. Restless legs syndrome (RLS) is associated with disagreeable leg sensations, such as pain, cramping and itching, at bedtime, which often interfere with the onset of sleep.

12.4.6 Circadian rhythm sleep disorder

Circadian rhythm disturbances result from a mismatch between the internal or endogenous circadian sleep–wake system and the external or exogenous demands on the sleep–wake system. Thus, the individual's tendency to sleep–wakefulness does not match that of her or his social circumstances or of the light–dark cycle. Although some individuals do not find this mismatch to be a problem, for others the circadian rhythm disturbance interferes with the ability to function properly at times when alertness or sleepiness is desired or required. For those individuals, insomnia, hypersomnia, sleepiness, and fatigue result in significant discomfort and impairment. The more common circadian rhythm disturbances include delayed and advanced sleep phase, shift work and jet lag. These will not be discussed in this chapter.

Clinical Vignette

Mr O was a 61-year-old married male attorney, seen alone, who presented for evaluation of complaints of snoring and observed pauses in breathing. His wife had reported to him her observation of very loud, continuous snoring and clear-cut sleep apnea episodes. On occasion, the snoring was loud enough that his wife needed to sleep in a guest bedroom. Mr O was aware, on occasion, of waking during the night due to snoring, but did not report awareness of any apneas. He had no difficulty initiating sleep at the start of the night, and would often fall asleep watching television in the evening.

Mr O reported that he did not feel fully restored or refreshed upon awakening in the morning, and that he would wake up several times during the night, usually with the need to go to the bathroom. He denied urinary frequency in the daytime,. He did report waking with a dry mouth during the night and in the morning, but not of a morning headache. He did report occasional problems with gastroesophageal reflux waking him during the night.

Mr O acknowledged some reductions in concentration, memory, and attention during the day. He reported that he had experienced some increase in irritability and that he felt that his energy level was somewhat reduced relative to the past. He acknowledged some tendencies to excessive sleepiness when sedentary. He completed an Epworth Sleepiness Scale questionnaire which resulted in a score of 12, which was in the mildly elevated range. However, this likely reflected an underestimation of the severity of actual sleepiness.

Mr O reported a benign medical history with no significant medical problems. However, his blood pressure had been observed to be "creeping up" when checked recently. He had a history of depression dating back many years, and was taking Wellbutrin with some benefit but without complete resolution of depressive symptoms. He denied taking any other medications on a regular basis. He did not smoke, and reported limited use of alcohol and caffeine-containing beverages. He acknowledged that use of alcohol made his snoring worse, and that he occasionally used caffeine to increase alertness during the day.

He denied any history of injuries to, or surgery involving, the nose, throat, neck, or jaw, or any history of allergies. He noted that his father probably had sleep apnea, and that other relatives had been loud snorers.

On physical examination, Mr O weighed 236 pounds fully clothed, carried on an approximate 70-inch frame. Body habitus was obese (body mass index = 34). The neck circumference was 18.5 inches, with a very full sub-mandibular space. Nasal flow was equal bilaterally without obvious constriction. Facial structure was not noteworthy for a foreshortened jaw. Examination of the oropharynx demonstrated a crowded airway outlet.

Mr O recognized that sleep apnea likely was present, but expressed concern about his ability to tolerate nasal CPAP if studies suggested that it would be appropriate therapy for him. Polysomnography was performed. Mr O demonstrated moderate obstructive sleep apnea–hypopnea, with an index (AHI) of 24.8 events per hour for total sleep time, 11.9 events per hour in NREM sleep, and 49.2 events per hour in REM sleep. Apnea was also more severe in the supine position (supine AHI = 32.5). Electrocardiogram showed mild acceleration–decelerations with obstructive breathing events, but otherwise was unremarkable.

After a review of the study results, Mr O agreed to a CPAP titration study, which documented that effective treatment of his sleep apnea could be attained at a CPAP pressure setting of $10\,cmH_2O$. He had little difficulty tolerating CPAP, indicated that the CPAP mask was properly fitted and that CPAP was comfortable, and stated that he would "absolutely" use it as therapy if prescribed. He rated his sleep quality with CPAP as much better than a normal night's sleep at home.

CPAP treatment was initiated, and Mr O was quite successful with his adaptation to CPAP, as measured by records of hours of use obtained from his CPAP unit. He reported an immediate improvement in his perceptions of sleep quality, energy, and cognitive function, and reported a progressive improvement in mood with functional absence of depressive symptoms.

He has continued to use nasal CPAP on a nightly basis for two years, with stability in mood, cognitive function and energy levels, and without continued increases in blood pressure. He has expressed a desire to work on weight reduction, but has not attained any persistent weight loss.

KEY POINTS

- Sleep disorders occur across the lifespan and across a variety of health states.

- Sleep disorders include dyssomnias and parasomnias.

- Insomnia, a perception of insufficient sleep or not feeling rested after a habitual sleep episode, is the most prevalent sleep disorder.

- Primary (idiopathic) insomnia occurs when no cause of a sleep disturbance (e.g., a mental health or medical diagnosis) can be identified.

- Treatment of insomnia is multidimensional, requiring behavioral and pharmacologic approaches.

- Sleep disorders occur commonly in patients who have psychiatric disorders (sleep disorders may contribute to the development of psychiatric conditions, and likewise psychiatric disorders may contribute to sleep disorders).

- Other sleep disturbances include narcolepsy, breathing-related sleep disturbance, periodic limb movement disorder, and circadian rhythm disturbances.

- Sleep disturbances can result in excessive daytime sleepiness or problem sleepiness, which can be a major risk factor for accidents and injuries.

Further Reading

Kryger, M.H., Roth, T.C., and Dement, W.C. (2005) *Principles and Practice of Sleep Medicine*, 4th edn, Saunders, Philadelphia.

National Sleep Foundation: Omnibus Sleep in America Poll (2000) (Available at: http://www.sleepfoundation.org/publication/2000pool.htm)

13 • • Bipolar Mood Disorders

13.1 Introduction

This chapter discusses various mood disorders: bipolar I disorder, bipolar II disorder, and cyclothymic disorder. These are characterized by mood episodes that can include irritability, intense euphoria (mania) and profound depression. Depression itself is covered more fully in Chapter 14.

Despite the fact that the DSM term is "bipolar disorders," implying that the characteristic mood states are polar opposites, the older term "manic–depressive disorder" is a more accurate term. Classically, mania has been considered to be the opposite of depression: manic individuals were said to be cheery, optimistic, and self-confident – hence the name bipolar disorder. However, in most descriptive studies, substantial proportions of hypomanic and manic patients actually exhibit dysphoric symptoms, while those with depressive episodes frequently exhibit manic symptoms. Although classically thought to be a desirable state, patients with mania or hypomania rate their preference for that state as equal to or less than their preference for euthymia, with depression and mixed states being rated less preferable. Thus the term *manic–depressive* is less misleading than *bipolar*.

13.2 The bipolar spectrum

At present the DSM bipolar diagnoses are those identified above, with all other mood disorders that fall outside the "normal" range considered in the category "not otherwise specified" (NOS). But there is actually a very large range in the presentation of patients within this category, and the present divisions have more to do with diagnostic convenience than a true clinical picture. The richness and complexity of mood disorders is not well captured by the present taxonomy.

13.2.1 Mood episodes

Major depressive episodes are defined by discrete periods of depressed or "blue" mood or loss of interest or pleasure in life that typically endures for weeks but must last for at least 2 weeks (see Chapter 14). These symptoms are often accompanied by an increase or decrease in sleep or appetite, decreased energy, and impaired cognition. *Depressive episodes* in manic–depressive disorder are indistinguishable from those in major depressive disorder. About 75% of people with manic–depressive disorder experience depressive episodes characterized by decreased sleep and appetite,

Fundamentals of Psychiatry, First Edition. Allan Tasman and Wanda K. Mohr.
© 2011 John Wiley & Sons, Ltd. Published 2011 by John Wiley & Sons, Ltd.
This chapter is based on Chapter 67 (Mark S. Bauer) of *Psychiatry, Third Edition*

while about 25% experience more "atypical" symptoms of increased sleep and appetite, rates that are indistinguishable from those in unipolar depression. Thus with regard to depressive episodes, the differential diagnosis between major depressive and manic–depressive disorders is made by longitudinal course not by cross-sectional symptom analysis.

Manic episodes are defined by discrete periods of abnormally elevated, expansive, or irritable mood accompanied by marked impairment in judgment and social and occupational function. These symptoms are frequently accompanied by unrealistic grandiosity, excess energy, and increases in goal-directed activity that frequently have a high potential for damaging consequences. Hypomanic and manic symptoms may be identical, but hypomanic episodes are less severe. A person is "promoted" from hypomania to mania (type II to type I) by the presence of one of three features: psychosis during the episode, sufficient severity to warrant hospitalization, or marked social or occupational role impairment. This is an imperfect set of criteria, however, because the phenomenologic differentiation between hypomania and mania is not always straightforward.

The DSM divides bipolar disorders into two types, "bipolar I" and "bipolar II."

13.2.2 Bipolar I disorder

Bipolar I disorder is characterized by one or more manic episodes, usually alternating with major depressive episodes. During the manic episode the patient may exhibit inflated self-esteem or grandiosity, decreased need for sleep, being more talkative than usual, flight of ideas, distractibility, increase in goal-oriented activity, and excessive involvement in risky activities.

The symptoms are severe enough to disrupt the patient's ability to work and socialize, and may require hospitalization to prevent harm to self or others. Manic episodes usually begin suddenly and last from a few days to a few months.

13.2.3 Bipolar II disorder

Bipolar II disorder is characterized by the patient having had a major depressive episode (either current or past) and at least one hypomanic episode over at least 4 days. Most hypomanic episodes in bipolar II disorder occur immediately before or after a major depressive episode. Bipolar II disorder differs from bipolar I in that the patient has never had a manic or mixed episode. Bipolar II patients may have had an episode in which they experienced a persistently elevated, expansive, or irritable mood (hypomania) that is clearly different from their usual mood. With Bipolar II, however, the patient ·does not experience hypomanic symptoms severe enough to cause marked social or occupational dysfunction or to require hospitalization. Bipolar II disorder can present diagnostic challenges, particularly if the patient presents for the first time with a depressive episode.

13.2.4 Cyclothymic disorder

Cyclothymia is a disorder resembling bipolar disorder, with less severe symptoms. Cyclothymic disorder presents as a "subclinical" bipolar I disorder. Patients with cyclothymic disorder experience repeated periods of non-psychotic depression and hypomania for at least 2 years (1 year for children and adolescents). The opposing manifestations of depression and hypomania are seen in the following pairs of symptoms: feelings of inadequacy (during depressed periods) and inflated self-esteem (during manic periods); social withdrawal and uninhibited social interaction; sleeping too much and too little; and diminished and increased productivity at work. Cyclothymic disorder is diagnosed only if a major depressive or manic episode has never been present.

13.2.5 Bipolar depression

At present, the DSM-IV criteria for major unipolar depression substitute for a genuine bipolar depression diagnosis. On the surface, there is little to distinguish between bipolar and unipolar depression, but certain "atypical" features may exist. People with bipolar depression are more likely to have psychotic features and more classic "slowed down" symptoms such as hypersomnia or fatigue, while those with unipolar depression are more prone to crying spells and significant anxiety (with difficulty falling asleep). Because bipolar II patients spend far more time depressed than hypomanic (50% depressed versus 1% hypomanic, according to a 2002 NIMH study) misdiagnosis is common. The implications for treatment are enormous insofar as misdiagnosis can result in inappropriate medication, which may confer no benefit, but which can drastically worsen the outcome of the illness, including switches into mania or hypomania and cycle acceleration. Bipolar depression calls for a far more sophisticated medications approach, which makes it absolutely essential that those with bipolar II be properly diagnosed.

13.2.6 Additional features: psychosis and rapid cycling

Psychosis is an episode modifier and can occur in either depression or mania. If psychotic symptoms are limited to the major mood episode, the individual is considered to have manic–depressive disorder with psychotic features. On the other hand, if psychotic symptoms endure significantly into periods of normal mood, the diagnosis of *schizoaffective disorder* is made.

For the formal DSM definition, 2 weeks of psychotic symptoms during normal mood is sufficient to convert a diagnosis of manic–depressive or major depressive disorder into schizoaffective disorder, because it is thought that such individuals have a clinical course midway between those with mood disorders or schizophrenia. However, this cut-off point is fairly arbitrary, and its validity is not well established. Rapid cycling as a longitudinal course specifier is defined by DMS-IV-TR as the occurrence of four or more mood episodes within 12 months. Despite the name, the episodes are not necessarily or even commonly truly cyclical; the diagnosis is based simply on episode counting.

Rapid cycling is of significance because it predicts a relatively poorer outcome and worse response to lithium and other treatments. Although rapid cycling was at one time considered by some to be an "end stage" of the disorder, empirical evidence indicates that it may have its onset at any time during the disorder and may come and go during the course of illness. Several specific risk factors may be associated with rapid cycling, each of which may give clues to its pathophysiology. These include female gender, antidepressant use, and prior or current hypothyroidism.

13.3 Etiology

No single paradigm can explain the occurrence, and variability in course and severity of manic–depressive disorder. Rather, an integrative approach to understanding the causes of manic–depressive disorder which recognizes the contributions of a variety of biologic, psychologic, and social factors is a better heuristic.

Available evidence indicates that familial factors are important determinants of who will develop manic–depressive disorder. A wide range of neurochemical, neuroendocrine, neuroanatomic, and neurophysiologic hypotheses have been put forward regarding the biological basis. The major hypotheses have been recounted in great detail in the literature (see Further Reading). While each has something of value to contribute regarding the pathologic basis of manic–depressive disorder, it is by no means clear whether the disorder is basically a disorder of a particular neurochemical system, a particular neuroanatomic locus, or a particular physiologic system. Integration of these hypotheses awaits development of new methodologies for clinical neurobiologic investigations. The psychological theories of mood disorders are wide ranging, including cognitive, behavioral, interpersonal, and psychoanalytic.

Unfortunately, the bulk of theory regarding the psychological basis of mood disorders concerns depression, with little attention as yet to mania or manic–depressive disorder. Data on the relationship between life events and the course of manic–depressive disorder have been reviewed. An association of episode onset with severe adverse life events, typically major losses, on symptoms or episodes has been fairly consistent across studies. This relationship appears to obtain for depressive but not manic episodes, though many depressive episodes have no identifiable stressor. There is less evidence that schedule-disrupting events trigger either type of episode, aside from sleep disruption being associated with mania.

13.4 Course and prognosis

Episodes of mania and depression typically recur across the lifespan. Between episodes, most people with bipolar disorder are free of symptoms, but as many as one-third of people have some residual symptoms. A small percentage of people experience chronic unremitting symptoms despite treatment. Without treatment the natural course of bipolar disorders tends to worsen. Over time a person may suffer more frequent (more rapid-cycling) and more severe manic and depressive episodes than those experienced when the illness first appeared. But in most cases, proper treatment can help reduce the frequency and severity of episodes and can help people with bipolar disorder maintain good quality of life.

13.5 Treatments

The most critical issue in establishing a clinician–patient relationship is coming to a shared understanding that manic–depressive disorder is a chronic condition that will require ongoing, anticipatory, and collaborative management.

Traditionally, treatment for manic–depressive disorder has been categorized as acute versus prophylaxis, or maintenance – that is, treatment geared toward resolution of a specific episode versus continued treatment to prevent further symptoms. Treatment should also be focused on improving clinical outcome (episodes and symptoms) or functional outcome (social and occupational function and health-related quality of life). As with all patients, treatment should be biopsychosocially oriented.

13.5.1 Pharmacologic treatment

Mood stabilizers, including lithium and the antiepileptics, are the first-line drugs of choice for patients with a bipolar disorder. Drugs in this class bring the depressive and manic mood cycles within a more normal range. Generally, however, they all have been shown more effective for mania than for depression within the bipolar spectrum. Patients with significant depressive symptoms during this phase of the bipolar spectrum or whose depressive symptoms do not respond well to mood stabilizers alone also often need antidepressant therapy. Use of combinations of mood stabilizers is common but requires extensive knowledge of potential pharmacokinetic interactions. In addition, close monitoring and frequent follow-up are critical elements of caring for patients taking these medications.

Although lithium is discussed elsewhere in this book (see Chapter 33), it is such an important medication that it bears repeating some information. Lithium is the only drug whose prophylactic activity in bipolar disorder has been proven unequivocally. It remains the first-line drug of choice in the long-term treatment of stabilizing mood in the bipolar disorders, and lithium has long been known to reduce suicidal tendencies in bipolar patients. Recent evidence, however, underscores that lithium therapy (even when supplemented by antidepressants and antipsychotics) is not adequate for most patients with bipolar disorder, particularly those who experience rapid cycling.

13.5.2 *Psychosocial treatment*

Improved social role function has been demonstrated with several psychotherapies. The major types of psychotherapy that have been investigated and shown to be efficacious include cognitive or cognitive–behavioral therapy, single- or multifamily therapy, and group and individual psychoeducation. It should be kept in mind that there are often not firm lines between the types of therapy, with cognitive techniques including substantial psychoeducational components and vice versa, and that there are no magic bullets that will address this complex disorder *in toto*.

Combined psychotherapy and pharmacotherapy is an optimistic strategy that has empirical support, but is tempered somewhat by evidence that more ill patients tend to do less well in at least cognitive psychotherapy than those who are higher functioning.

With respect to research on specific psychotherapies, bipolar depressed patients seem to achieve similar levels of reduction in depressive symptoms following cognitive–behavioral therapy as do a unipolar depressed group. But, on measures of more pervasive dysfunctional attitudes, bipolar patients did not improve to the same degree. Consensus on psychosocial and psychotherapeutic approaches for treatment of bipolar disorder indicate that treatment should include a strong education component, a focus on teaching the signs of relapse and planning for that eventuality, an emphasis on normalizing regular rhythms of sleep and activity and, to the extent possible, direct family involvement.

The National Institute of Mental Health (NIMH) maintains a website that describe best practices and current clinical trials on a variety of treatments for psychiatric disorders (available at: http://www.nimh.nih.gov/trials/index.shtml).

Chronic care models (CCMs) have been applied to the management of chronic psychiatric illnesses. The central focus of CCMs, which are based on principles of social learning and self-regulation theories, is to reorganize medical care to support an effective partnership between clinicians and patients to improve outcomes relevant to patients. Substantial evidence indicates that CCMs improve process and outcome measures for a variety of chronic medical illnesses and may be cost-effective. CCMs likely have a role in optimizing outcome for individuals with manic–depressive disorder, including those with severe illness. Based on these studies, at least one major practice guideline has endorsed their use in this disorder. Notably, CCMs involve psychotherapeutic components, and psychotherapeutic interventions involve some (usually implicit) care coordination; thus both may be considered along a continuum of psychosocial interventions. CCMs provide a care-organization platform through which medications and psychotherapies may be more effectively delivered.

13.5.3 *Treatment refractoriness*

Issues of treatment refractoriness are discussed in Chapter 33. A complementary approach to understanding refractoriness is to consider characteristics that coexist with the illness that increase difficulty in treatment. Such contributors include comorbid psychiatric disorders, comorbid medical disorders that limit treatment choice or contribute to depressive symptoms and functional deficits, and non-adherence.

Additionally, when an individual does not respond to a variety of treatments, the diagnosis itself should be reconsidered, and investigation undertaken in particular for medical and substance-related causes of the symptoms.

13.5.4 Special features influencing treatment

Regarding comorbid psychiatric disorders, the choice of approach to management may be driven by a variety of implicit assumptions. Psychiatrists may assume that the comorbid disorder is caused by the manic–depressive disorder and consequently believe that treatment of the manic–depressive disorder will lead to resolution of the comorbidity. Others may assume that the mood instability of manic–depressive disorder is due to the comorbid illness, such as alcohol or drug intoxication or withdrawal, or intrapsychic or psychophysiological effects of prior trauma.

Parallel (simultaneous) treatment is preferable to *sequential* treatment (treating one disorder until resolution and then attending to the other), as the prognosis of manic–depressive disorder is worse when complicated by substance use and the course of alcoholism is worse when complicated by mood disorders.

It is also likely that the highly confrontational approaches of some traditional treatment programs for substance dependence will not serve the needs of often highly impaired depressed or manic persons. Similarly, the presence of anxiety disorders is associated with worse outcome.

Clinical Vignette

Ms B, a 59-year-old woman with type I disorder, enrolled in a collaborative chronic care model (CCM) after hospitalization for an acute manic episode with psychotic features. She was retired, separated, and had few social contacts.

Although diagnosed with manic–depressive disorder 19 years earlier, Ms B had inconsistent mental health treatment. Episodes had been dramatic for her, often involving police bringing her to the hospital. Medical records documented that her denial of illness was the greatest barrier to treatment.

Initially she presented as distrustful and engaged in only limited discussion of her mood disorder. Gradually, psychoeducation group participation provided her with a sense of support and an ability to identify her own illness characteristics. She became proficient in identifying early warning symptoms of mood episodes and the benefits of consistency in taking medications. She used personal cost–benefit analysis to address medication side-effects, and used easy-access CCM appointments to remain in treatment rather than stopping medications as she had in the past.

Although Ms B had two more hospitalizations over the next 3 years, her daughter reported to the CCM staff, saying: "This program is the best thing that has happened to her, she has been so much better."

KEY POINTS

- Bipolar disorders are characterized by mood episodes, which can include irritability, intense euphoria (mania) and profound depression; psychotic features may also be present.

- Depressive episodes in manic–depressive disorder are indistinguishable from those in major depressive disorder.

- Manic episodes are defined by discrete periods of abnormally elevated, expansive, or irritable mood accompanied by marked impairment in judgment and social and occupational function.

- Bipolar I disorder is characterized by one or more manic episodes, usually alternating with major depressive episodes.

- Bipolar II disorder is characterized by the patient having had a major depressive episode (either current or past) and at least one hypomanic episode over at least 4 days.

- Cyclothymia is a disorder resembling bipolar disorder, with less severe symptoms.

- People with bipolar depression are more likely to have psychotic features and more classic "slowed down" symptoms such as hypersomnia and fatigue, while those with unipolar depression are more prone to crying spells and significant anxiety.

- Without treatment the natural course of bipolar disorders tends to worsen.

- Treatment of bipolar disorders should be focused on improving clinical outcome (episodes and symptoms) or functional outcome (social and occupational function and health-related quality of life).

- Mood stabilizers, including lithium and antiepileptics, are the first-line drugs of choice for patients with bipolar disorders.

Further Reading

Bauer, M.S. (2001) The collaborative practice model for bipolar disorder: design and implementation in a multi-site randomized controlled trial. *Bipolar Disorders*, **3**, 233–244.

Bauer, M.S. (2001) An evidence-based review of psychosocial interventions for bipolar disorder. *Psychopharmacology Bulletin*, **35**, 109–134.

Johnson, S. and Roberts, J.R. (1995) Life events and bipolar disorder: implications from biological theories. *Psychological Bulletin*, **117**, 434–449.

Johnson, S.L. (2005) Life events in bipolar disorder: towards more specific models. *Clinical Psychology Review*, **25**, 1008–1027.

Scott, J. and Colom, F. (2005) Psychosocial treatments for bipolar disorders. *Psychiatric Clinics of North America*, **28**, 371–384.

Scott, J., Paykel, E., Morriss, R. *et al.* (2006) Cognitive–behavioural therapy for severe and recurrent bipolar disorders: randomised controlled trial. *British Journal of Psychiatry*, **188**, 313–320.

Simon, G.E., Ludman, E.J., Bauer, M.S. *et al.* (2006) Long-term effectiveness and cost of a systematic care management program for bipolar disorder. *Archives of General Psychiatry*, **63**, 500–508.

Stahl, S.M. (2008) Mood disorders, in *Essential Psychopharmacology*, 3rd edn, Cambridge University Press, Cambridge, UK

Depression

14.1 Introduction

The term "mood" refers to a pervasive, sustained emotional coloring of one's experiences. Extreme changes in mood can signal a mood disorder. These disorders have been described for more than 40 centuries.

The mood disorders include major depressive disorder, dysthymic disorder, bipolar I and II disorders, and cyclothymic disorder. Each disorder is associated with disturbances in functioning across many domains. All are characterized by many symptoms, of which mood is only one.

Because mood is an unseen entity, mood disorders often go undetected. If untreated, patients may suffer for months or even years with an illness that is treatable. The economic costs to society and personal costs are enormous. The World Health Organization (WHO) estimates that depressive disorders are the leading cause of disability in the United States and other economies worldwide. This chapter deals with the depressive disorders, their assessment, differential diagnoses, and treatment. Chapter 13 covers dysthymic disorder, bipolar I and II disorders, and cyclothymic disorder.

14.2 Epidemiology

Global epidemiologic studies of depression show considerable variations across and within countries, to a large extent due to the cross-cultural unsuitability of assessment instruments. About 18.8 million adults, or about 9.5% of the US population aged 18 years or older, have a depressive disorder in a given year. Nearly twice as many women (6.5%) as men (3.3%) suffer from a major depressive disorder every year, with the average age of onset being the mid-20s. Dysthymic disorder affects about 5.4% of the US population.

Patients at highest risk for recurrent depressive disorders include those whose first depression was before age 25, those who have had more than 16 weeks of depression in their lifetime, and those who have had a recurrence of depression within 2 months of discontinuing an antidepressant.

Mood disorders in children and teenagers are a significant problem in the US. Studies have reported that up to 2.5% of children and up to 8.3% of adolescents in the US suffer from mood disorders. One longitudinal prospective study found that early-onset depression often continues into adulthood, which indicates that mood disorders in youth may also predict more severe illness in adult life.

Mood disorders in older adults also are a significant problem. A conservative estimate is that about 6% of the US population aged 65 years or older have a diagnosable depressive illness (major depressive disorder or dysthymic disorder). Depression in older adults often co-occurs with other illnesses. Suicide is a frequent companion to mood disorders and has been identified recently as an

Fundamentals of Psychiatry, First Edition. Allan Tasman and Wanda K. Mohr.
© 2011 John Wiley & Sons, Ltd. Published 2011 by John Wiley & Sons, Ltd.
This chapter is based on Chapter 66 (Heinz Grunze, Cornelius Schüle) of *Psychiatry, Third Edition*

emergent national public health priority (see Chapter 38). Older Americans are disproportionately likely to commit suicide.

14.3 Etiology

Although the anatomical and physiological basis of depression is far from being completely understood, a major depressive disorder most likely involves the limbic structures in circuits involving the cingulate, hippocampus, mamillary bodies, and anterior thalamus, reward circuits (nucleus accumbens, sublenticular extended amygdala, amygdala, ventral tegmentum, cingulate, insula, thalamus, parahippocampal gyrus, and prefrontal cortex), hypothalamus, and anterior temporal cortex. Deficiencies of neurotransmitters involved in these circuitries, as well as damage to neurons and loss of connectivity (e.g., by enduring hypercortisolemia), can underlie what manifests clinically as depression.

Three principal neurotransmitters have been implicated in the pathophysiology and the treatment of depression: norepinephrine (noradrenaline), dopamine, and serotonin. They comprise what is known as the "trimonoaminergic neurotransmitter system." These three monoamines often work in concert. Many of the symptoms of all mood disorders are hypothesized to involve dysfunction of various combinations of these three, and essentially all known treatments of mood disorders act on one or more of them.

The monoamine hypothesis of depression represents an oversimplified idea about depression that was valuable in focusing attention on the three neurotransmitters. However, the focus of hypotheses for the etiology of depression has shifted from the monoamine neurotransmitters themselves to their receptors and the downstream molecular events that these receptors trigger, including the regulation of gene expression.

Family studies have reported an approximately threefold increased risk for a major depressive disorder (MDD) in the first-degree relatives of individuals with MDD as compared to the general population. Family studies, however, do not allow one to distinguish the effects of genetic factors versus family environment. Extensive research continues in the area of behavioral genetics, or how genes influence human behavior. Depression is a complex disorder and as such is likely to involve a relatively large number of individual genes, none of which may themselves have a major impact on risk, as well as interactions with environmental factors.

14.4 Signs, symptoms, and diagnostic criteria

The mood disorders can be categorized in various ways, depending on the number of symptoms, their severity, and persistence. Clinically significant depressive disorders can be grouped by their severity and distance from the euthymic state.

14.4.1 Dysthymic disorder

The word *dysthymia* comes from the Greek prefix *dys*, meaning difficult or bad, and *thymos*, meaning mind. DSM-IV-TR considers dysthymia a mild form of depressive illness in which the symptoms – poor appetite, overeating, difficulty falling asleep, excessive sleep, low energy, fatigue, low self-esteem, poor concentration, or difficulty making decisions – are less severe than in depressive disorder but are chronic. Diagnostic criteria for dysthymic disorder include depressed or irritable mood most of the day, occurring more days than not for at least 2 years (1 year in children and adolescents). During this time, the patient has had no more than 2 months in which symptoms are not present and has not experienced a manic or depressive episode.

The chronic nature of dysthymia is a cause for concern, because it often presents as a lifelong struggle against depression, which can assume various forms and cause significant distress. In an attempt to escape negative self-esteem, feelings of self-depreciation, emptiness, low energy and fatigue, pessimism about the future, and hopelessness with suicidal ideations, the patient may engage in certain activities to generate excitement. He or she may focus heavily on work, spend money, engage in sexual behavior, or become preoccupied with religious and mystic involvement in the struggle against depression. The patient with dysthymia may turn to substance abuse or food to dull or escape psychic pain. Many times, the patient with dysthymia has become accustomed to the chronic, negative, oppressive effect of the disorder and, therefore, does not readily recognize symptoms as being abnormal.

The treatment for dysthymic disorder includes the same psychotherapies and medications that are discussed below for MDD. Treatment plans should be guided by the severity of the patient's symptoms.

14.4.2 Major depressive disorder

According to DSM-IV-TR, a patient diagnosed with major depressive disorder must have either a depressed mood or a loss of interest or inability to derive pleasure from previously enjoyable activities. Other symptoms include recurrent thoughts of suicide, decreased or increased appetite, inability to concentrate, difficulty making decisions, feelings of worthlessness and self-blame, decreased energy, motor disturbances (agitation or severe slowness), disturbed sleep (insomnia or excessive sleeping), substance abuse, and social withdrawal. Also, the patient with depression often disregards grooming, cleanliness, and personal appearance. These patients may present disheveled, downcast, without eye contact, and tearful. Conversely, they may be agitated but *usually* do not exhibit bizarre or unusual behaviors. Many patients with depression tend to exhibit withdrawn behavior and they resist attempts by others to engage them in the environment.

Diagnosis of depression in older adults can be difficult because many of them suffer from comorbid physical conditions, such as heart disease, diabetes, cancer, and Parkinson's disease. Because depression often accompanies these, and older adults often face losses and may experience physical, psychological, and social difficulties, healthcare professionals may mistakenly conclude that depression is a normal consequence of these problems – an attitude often shared by the patients themselves.

For diagnostic purposes, symptoms must be present most of the day nearly every day for at least 2 weeks, and they must cause significant distress or impair functioning. Major depressive disorder is further classified according to severity, longitudinal course of recurrent episodes, and descriptions of the most recent episode. Typically, major depressive episodes last several weeks to several months and are followed by periods of relatively normal mood and behavior. The average major depressive episode lasts about 4 months; however, it can last for 12 months or more without remitting.

14.5 Other clinical features in depressive disorders and subtypes

14.5.1 Depression with psychotic features

Psychotic features of depression such as hallucinations or delusions (e.g., delusional hypochondria, feelings of guilt, nihilistic thoughts) are predominantly mood congruent, but may rarely be incongruent. Psychotic symptoms are in most cases an indicator of the particular severity of depression, including suicide risk.

14.5.2 Catatonic features

Severe psychomotor retardation, stupor, immobility, or (in contrast) severe agitation can be observed in depressed patients. These are sometimes labeled as catatonic features.

14.5.3 Melancholic features

According to DSM-IV-TR, melancholia is characterized by a loss of the ability to feel pleasure and a variety of somatic symptoms and psychomotor alterations. Therapeutic consequences of melancholic features are similar to those for severe depression.

14.5.4 Atypical features

According to DSM-IV-TR, atypical depression is characterized by the presence of at least two of the following criteria: increase in appetite and weight gain, hypersomnia, leaden paralysis, and a longstanding pattern of interpersonal rejection sensitivity. Patients with atypical depression are more likely to have an earlier age at onset, a greater comorbidity with anxiety symptoms, and greater symptom severity compared with typical depression.

14.5.5 Seasonal pattern

Seasonal affective disorder (SAD) or seasonal depression is a condition that appears during the colder months when there are also fewer hours of sunlight. Depression symptoms can be moderate or severe. They may be accompanied by fatigue, lack of interest in normal activities, weight gain, hypersomnia, craving for foods high in carbohydrates, and social withdrawal. Symptoms typically begin to dissipate when spring begins and the daylight hours are longer.

14.5.6 Depression in the postpartum period

During the postpartum period, up to 85% of women experience some type of mood disturbance. For most women, symptoms are transient and relatively mild (i.e., postpartum blues); however, 10–15% of women experience a more disabling and persistent form of mood disturbance (e.g., postpartum depression, postpartum psychosis).

Postpartum blues is typically mild and remits spontaneously, requiring nothing other than support and reassurance. On the other hand, puerperal psychosis is a psychiatric emergency that typically requires inpatient treatment. The severity of the condition should guide treatment. Early intervention is associated with better prognosis. Treatment for severe postpartum depression should continue for 6–12 months or longer if necessary. Clinicians should note that risk factors for postpartum depression include prior episodes of depression after childbirth.

14.5.7 Depressive syndromes in pain conditions

Depressive syndromes and chronic pain are frequent comorbid conditions. Approximately 70% of patients with major depression present with physical complaints. Somatization disorders, fibromyalgia, and similar conditions with predominant pain are often accompanied by depressed mood.

14.5.8 Adjustment disorders

Adjustment disorder with depressed mood, and mixed anxiety and depressed mood, are covered in Chapter 21.

14.5.9 Dysthymic disorder and MDD in combination with dysthymic disorder

Diagnostic criteria for dysthymia and depressive disorders differ as far as the severity and duration of the symptoms are concerned. Dysthymic disorder is characterized by a period of at least 2 years with depressed mood, but having fewer than the five core symptoms of depression demanded by DSM-IV-TR for the diagnosis of MDD. As mentioned earlier, dysthymic disorder is characterized by a chronic depressive syndrome of lower intensity of symptoms than in major depression, although it produces very similar levels of disability and loss of quality of life. A superimposing major depressive episode can occur in patients suffering from dysthymic disorder, named "double depression." The differential diagnosis of both disorders is difficult when dysthymic disorder follows a depressive episode, because the symptoms of the former are then indistinguishable from MDD with incomplete remission. Only after achieving full remission for at least 6 months can any subsequent dysthymic symptoms be diagnosed with some confidence as dysthymic disorder.

14.6 Differential diagnosis

As with all psychiatric disorders, physical disease should be ruled out by way of thorough history and physical assessment, including laboratory studies and imaging if needed. Clearly if positive results are obtained the patient should be treated for the primary organic disorder. Table 14.1

Table 14-1   Possible organic factors underlying depressive disorders

Disorders	Organic Factors
Neurological disorders	• Stroke • Dementia • Epilepsy • Huntington's chorea • Hydrocephalus • CNS infectious diseases • CNS neoplasias • Parkinson's disease • Narcolepsy • Sleep apnea • Trauma • Wilson's disease
Endocrine disorders	• Adrenal disorders (Cushing's disease, Addison's disease) • Hyperaldosteronism • Hyper- or hypoparathyroidism • Hyper- or hypothyroidism • Postpartum hormonal changes
Other medical disorders	• Neoplasias and paraneoplastic syndromes • Cardiopulmonary diseases • Autoimmune disorders (e.g., lupus erythematodes) • Porphyria • Uremia • Avitaminoses (vitamins B12, C, folate, niacin or thiamin)
Pharmacogenic depression	• Analgesics (ibuprofen, indomethacin, opiates, phenacetin) • Antibiotics (streptomycin, sulfonamides, tetracyclines) • Antihypertensives (reserpin, clonidine, digitalis) • Chemotherapeutics (asparaginase, azathioprine, bleomycin, trimethoprime, vincristine) • Hormones (high-estrogen oral contraceptives) • Immune system therapy/suppression (corticosteroids, interferons, mycophenolatmofetile, tacrolimus)

illustrates a partial list of medical conditions that can induce depression or look very much like a depression.

If organic factors can be ruled out as the underlying cause for depressive symptoms, MDD still needs to be separated from other mental disorders that show features and symptoms of depression, without fulfilling full DSM-IV-TR criteria for MDD. The DSM-IV-TR heading "Depressive disorder not otherwise specified" summarizes further depressive syndromes that fall short of the threshold for MDD or dysthymic disorder. These syndromes include recurrent brief depression and minor depression, but also premenstrual dysphoric disorder, postnatal depression, and post-psychotic depressive disorder in schizophrenic patients. In those instances, depression can be conceived as secondary to another somatic condition or psychiatric illness. The treatment of post-psychotic depression has attracted little attention; however, the occurrence of depression after psychosis is frequent (in up to 40% of patients), constitutes one of the most worrisome predictors for a poor functional outcome, and therefore needs intense treatment.

Furthermore, mood symptoms are common in substance abusers, and can usually be directly related to the intake of drugs. They may be transient as a direct action of the substance, or lasting as a consequence of toxic brain impairment. Substance-induced mood symptoms can also occur as a side-effect of prescribed medication.

A depressive episode, fulfilling MDD criteria, can also manifest itself as part of a bipolar or a schizoaffective disorder.

14.7 Depressive disorders with comorbid psychiatric disorders

Frequently, depression does not occur alone but as a psychologic or biologic consequence of a somatic or psychiatric disorder. In this chapter we deal only with the most frequent comorbidity patterns. It should be noted that pharmacotherapeutics with individuals having comorbid disorders with depression can be challenging and unlike treatment of primary depression in the absence of comorbidity. However, the permutations of these are beyond the scope of this chapter and readers are advised to avail themselves of the sources at the end of this chapter for more detailed information.

Psychiatric comorbidities negatively impact on treatment outcomes and long-term prognosis, and need to be treated simultaneously with the same effort as the depressive episode.

Comorbidity of depressive disorders with other psychiatric disorders is common and significantly affects treatment outcomes. Greater numbers of concurrent comorbid conditions are associated with increased severity, morbidity, and chronicity of depressive disorders.

14.7.1 Anxiety disorders

A lifetime prevalence of more than 40% for comorbid anxiety disorders (panic disorder, phobias, and generalized anxiety disorder) has been reported in patients suffering from depressive disorders, but it is not clear whether the diagnostic entities can be separated or represent a mixed anxiety–depression syndrome. Patients with comorbid MDD and panic disorder show a greater severity of syndromes in comparison to patients suffering from MDD alone.

14.7.2 Substance abuse

Abuse of and addiction to alcohol, nicotine, and other drugs are often accompanied by depression. Depressed patients with comorbid substance abuse are more likely to have an earlier age of onset of depression, more depressive symptoms, a greater functional impairment, and a history of more previous suicide attempts than patients with depression alone.

14.7.3 Personality disorders

At least one-third of depressed patients fulfill the diagnostic criteria of a personality disorder. It has been estimated that 6% of depressed patients also display features of borderline personality disorder (BPD)

14.8 Depressive disorders with comorbid general medical conditions

Depressive syndromes are frequently present in people with severe or chronic general medical conditions. Slowly progressing illnesses leading irrevocably to severe incapability show a high percentage of comorbid MDD. General medical conditions or their treatment may also be directly responsible for depressive symptoms (see Table 14.1). Medical comorbidity will affect both treatment responsiveness of depressive syndromes and the choice of medication.

14.8.1 Cardiovascular disorders

An exceptionally high comorbidity of depressive symptoms and cardiovascular disease (CVD) has been described in studies, but depression is rarely diagnosed in patients suffering from CVD in routine clinical settings. Comorbid MDD worsens the outcome of coronary heart disease or a myocardial infarction, especially in treatment-refractory depressed patients. Depression, especially MDD, increases cardiovascular mortality independently of other cardiovascular risk factors.

14.8.2 Endocrinological disorders and diabetes mellitus

Depression is a risk factor for type II diabetes mellitus and a bidirectional positive association has been assumed. MDD may impact negatively on therapeutic adherence with a subsequent risk for vascular complications. By the same token, hypercortisolism during MDD may facilitate the onset of diabetes.

14.8.3 Renal disorders

Having a severe acute or chronic renal disease predisposes to an adjustment disorder with marked depressive syndromes or major depressive disorder.

14.8.4 Hepatic disorders

Patients suffering from chronic hepatitis have an enhanced risk for developing depression, especially those receiving interferon treatment. Patients with a history of depression may even require prophylactic antidepressant treatment when starting interferons. Treatment of comorbid depression and hepatic disorders requires specific precautions.

14.8.5 Infections

Viral or bacterial infections are often accompanied by psychiatric syndromes, frequently depression, which may require specific treatment. Infections of the nervous system, in particular, such as Lyme disease or neurosyphilis (neurolues), may provoke psychiatric disorders including MDD. Infection with the human immune deficiency virus (HIV) is highly associated with depression and suicidal behavior, and HIV risk behaviors endangering others occur more frequently with comorbid depression. Hepatitis C-infected patients are also more likely to have psychiatric comorbidities such as depressive disorders. Finally, treatments directed against infections, such as interferons or antibiotics, may increase the risk of developing depressive symptoms.

14.8.6 Neurological disorders

Depression is a relatively common psychiatric comorbidity of most neurological disorders, with prevalence rates ranging between 20% and 50% among patients with epilepsy, stroke, dementia, Parkinson's disease, or multiple sclerosis. In addition, some treatments of neurological disorders (e.g., corticosteroids) enhance the risk for depression as a treatment-related adverse event.

14.8.7 Neoplasias and paraneoplastic syndromes

Depression is frequent in patients suffering from cancer; rates of 19% for depressive symptoms and 8% for MDD have been reported. In addition, most chemotherapeutics used in the treatment of cancer may provoke depression.

14.9 Treatments

The goals of clinical management of MDD can be divided into acute, intermediate, and long-term.

The goal of acute treatment is to achieve remission, meaning not only being asymptomatic (in the sense of not meeting the criteria for diagnosis of the disorder and having no or only minimal residual symptoms), but also showing improvement in psychosocial and occupational functioning. From the patient's perspective, remission means the presence of features of positive mental health such as optimism and self-confidence, and a return to one's usual, normal self.

The intermediate goal of treatment is stabilization and prevention of a relapse, elimination of sub-syndromal symptoms, and restoration of the prior level of functioning. The long-term goal is full recovery, to prevent further episodes, maintain functioning, and ensure a satisfactory quality of life.

14.9.1 Acute treatment

At least in severe depression and depression previously unresponsive to psychotherapy alone, initiation of antidepressant therapy is a regular part of the overall treatment plan. If not already ongoing, the treatment plan should also include psychotherapy, psychoeducation, and psychosocial support.

The choice of medication depends on several factors, including proven efficacy, tolerability and safety, previous experience, and preference of the patient. Titrating medication usually starts with the lowest effective dose, derived from clinical studies, to ensure good tolerability. If side-effects do not occur or fade within a few days, stepwise dosage increases up to the usual standard dose as recommended by the manufacturer can be made until relief from depressive symptoms begins. A delay of several weeks may occur until sufficient antidepressant effects can be observed (see Chapter 33). When switching from one medication to another, overlapping tapering is recommended unless a specific medication demands a washout phase.

Expectations about the potential efficacy of a given treatment are not uniform across guidelines. Antidepressants currently in use achieve treatment response rates of 50–75% in moderately to severely depressed patients. This means that, despite sufficient dosage, up to one-half of patients do not respond sufficiently to the initial treatment choice. Concurrent pain and somatization indicate a longer time course until remission is achieved; especially the presence of bodily pain predicts difficulties in treating depression. These patients may require more intensive treatment right from the start, such as the use of dual-mechanism antidepressants that also address pain and thus increase the chances of achieving remission.

The decision concerning whether a response is sufficient can be made clinically or, especially in research settings, be guided by the administration of established rating scales (see Chapter 31). "No response" is usually defined as a 0–25% decrease in baseline symptom severity, "partial response" as a 26–49% decrease, and "response" as a 50–100% decrease. In cases of non-response after 4 weeks of treatment, a switch of medication is usually recommended. Patients with a partial response after 6–8 weeks should receive a dose escalation, followed by augmentation or a switch of strategy.

14.9.2 General principles of maintenance treatment

The ultimate goal in any psychiatric disorder is to prevent recurrence of acute symptomatology and improve functionality and quality of life. Prophylactic treatment of unipolar depression is not restricted to pharmacotherapy. Psychotherapy, especially IPT and CBT (see Chapter 32), should be included in the overall treatment plan. Maintaining a good therapeutic relationship, monitoring adherence, and psychoeducation are important as well. To prepare patients and their relatives for long-term prophylactic treatment, they should be informed about topics such as the expected course of the illness, treatment options, medication efficacy and side-effects, use of a daily self-reporting instrument for mood to detect early signs of relapse or recurrence, long-term perspectives, and, if applicable, the projected end of treatment. Patients should be told how to distinguish between spontaneous and short mood fluctuations ("blips") and the true emergence of a new episode that should be treated as soon as possible.

14.9.3 Continuation treatment

After the initial remission from acute depression, continuation treatment should ensure stabilization, the prevention of early relapse, and further improvement in functionality and promotion of reintegration.

When antidepressant treatment has been effective and the primary goal of symptomatic remission has been achieved, it is usually recommended to continue the antidepressant in unchanged dosage for continuation treatment, unless side-effects force tapering of the medication. The prophylactic effect of continuing antidepressant medication has been shown in a multitude of studies. Up to 50% of patients successfully stabilized in acute-phase treatment will relapse if medication is not sustained throughout the continuation period, whereas only 10–15% relapse if medication is continued. Thus, the often applied clinical practice of dose reduction during maintenance treatment lacks evidence and may put the patient at an increased risk of relapse.

When full response is achieved with low-dose acute antidepressant treatment, it may be justified to continue treatment in the lower dose range. It is generally recommended to continue the effective antidepressant monotherapy or combination treatment for at least another 3–6 months, but at least until all symptoms have totally subsided, as residual symptoms are predictive for early relapse. Patients with a history of previous long-lasting episodes or several risk factors of recurrence may be candidates for longer continuation treatment.

14.9.4 Dealing with treatment refractoriness

A general problem in the therapy for depression is the likelihood of non-response to the first antidepressant treatment. Up to 50% of depressed patients do not respond sufficiently to a first course of an adequate antidepressant treatment (about 30% do not show sufficient improvement; about 20%

drop out due to tolerability problems). Half of patients also fail to respond to a second antidepressant treatment trial. If several antidepressant treatment trials have been unsuccessful, response rates after switching to another drug are likely to decrease further and long-term prognosis worsens.

Patients who do not respond to at least two antidepressant monotherapies are often defined as "treatment resistant." Reasons may vary and often do not reflect true resistance to treatment. Two biological hypotheses for therapy resistance are undiagnosed medical conditions maintaining depression, or an abnormal drug metabolism. Other factors that may lead to less favorable outcomes include alcohol and substance abuse, personality disorder, and anxiety and panic disorder. Several other factors have been predictive for poor response, including a family history of affective disorders, severity of depression, suicide attempts, number of previous episodes, long duration of depression prior to treatment, negative life events, and poor social support.

Several pharmacologic treatment strategies are used to deal with treatment refractoriness, including increase of dosage, switching to an antidepressant of the same class, switching to an antidepressant of another class, combination therapies with more than one antidepressant, and pharmacologic and non-pharmacologic augmentation strategies. However, it is impossible to predict the most effective treatment strategy for an individual patient.

If a patient is not responsive to antidepressant treatment, it is strongly recommended that generalist clinicians seek a second opinion or consultation. Some alternative medications to antidepressants or augmentation strategies have appeared in the literature, but these require a certain level of expertise and experience.

With a partial response it may be unwise to discontinue the medication and risk worsening of symptoms. Thus, combination with another antidepressant or augmentation should be considered, and there is now sufficient evidence that combinations of antidepressants or augmentation strategies are more effective than monotherapy in some patients. Combination treatment is defined as the addition of another medication without expecting potentiation of efficacy of the previous drug. Benefits as well as side-effects are additive. Usually, a medication with a different pharmacology or a drug with a dual mechanism of action is chosen for combination treatment. In contrast, augmentation means the addition of another agent which by itself may be not specifically helpful as a primary treatment of depression, but may enhance responsiveness to a given antidepressant. Such agents include lithium, thyroid hormones, pindolol, buspirone, and some atypical antipsychotics.

One alternative maintenance treatment is long-term lithium therapy. Although it may be even more efficacious in bipolar disorder, and despite some negative published results in unipolar disorder, the efficacy of lithium in preventing relapses in unipolar recurrent depression has been well established. Besides preventing new episodes, lithium has been demonstrated to normalize the mortality rates for cerebrovascular and cardiovascular disorders in affectively ill patients. Combined lithium and antidepressant treatment reduces the risk of suicide to a significantly larger extent than antidepressants alone.

Pharmacotherapy is not always mandatory for less severe forms of depression, whereas severe depression usually requires pharmacotherapy or electroconvulsive therapy (see Chapter 37).

In addition, a variety of other biologic interventions such as sleep deprivation and bright-light therapy may be effective in certain patient subgroups. Phototherapy for depression has been shown to be effective for some individuals who have mild to moderate symptoms of mood disorder with a seasonal pattern. This treatment consists of using artificial light therapy for one or two 30-minute to 3-hour daily sessions. Recent studies support the use of phototherapy as an efficacious *adjunctive* treatment in non-seasonal unipolar and bipolar depression as well.

Total sleep deprivation is a non-pharmacologic intervention, which exerts rapid antidepressant effects in about 60–70% of depressed patients who stayed awake for one night and the consecutive day. Partial sleep deprivation means that patients get up at between 1 a.m. and 2 a.m. and stay awake for the second half of the night and the consecutive day at least until 8 p.m. This is as effective as total sleep deprivation and usually better accepted by depressed patients. The clinical usefulness of total sleep deprivation is limited since relapse is observed in most patients when returning to a normal sleep pattern, or even after a short nap on the next day.

14.9.5 Psychosocial treatments

Several specific forms of psychotherapy have been developed for the treatment of depression, including CBT and IPT (see Chapter 32). In addition, various other forms of psychotherapy have been adapted for depression treatment. These include supportive psychotherapy, psychodynamic psychotherapy, and marital and family therapy.

In general, empirically supported psychotherapies have demonstrated similar response and remission rates to pharmacotherapy for outpatients with depressive disorders, who, on average, may be less severely ill than inpatients. They treat mood and demoralization more quickly than neuro-vegetative symptoms of depression, the reverse of the pattern seen for most antidepressant medications. IPT and CBT also provide prophylaxis against relapse and recurrence when prescribed as less frequent (e.g., monthly) maintenance treatments.

However, the use of these psychotherapies clearly has its limitations. Some severely depressed patients may be too depleted to engage in psychotherapy effectively. They are also not intended to treat depression with psychotic features, nor as monotherapy for bipolar I depression.

14.10 Treatment-related suicidality

The effect of antidepressants on suicidality needs further evaluation. If at all, there may be more compelling evidence for an association in adolescents than in adults. A possible explanation for this might be a higher rate of substance abuse or an undetected bipolar disorder with mixed symptomatology. Both underlying conditions may become harmful in the presence of the activating, sometimes agitating, effects of antidepressants. In adults, the more compelling evidence is for an antisuicidal effect of antidepressant treatment, derived mainly from large observational databases and partially from meta-analysis of controlled trials.

Clinical Vignette

Mrs D is a 62–year-old former teacher, living alone, who retired from work 6 months ago. She presented to her general practitioner complaining about loss of appetite, constipation, abdominal cramps, and a general feeling of weakness and loss of energy. Abdominal sonography and an abdominal CT scan were without pathological findings, but there were moderate signs of dehydration with an increase in creatinine and hematocrit as well as low serum iron and serum ferritin. She was prescribed a combined iron sulfate and folic acid preparation and advised to drink at least 1.5 liters a day. No improvement in symptoms was observed after 1 month, and then Mrs D also mentioned an increasing loss of pleasure. She was referred to a psychiatrist.

At presentation Mrs D reported low self-esteem after retirement and difficulties structuring her daily routine; also, she didn't feel challenged by it. Diagnosis of a MDD was made and she was started on fluoxetine 20 mg/day. She was sent to a CBT therapist. Her low self-esteem after retirement and consecutive thoughts of being now worthless became the focus of the CBT. After having 12 sessions of CBT and fluoxetine at a final daily dose of 40 mg for 8 weeks she started to improve slowly but constantly and reached full recovery after 3 months. For the next 2 years, CBT was continued at low frequency with one session per month and she continued to take fluoxetine for another year before it was tapered off over a 6-month period.

KEY POINTS

- Extreme changes in mood can signal a mood disorder that can be grouped by its severity and distance from the euthymic state.

- Mood disorders include major depressive disorder, dysthymic disorder, bipolar I and II disorders, and cyclothymic disorder.

- Mood disorders can occur across the lifespan and are associated with disturbances in functioning across multiple domains.

- Suicidal ideation is a frequent companion to mood disorders.

- Many medical conditions can result in mood disorders and should be ruled out prior to initiating treatment.

- The treatment plan for major depressive disorder should include psychotherapy, psychoeducation, and psychosocial support, as well as pharmacotherapy.

- The choice of medication depends on several factors including proven efficacy, tolerability and safety, previous experience, and preference of the patient.

Further Reading

Leahy, R.L. and Holland, S.J. (2000) *Treatment Plans and Interventions for Depression and Anxiety Disorders*, Guilford, New York.

Tatano, B.C. and Driscoll, J.W. (2005) *Postpartum Mood and Anxiety Disorders: A Clinican's Guide*, Jones & Bartlett, New York.

Schou, M. (2004) *Lithium Treatment of Mood Disorders: A Practical Guide*, Karger S. Inc., Denmark.

Stahl, S. (2008) *Depression and Bipolar Disorder*, Cambridge University Press, Cambridge, UK.

15   •_••   Anxiety Disorders

The experience of fear and the related emotion of anxiety are universal. This chapter discusses fear, its relation to anxiety, and their expression as nonadaptive responses as manifested in the various anxiety disorders.

15.1 Fear and anxiety

Fear exists in all cultures and appears to exist across species. Presumably, the purpose of fear is to protect an organism from immediate threat and to mobilize the body for quick action to avoid danger. Fear is often referred to as a fight-or-flight response. All the manifestations of fear are consistent with its protective function. For example, heart rate and breathing rate increase to meet the increased oxygen needs of the body, increased perspiration helps to cool the body to facilitate escape, and pupils dilate to enhance visual acuity.

Anxiety, on the other hand, is a future-oriented mood state in which the individual anticipates the possibility of threat and experiences a sense of uncontrollability focused on the upcoming negative event. If one were to put anxiety into words, one might say, "Something bad might happen soon. I am not sure I can cope with it but I have to be ready to try." Anxiety is primarily mediated by the gamma-aminobutyric acid–benzodiazepine system.

Fear and anxiety are not always adaptive. At times, the responses can occur in the absence of any realistic threat or out of proportion to the actual danger. Almost everyone has situations that arouse anxiety and fear despite the fact that the actual risk is minimal. For some people, these fears reach extreme levels and may cause significant distress or impairment in functioning.

Anxiety becomes pathological if a person feels anxious when no real threat exists, when a threat has passed long ago but continues to impair the person's functioning, or when a person substitutes adaptive coping mechanisms with maladaptive ones. Other signs suggesting that a person needs treatment include the following:

- Anxiety of greater-than-expected intensity
- Anxiety that prevents fulfillment of professional, personal, or social roles
- Anxiety accompanied by flashbacks, obsessions, or compulsions
- Anxiety that causes a curtailment of daily or social activities
- Anxiety that lasts longer than expected.

Unrelieved anxiety causes physical and emotional problems, and people may use a variety of coping mechanisms (adaptive or maladaptive) to try to manage the anxiety. Persistent or recurrent anxiety should be evaluated to determine whether the person is suffering from an anxiety disorder.

Fundamentals of Psychiatry, First Edition. Allan Tasman and Wanda K. Mohr.
© 2011 John Wiley & Sons, Ltd. Published 2011 by John Wiley & Sons, Ltd.

The term "anxiety disorders" refers to a group of conditions in which people experience persistent anxiety that they cannot dismiss and that interferes with their activities of daily life. Anxiety disorders include panic disorder, obsessive–compulsive disorder, post-traumatic stress disorder, generalized anxiety disorder, and phobias (social phobia, agoraphobia, and specific phobia). Each of these will be discussed briefly in this chapter.

15.2 Epidemiology

Anxiety disorders are very common. Approximately 40 million US adults aged 18 years and older, or about 18.1% of people in this age group in a given year, have an anxiety disorder. They frequently co-occur with depressive disorders or substance abuse, and most people with one anxiety disorder also have another anxiety disorder. Nearly three-quarters of those with an anxiety disorder will have their first episode by age 21.

15.3 Etiology

Anxiety disorders have several possible etiologies and there are a number of theories, from the biologic to the psychodynamic, that contribute to our understanding. They are discussed in very general terms below.

The fear network is thought to be influenced by genetic factors and stressful life events, particularly events in early childhood. Genetic variants of several candidate genes of neurotransmitter or neurohormonal systems, each with a small individual effect, may contribute to the susceptibility to anxiety and mood disorders. The biologic vulnerability to certain anxiety disorders varies from person to person. This vulnerability may never be stressed, however, and a person with the same family history may not develop the disorder. Brain chemistry and developmental factors also play a role. Studies have shown that variations in the autonomic nervous system or noradrenergic system may cause some people to experience anxiety to a greater degree than others. Other studies suggest abnormalities in the regulation of substances such as serotonin and gamma-aminobutyric acid (GABA) may play a role in the development of anxiety disorders.

Fear and anxiety are also influenced and mediated by several interacting brain structures, such as the amygdala, hippocampus, striatum and locus coeruleus, which may play a role in making individuals more vulnerable to an anxiety disorder.

Psychological factors appear to play a part in the development of anxiety disorders. Long-term exposure to abuse, violence, or poverty may affect a person's susceptibility. According to learning theory, anxiety may result from conditioning, by which a person develops an anxious response by linking a dangerous or fear-inducing event (e.g., a house fire) with a neutral event (e.g., watching someone light a match). In cases of general anxiety, a person may learn the anxiety response when he or she begins to liken any anxious symptoms with a full-fledged anxiety attack, causing a vicious anxiety cycle to continue.

Cognitive theories explain anxiety as a manifestation of distorted thinking and suggest that the individual's perception or attitude overestimates the danger of the stimulus that evokes their anxiety response. According to cognitive theorists, many people with anxiety disorders have a tendency to *catastrophically misinterpret* autonomic arousal sensations that occur in the context of no pathological anxiety.

There is a great deal of overlap between the symptoms of anxiety disorders and major depression, although the core symptoms (worry, anxiety and fear versus depressed mood) differ. Overlapping symptoms include problems with sleep, concentration, fatigue, and psychomotor/arousal symptoms. From a diagnostic standpoint, it might make little difference whether a patient has anxiety or depression insofar as pharmacologic treatments are similar.

15.4 Panic disorder

The essential features of panic disorder are recurrent, unexpected panic attacks that cause the affected person to persistently worry about recurrences or complications from the attacks or to undergo behavioral changes in response to the attacks for at least 1 month. Panic disorder may be with or without agoraphobia.

Panic attacks typically are characterized by a discrete period of intense apprehension or terror without any real accompanying danger. The clinical picture involves a physiologic and psychologic over-response to stressors. A person experiencing a panic attack may perceive the circumstances to be life-threatening and experience such reactions as chest pain, choking or smothering sensations, dizziness, dyspnea, fainting, hot and cold flashes, palpitations, paresthesias, sweating, and vertigo. The person may also report feelings of depersonalization or derealization, feelings of dread or doom, fears of dying or losing their mind, or fears of engaging in some sort of uncontrollable behaviors. Attacks typically last for several minutes, reaching a peak within 10 minutes.

Panic attacks are frightening and uncomfortable and people may make extreme efforts to escape from what they believe to be causing the panic and their behavior may appear strange or erratic to others. Between panic attacks, the person often remains moderately to severely anxious in anticipation of the next episode.

Although panic attacks are unpredictable in onset, they may occur in specific situations, such as driving an automobile, but not necessarily every time the patient engages in the activity. Panic attacks may occur in other circumstances and this feature is helpful in distinguishing panic attacks from phobias.

Panic disorder can occur with agoraphobia, which is a marked fear of being alone or in a public place from which escape would be difficult or help would be unavailable in the event of becoming disabled. Recent data suggest that the prevalence of lifetime comorbidity in panic disorder with agoraphobia is 100%. Agoraphobia is the most severe and persistent phobic disorder. People with agoraphobia often fear such scenarios as being outside the house alone, using public or mass transportation, and being in a crowd. As a response, many people with agoraphobia avoid such situations or endure them with such agony that they rearrange their lifestyles to minimize these occurrences (e.g., restrict their travel, stop leaving the house). Eventually, the limitations that agoraphobia imposes may diminish the person's enjoyment of life and lead to depression.

This/these disorders are highly comorbid with other anxiety disorders, major depression, somatoform disorders, pain-related disorders, substance-abuse disorders, and personality disorders. Panic disorder symptoms may wax and wane but, if left untreated, the typical course is chronic. In general, among those receiving tertiary treatment, approximately 30% of patients have symptoms that are in remission, 40–50% are improved but still have significant symptoms, and 20–30% are unimproved or worse at 6- to 10-year follow-up.

Treatment goals as they pertain to panic disorder with and without agoraphobia are, in general, to reduce the frequency and severity of panic attacks, avoidance behaviors, and panic-related disability in social and occupational functioning. There are a number of approaches that can be taken in treating panic disorder with and without agoraphobia. Interventions with the most enduring treatment effects include cognitive–behavioral therapy and particular pharmacotherapies (e.g., a selective serotonin-reuptake inhibitor, imipramine, clomipramine). Serotonin/norepinephrine-reuptake inhibitors are another promising treatment. High-potency benzodiazepines are effective in the short term but are less effective in producing long-term remission of panic disorder.

15.5 Obsessive–compulsive disorder

Obsessive–compulsive disorder (OCD) is an often debilitating syndrome characterized by the presence of two distinct phenomena: obsessions and compulsions. Obsessions are intrusive, recurrent, unwanted ideas, thoughts, or impulses that are difficult to dismiss despite their disturbing nature. Compulsions are repetitive behaviors, either observable or mental, that are intended to reduce the anxiety engendered by obsessions. Obsessions or compulsions that clearly interfere with functioning and/or cause significant distress are the hallmark of OCD.

Most affected patients have multiple obsessions and compulsions over time, with a particular fear or concern dominating the clinical picture at any one time. The presence of obsessions without compulsions, or compulsions without obsessions, is unusual.

The disorder is characterized of common obsessions. Contamination obsessions are the most frequently encountered, usually characterized by a fear of dirt or germs. Contamination fears may also involve toxins or environmental hazards (e.g., asbestos or lead) or bodily waste or secretions. Excessive washing is the compulsion most commonly associated with contamination obsessions.

The need for symmetry describes a drive to order or arrange things perfectly or to perform certain behaviors symmetrically or in a balanced way. Patients describe an urge to repeat motor acts until they achieve a "just right" feeling that the act has been completed perfectly. Patients with a prominent need for symmetry may have little anxiety but rather describe feeling unsettled or uneasy if they cannot repeat actions or order things to their satisfaction. Patients with a need for symmetry frequently present with obsessional slowness, taking hours to perform acts such as grooming or brushing their teeth.

Patients with somatic obsessions are worried about the possibility that they have or will contract an illness or disease.

People with sexual or aggressive obsessions are plagued by fears that they might harm others or commit a sexually unacceptable act such as molestation. Often, they are fearful not only that they will commit a dreadful act in the future but also that they have already committed the act. Patients are usually horrified by the content of their obsessions and are reluctant to divulge them. Patients with these highly distressing obsessions frequently have checking and confession or reassurance rituals.

Pathological doubt is a common feature of patients with OCD who have a variety of different obsessions and compulsions. Individuals with pathological doubt are plagued by the concern that, as a result of their carelessness, they will be responsible for a dire event.

Comorbidity includes major depression, and OCD is highly comorbid with the other anxiety disorders. Although findings have varied, the generally accepted frequency of tic disorders in patients with OCD is far higher than in the general population, with a rate of approximately 5–10% for Tourette's disorder and 20% for any tic disorder. Conversely, patients with Tourette's disorder have a high rate of comorbid OCD, with 30–40% reporting obsessive–compulsive symptoms. Finally, it has long been noted that the co-occurrence of OCD symptoms in patients with psychotic disorders is more than would be expected by chance.

Age at onset usually refers to the age when OCD symptoms (obsessions and compulsions) reach a severity level wherein they lead to impaired functioning or significant distress or are time-consuming (i.e., meet DSM-IV-TR criteria for the disorder). Reported age at onset is usually during late adolescence.

Earlier age at onset has been associated with an increased rate of OCD in first-degree relatives. These data suggest that there is a familial type of OCD characterized by early onset. Age at onset of OCD may also be a predictor of course. The vast majority of patients report a gradual worsening of obsessions and compulsions prior to the onset of full-criteria OCD, which is followed by a chronic course. A subtype of OCD that begins before puberty has been described in the literature. It is characterized by an episodic course with intense exacerbations. Exacerbations of OCD symptoms in this subtype have been linked with group A beta-hemolytic streptococcal infections, which has led to the subtype designation of pediatric autoimmune neuropsychiatric disorders associated with streptococcal infections (PANDAS). In a study of 50 children with PANDAS, the average age of onset was 7.4 years.

In terms of prognosis, a recent meta-analysis pooled 16 study samples comprising 521 children followed for between 1 and 15.6 years. The persistence of OCD was lower than previously believed. The authors reported that two-thirds of studies showed that OCD did not persist as a full clinical syndrome in the majority of subjects. The pooled mean rate of persistence of full-threshold OCD was 41%. The persistence of OCD was predicted by inpatient treatment, longer duration of illness at baseline, and an earlier age at onset of OCD. However, gender, age at assessment, and length of follow-up may also be related to the persistence of OCD.

OCD is sometimes difficult to distinguish from certain other disorders. Obsessions and compulsions may appear in the context of other syndromes, which can raise the question whether the obsessions and compulsions are a symptom of another disorder or whether both OCD and another disorder are present. A general guideline is that, if the content of the obsessions is not limited to the focus of concern of another disorder (e.g., an appearance concern, as in body dysmorphic disorder, or food concerns, as in an eating disorder) and if the obsessions or compulsions are preoccupying as well as distressing or impairing, OCD should generally be diagnosed.

Both pharmacologic and behavioral therapies have proved effective for OCD. The majority of controlled treatment trials have been performed with adults aged 18–65 years. However, these therapies have been effective for patients of all ages. In general, children and the elderly tolerate most of these medications well. The most extensively studied agents for OCD are medications that affect the serotonin system. Clomipramine and the selective serotonin-reuptake inhibitors are the treatments of choice, with the SSRIs being better tolerated due to a more favorable side-effect profile.

Behavioral treatment is a powerful adjunct to pharmacotherapy. A meta-analysis has demonstrated that combined behavioral therapy and SSRI treatment is superior to either behavioral therapy or pharmacotherapy alone. From a clinical perspective, it may be useful to have patients begin treatment with medication to reduce the intensity of their symptoms or comorbid depressive symptoms if present; patients may then be more amenable to participating in behavioral therapy and experiencing the anxiety that will be evoked by the behavioral challenges they perform. Behavioral therapy has been used successfully in all age groups, although when treating children with this modality it is usually advisable to use a parent as a co-therapist. In general, the goals of treatment are to reduce the frequency and intensity of symptoms as much as possible and to minimize the amount of interference the symptoms cause.

It should be noted that few patients experience a cure or complete remission of symptoms. Instead, OCD should be viewed as a chronic illness with a waxing and waning course. Symptoms are often worse during times of psychosocial stress.

15.6 Post-traumatic stress disorder

Post-traumatic stress disorder (PTSD) is defined in DSM-IV-TR by six different criteria. First, the disorder arises in a person who has been exposed to a traumatic event in which he or she experienced, witnessed, or was confronted with actual or threatened death or serious injury or a threat to the physical integrity of self or others. A wide range of traumatic events may meet this criterion, including military combat exposure, natural disasters, serious accidents, childhood physical, sexual, or emotional abuse, adult physical and sexual assault, domestic violence, and terrorist incidents.

Furthermore, the emotional response to this traumatic event must have involved intense fear, helplessness, or horror. In children, the response may take the form of disorganized or agitated behavior.

Second, there must have been at least one of five possible intrusive symptoms focused on the re-experiencing or recollection of the trauma. The first includes distressing recollections, images, thoughts, or perceptions of the traumatic event. For instance, a rape survivor may have disturbing recollections of details of the assault that come to mind unexpectedly when she does not expect to think about the event; these memories may evoke similar feelings of fear and helplessness as when the event occurred. A second re-experiencing symptom may include recurrent distressing nightmares, where trauma survivors may struggle at night reliving the trauma in their dreams. Third, trauma survivors may act or feel as if the trauma were recurring, also known as "flashbacks." These are very vivid reliving experiences in which they may have sensory experiences, including sights, sounds, and smells, related to the trauma. Fourth, trauma survivors may have intense psychological distress when exposed to internal or external cues resembling the trauma (e.g., a rape survivor acutely distressed when seeing a man who looks like the perpetrator). The last intrusive symptom includes physiological reactivity (e.g., increased heart rate and sweating) when exposed to trauma-related cues. Allowance is made for a different set of reactions in children, in whom re-experiencing symptoms may take the form of repetitive play, frightening dreams without recognizable content, or re-enactment of the trauma.

Third, persistent avoidance of stimuli associated with the trauma and numbing of general responsiveness must occur as evidenced by at least three out of seven symptoms. Although grouped together as one criterion, it is likely that phobic avoidance, emotional numbing, and withdrawal do not reflect the same underlying phenomenon. These seven symptoms include avoidance of thoughts, feelings, or conversations about the trauma; avoidance of activities, places, or people that cause remembrance of the trauma; difficulty recalling important details of the traumatic stressor; decreased interest in significant life activities; feeling detached or distant from others; a restricted range of affect; and sense of a foreshortened future.

Fourth, there must be at least two out of five symptoms of increased arousal following exposure to the traumatic event. Arousal symptoms may include sleep disruption, irritability or anger outbursts, problems concentrating, hypervigilance, and exaggerated startle responses. Diagnostically, all of these symptoms should have an onset temporally related to the traumatic event.

Symptoms of PTSD should last at least 1 month, and it is necessary that the symptoms cause clinically significant distress or impairment in social, occupational, or other areas of functioning. PTSD is considered to be "acute" if the duration of symptoms is between 1 and 3 months or "chronic" if the symptoms persist for 3 months or longer. If symptoms do not occur until at least 6 months have passed since the stressor occurred, the "delayed-onset" subtype is given.

Comorbidity is the rule rather than the exception in PTSD. Comorbid conditions include major depressive disorder, all of the anxiety disorders, alcohol and other substance use disorders, somatization disorder, and schizophrenia and schizophreniform disorder.

Immediately following traumatic exposure, a high percentage of individuals develop a mixed symptom picture, which includes disorganized behavior, dissociative symptoms, psychomotor change, and sometimes, paranoia. The diagnosis of ASD, as described later in this chapter, accounts for many of these reactions. These reactions are generally short-lived, although by 1 month the symptom picture often settles into a more classic PTSD presentation, such that after rape, for example, as many as 90% of individuals may qualify for the diagnosis of PTSD. Approximately 50% of people with PTSD recover, and approximately 50% develop a persistent, chronic form of the illness still present 1 year following the traumatic event. The longitudinal course of PTSD is variable in both child and adult samples.

General principles of treating PTSD involve explanation and destigmatization, which can be provided to both the patient and the family members. This often includes psychoeducation about basic PTSD symptoms and the way in which the condition can affect behaviors and relationships. Information can be given about general treatment principles, pointing out that sometimes cure is attainable but that at other times symptom containment is a more realistic treatment goal, particularly in chronic and severe PTSD.

Despite theoretical differences, most schools of psychotherapy recognize that cognitively oriented approaches to the treatment of anxiety must include an element of exposure. Anxiety management techniques are designed to reduce anxiety by providing patients with better skills for controlling worry and fear. Among such techniques are muscle relaxation, self-distraction (thought stopping), control of breathing and diaphragmatic breathing, guided self-dialog, and stress inoculation training. These techniques focus on enhancing a trauma survivor's ability to manage negative affect, especially anxiety and anger, and improve everyday functioning. Although these interventions have less empirical evidence regarding treatment efficacy for PTSD, generally the results are positive. Further, cognitive approaches to the treatment of PTSD have also gained empirical support. Overall, cognitive therapy for PTSD focuses on challenging dysfunctional, automatic thoughts that may develop following trauma exposure.

Other recent approaches have focused on efficaciously treating specific aspects of PTSD symptomatology, such as anger and nightmares. Some approaches have focused on specific interpersonal difficulties, such as difficulty dealing with authority figures following combat trauma.

With regard to medication, selective serotonin-reuptake inhibitors have demonstrated superiority over placebo in multiple well-controlled, double-blind trials in the past decade, and sertraline and paroxetine are two SSRIs officially indicated for the treatment of PTSD in the United States and elsewhere. Overall, the antidepressants and, to a lesser extent, the atypical antipsychotics are the most useful, and best studied, medication groups in treating PTSD. Mood stabilizers, hypnotics, beta- blockers, alpha-2-agonists, alpha-1- antagonists, and anxiolytics have a less clearly defined place.

15.7 Acute stress disorder

Acute stress disorder (ASD) occurs within the first month of exposure to extreme trauma: combat, rape, physical assault, near-death experience, or witnessing a murder. The general symptoms begin during or shortly following the event. The symptom of dissociation, a state of detachment in which the person experiences the world as dreamlike and unreal, is a primary feature. Poor memory of specific events surrounding the trauma also may accompany the dissociative state, a condition referred to as *dissociative amnesia*. Usually, ASD resolves within 2 days to 4 weeks after exposure to the trauma.

Little is known about the etiology of ASD specifically, but it is likely that many of the same factors that apply to PTSD are relevant for ASD; that is, trauma intensity, pre-existing psychopathology, family and genetic vulnerability, abnormal personality, lack of social supports at the time of the trauma, and physical injury are all likely to increase vulnerability for ASD.

A recent review of prospective studies of ASD suggests that approximately three-quarters of individuals who meet criteria for ASD will later develop full-blown PTSD. Therefore, the ASD diagnosis is strongly predictive of the development of PTSD over time.

Six general principles are involved in administering any treatment immediately after trauma. These include principles of brevity, immediacy, centrality, expectancy, proximity, and simplicity. That is, treatment of acute trauma is generally aimed at being brief, provided immediately after the trauma whenever possible, administered in a centralized and coordinated fashion with the expectation of the person's return to normal function and as proximately as possible to the scene of the trauma, and not directed at any uncovering or explorative procedures. Different components of treatment include providing information, psychological support, crisis intervention, and emotional first aid.

15.8 Social and specific phobias

A phobia is a persistent, irrational fear attached to an object or situation that objectively does not pose a significant danger. The affected person experiences anticipatory anxiety followed by a compelling desire to avoid the dreaded object or situation, even though he or she usually recognizes that the fear is unreasonable or excessive in proportion to the actual threat.

Unlike panic attacks (discussed earlier in this chapter), phobias are always anticipated and never manifest unexpectedly. They may be simple and specific to certain situations, events, or objects. They may also be globally incapacitating, as in the case of severe agoraphobia. When phobias accompany panic attacks, the condition is diagnosed as a panic disorder. The degree to which phobias are disabling depends largely on how central the phobia is in the person's life.

Specific and social phobias have both overlapping and distinguishing diagnostic and clinical features. In DSM-IV-TR, social phobia (also known as social anxiety disorder) is defined as a "marked and persistent fear of one or more social or performance situations in which the person is exposed to unfamiliar people or to possible scrutiny of others." Typical situations feared by individuals with social phobia include meeting new people, interacting with others, attending parties or meetings, speaking formally, eating or writing in front of others, dealing with people in authority, and being assertive. Specific phobia is defined as a "marked and persistent fear that is excessive or specific to an object or situation (e.g., flying, heights, animals, receiving an injection, seeing blood)."

The diagnostic criteria for specific and social phobias share many features. For both disorders, the phobic situation must almost invariably lead to an anxiety response (immediately, in the case of specific phobias), which may take the form of a panic attack. In addition, the individual must recognize that the fear is excessive or unreasonable (although this feature may be absent in children), avoid the phobic situation or endure it with intense distress, and experience marked distress or functional impairment as a result of the phobia. In the case of social phobia, the fear must not be related to another mental disorder or medical condition. For example, if an individual develops difficulties communicating after suffering a stroke, the fear must be unrelated to having other people notice one's problems in speaking. However, if the clinician judges that social anxiety is substantially in excess of what most individuals with this disability would experience, a diagnosis of anxiety disorder not otherwise specified may be appropriate. Finally, for both disorders the fear must not be better accounted for by another problem. Each diagnosis has specifiers or subtypes to allow for the provision of more specific diagnostic information. For social phobia, the clinician can specify whether the phobia is generalized (i.e., includes most social situations). For specific phobias, the clinician can indicate which one of five types best describes the focus of the phobia: animal, natural environment, blood – injection–injury, situational, or other.

Specific phobias tend to co-occur with other specific phobias. In addition, specific phobias often co-occur with other DSM-IV-TR disorders, such as mood or anxiety disorders. The mean onset of social phobias is in adolescence. Although many phobias begin after a traumatic event, many patients do not recall the specific onset of their fear, and few empirical data exist regarding the initial period after the fear onset. Clinically, however, some patients report a sudden onset of fear, whereas others report a more gradual onset. It is estimated that 50–80% of patients with social phobia have at least one other mental disorder, most commonly another anxiety disorder, major depressive disorder, or substance abuse disorder.

Other diagnoses that should be considered before a diagnosis of specific phobia is assigned include post-traumatic stress disorder (if the fear follows a life-threatening trauma and is accompanied by other PTSD symptoms such as re-experiencing the trauma), obsessive–compulsive disorder (if the fear is related to an obsession, such as contamination), hypochondriasis (if the fear is related to a belief that he or she has some serious illness), separation anxiety disorder (if the fear is of situations that might lead to separation from the family, such as traveling on a plane without one's parents), eating disorders (if the fear is of eating certain foods but not related to a fear of choking), and psychotic disorders (if the fear is related to a delusion).

Social phobia should not be diagnosed if the fear is related entirely to another disorder. For example, if an individual with obsessive–compulsive disorder avoids social situations only because of the embarrassment of having others notice her or his excessive hand washing, a diagnosis of social phobia would not be given. Furthermore, individuals with depression, schizoid personality disorder, or a pervasive developmental disorder may avoid social situations because of a lack of interest in spending time with others.

The main goal of treatment is to decrease fear and phobic avoidance to a level that no longer causes significant distress or functional impairment. Numerous studies have shown that exposure-based treatments are effective for helping patients to overcome. a variety of specific phobias. The way in which exposure is conducted appears to make a difference. Exposure-based treatments can vary on a variety of dimensions including the degree of therapist involvement, duration and intensity of exposure, frequency and number of sessions, and the degree to which the feared situation is confronted in imagination versus in real life. Adding various panic management strategies (e.g., cognitive restructuring, exposure to feared sensations) may help to increase the efficacy of behavioral treatments for certain specific phobias. In some cases, treatment includes strategies for improving specific skill deficits as well. For example, individuals with social phobia may lack adequate social skills and can sometimes benefit from social skills training. Likewise, some individuals with specific phobias of driving may have poor driving skills if their fear has prevented them from learning how to drive properly.

Typically, effective treatment for social phobia lasts several months, although treatment of discrete social phobias (e.g., public speaking) may take less time. Specific phobias can usually be treated relatively quickly. In fact, for certain phobias (e.g., animals, blood, injections), the vast majority of individuals are able to achieve clinically significant, long-lasting improvement in as little as one session of behavioral treatment.

Pharmacotherapy is generally thought to be ineffective for specific phobias, although it is not uncommon for phobic patients occasionally to be prescribed low dosages of benzodiazepines to be taken in the phobic situation (e.g., while flying).

In contrast to specific phobias, social phobia has been treated successfully with a variety of pharmacologic interventions. They include selective serotonin-reuptake inhibitors (e.g., sertraline, fluvoxamine, fluvoxamine CR, fluoxetine, citalopram, escitalopram, paroxetine), benzodiazepines (e.g., clonazepam, alprazolam), traditional monoamine oxidase inhibitors, serotonin/norepinephrine-reuptake inhibitors (e.g., venlafaxine), and reversible inhibitors of monoamine oxidase A (e.g., moclobemide, brofaromine).

With regard to specific phobia, it is common for some return of fear to occur in the presence of the phobic stimulus, although relapse following treatment of a specific phobia is believed to be rare.

15.9 Generalized anxiety disorder

Generalized anxiety disorder (GAD) is a category that has a history of disputation in the psychiatric community, as criteria in the DSMs have changed over time, with some scholars arguing that the present criteria are vague.

The condition as currently described is characterized by chronic and excessive worry and anxiety more days than not, occurring for at least 6 months and involving many aspects of the person's life. The worry and anxiety of this disorder cause such discomfort that they interfere with the client's daily life and relationships. Seldom do people suffering from this disorder experience eruptions of acute anxiety. Rather, they persistently exhibit signs of severe anxiety, such as motor tension, autonomic hyperactivity, and apprehensive expectation. Some clients may also exhibit chronic hypervigilance for potential threats. Displays of impatience and irritability and complaints of feeling "on edge" are common.

Because of this tense hyperarousal, the person may be unable to concentrate, suffer chronic fatigue, and experience sleep pattern disturbances. Additionally, he or she may exhibit tenseness and distractibility in social situations. For these reasons, this disorder eventually may lead to depression.

Many patients with GAD have difficulty pinpointing a clear age of onset or report that their symptoms began in childhood, suggesting a chronic course similar to that observed in personality disorders. Several studies, however, have indicated that GAD often begins in adulthood.

GAD shares several diagnostic features with both MDD and dysthymic disorder, including impaired concentration and sleep disturbance. Because of the substantial overlap between GAD and depression, a DSM-IV-TR hierarchy rule stipulates that GAD is not diagnosed if the symptoms have occurred within the context of a mood disorder. Therefore, the clinician must determine when the symptoms of GAD appeared relative to depression in order to make an accurate diagnosis. Measures of worry and the associated symptoms of GAD have not been effective at differentiating GAD from depression.

Several medical conditions are associated with prominent symptoms of anxiety. Self-reported anxiety is a significant predictor of functional impairment in a variety of medical conditions, although it is most common in individuals with digestive ailments. Thyroid dysfunction, particularly hyperthyroidism, has long been associated with increased risk of generalized anxiety and panic attacks. Although the magnitude of this increased risk is unclear, practitioners may consider thyroid function testing in previously unscreened patients. Many patients with GAD present to their primary-care physician for treatment of somatic problems, which may include headache, muscle tension, gastrointestinal problems, and fatigue. Unfortunately, these physicians infrequently recognize GAD and rarely prescribe psychotherapy or pharmacotherapy, although empirically supported treatments are available.

The most common pharmacologic treatments for GAD include benzodiazepines, azapirones, and selective serotonin-reuptake inhibitors. Benzodiazepines, which produce short-term sedation, muscle relaxation, and decreased physiological arousal, may provide relief from the somatic symptoms of GAD. Concerns have emerged, however, about the long-term use of benzodiazepines, which may lead to dependence. Azapirones, which include buspirone, are associated with less risk of dependence, although evidence for their efficacy in the treatment of GAD is equivocal.

Numerous antidepressants have been evaluated in the treatment of GAD. Several trials with newer antidepressants, including SSRIs and SNRIs, have produced promising findings. Venlafaxine, a serotonin/norepinephrine-reuptake inhibitor, was the first antidepressant approved by the US Federal Drug Administration for the treatment of GAD based on the results of several large, placebo-controlled trials.

With regard to psychosocial interventions, a 2005 meta-analysis of cognitive–behavioral therapy for GAD, found that it was more efficacious than control conditions, yielding medium to large effect sizes when compared to pill or psychologic placebo. In studies directly comparing CBT with pharmacotherapy (most often benzodiazepines), there was no difference in effect sizes between the two treatments. In contrast, an indirect comparison of CBT and pharmacotherapy (which included studies comparing each treatment to a control condition) suggested the superiority of drug treatment. However, attrition was lower for individuals receiving CBT (9%) than for those receiving pharmacotherapy (25%). Currently, neither mode of treatment is unequivocally superior to the other, and there are no large trials comparing combination therapy to either CBT or pharmacotherapy alone.

Clinical Vignette

Mr R, a 34-year-old married man, was referred for medication management by his counselor. He had been healthy until a life-endangering plane accident 2 years earlier, in which all passengers were killed except for him. He was still experiencing intrusive memories and reliving of the event when seen, despite having had helpful individual counseling. The events of the accident were engraved in his memory with clarity, and he could not understand how he survived. He was physically injured, with a broken ankle, severe lacerations of his arm, and damage to his back and face.

Whenever he saw a plane, he experienced a resurgence of symptoms, and he was unable to take plane trips. Whenever he rode in an elevator, the sensations he experienced while ascending or descending reminded him of the incident, and he became upset. He experienced hundreds of nightmares relating to the accident, felt as if he were constantly waiting for something bad to happen, and often found it impossible to direct his attention and his mind away from trauma images and memories. He had become fearful of even going to sleep. There was a general reduction of interest in things, and many of his former hobbies no longer gave him any pleasure. He found doing his job to be extremely difficult and thought about quitting. He revisited the site of the accident on each anniversary.

The initial treatment plan recognized that he had already received helpful individual counseling, the focus of which had been on reliving and retelling the story, accepting the painful consequences, and dealing with feelings of guilt because of his survival. Although he recognized the usefulness of these approaches, the intensity of his symptoms continued to be distressing and troublesome. It was agreed to initiate treatment with sertraline (25 mg/day), increasing to 50 mg daily after a week. This was supplemented by clonazepam (0.25 mg at night) largely to facilitate sleep and reduce hyperarousal and startle response. It was explained to Mr R that the sertraline would be expected to help more with the intrusive and avoidant and numbing symptoms.

He also completed two self-rating scales for PTSD, the Impact of Events Scale (IES) and the Davidson Trauma Scale (DTS). The baseline IES score was 47 (range of scores is 0–88), and the baseline DTS score was 101 (range 0–136). After 5 weeks, the dose of sertraline was increased to 100 mg/day and the dose of clonazepam remained at 0.25 mg at night. By the sixth week, his symptom distress was much less, with an IES score of 22 and a DTS score of 49. In other words, there was a greater than 50% reduction of symptoms. Mr R noticed much less avoidance of going into situations reminding him of the trauma, reduced frequency and severity of nightmares and daytime recollections, and greater ability to focus on important tasks related to his work and family. However, he continued to describe persistent startle response.

Mr R did not continue his individual therapy, feeling that he had maximal benefit after receiving this form of treatment for more than a year. He continued with his medication for another year and noticed improved ability to deal with situations that might have been extremely distressing to him, including being a direct witness to a fatal traffic accident. He was still unable to take air trips.

At one point during his medication management he unilaterally opted to discontinue his medication without discussing it. This was because he had experienced sexual difficulties, including a loss of sex drive, which was particularly vexing as he and his wife were attempting to start a family. The use of cyproheptadine proved to be helpful in counteracting this side-effect.

Mr R was also involved in litigation after the traffic accident and recognized that it was going to be extremely protracted. The litigation also brought with it a whole new set of problems, in which he felt himself being put in the victim position. He acknowledged that, although much progress had been made and he was much more highly functional, "nothing is quick with this condition" and that he still had a number of symptoms. He was willing to consider the possibility of additional treatment focused on his year of flying. He also recognized that when he had stopped his medicine, the symptoms came back with a vengeance, and he became more compliant in taking his antidepressant and anxiolytic medications.

KEY POINTS

- Anxiety disorders are the most common of all psychiatric syndromes. They affect humans across the lifespan and are often misdiagnosed and undertreated.

- While anxiety is a normal response to a threatening situation, prolonged anxiety in the absence of threat, exaggerated reactions, or reactions that impair functioning are not adaptive.

- Anxiety disorders include phobic disorders, panic disorder, generalized anxiety disorder, obsessive–compulsive disorder, and post-traumatic stress disorder.

- Treatments of anxiety disorders include non-pharmacologic and pharmacologic interventions.

- Non-pharmacologic methods include cognitive–behavior therapy and interventions grounded in behavior therapy such as relaxation techniques, systematic desensitization, and problem-solving strategies.

- Medications most often used are selective serotonin-reuptake inhibitors, benzodiazepines, buspirone, beta-blockers, and tricyclic antidepressants.

This chapter contains material from the following chapters in *Psychiatry, Third Edition*: Chapter 69 (Gordon J. G. Asmundson, Steven Taylor); Chapter 70 (Randi E. McCabe, Martin M. Antony); Chapter 71 (Michele T. Pato, Ayman Fanous, Jane L. Eisen, Katharine A. Phillips); Chapter 72 (Amanda M. Flood, Jonathan R. T. Davidson, Jean C. Beckham); and Chapter 73 (Amy E. Lawrence, Timothy A. Brown).

Further Reading

Kase, L., Ledley, D.R., and Weiner, I.B. (2007) *Anxiety Disorders*, John Wiley & Sons, New York.
Leahy, R.L. and Holland, S.J. (2000) *Treatment Plans and Interventions for Depression ad d Anxiety Disorders*, Guilford, New York.

16 Eating Disorders

16.1 Introduction

This chapter discusses eating disorders. In the current psychiatric nomenclature of DSM-IV-TR the eating disorders consist of two clearly defined syndromes, anorexia nervosa and bulimia nervosa, but many individuals presenting for treatment of an eating disorder fail to meet the formal criteria for either. It is likely that eating disorders are more heterogeneous than the DSM indicates and the categories may be too restrictive. A broader approach is to think of an eating disorder as a persistent disturbance of eating behavior intended to control weight that impairs psychological functioning and/or physical health.

16.2 Anorexia nervosa

The DSM-IV-TR criteria for anorexia nervosa (AN) require the individual to be significantly underweight for age and height. Although it is not possible to set a single weight-loss standard that applies to all individuals, DSM-IV-TR provides a guideline of 85% of the weight considered normal for age and height. Despite being of an abnormally low body weight, individuals with anorexia nervosa are intensely afraid of gaining weight and becoming fat, and this fear typically intensifies as the weight falls.

DSM-IV-TR criterion C requires a disturbance in the person's judgment about his or her weight or shape. Despite being underweight, individuals with anorexia nervosa often view themselves or a part of their body as being too heavy. Typically, they deny the grave medical risks engendered by their semi-starvation and place enormous psychological importance on whether they have gained or lost weight. Patients with anorexia nervosa may feel intensely distressed if their weight increases by half a pound. Criterion D of DSM-IV-TR additionally requires that women with anorexia nervosa be amenorrheic.

Although the criteria seem relatively straightforward, the greatest problem in the assessment of patients with anorexia nervosa is their denial of the illness and their reluctance to participate in an evaluation. A straightforward but supportive and non-confrontational style is probably the most useful approach to making a diagnosis and treatment, but it is likely that the patient will not acknowledge significant difficulties in eating or with weight and will rationalize unusual eating or exercise habits. It is therefore helpful to obtain information from other sources, such as the patient's family.

There are two types of anorexia nervosa:

- **Restricting type:** The person restricts food intake and does not engage in binge-eating or purging behavior.

Fundamentals of Psychiatry, First Edition. Allan Tasman and Wanda K. Mohr.
© 2011 John Wiley & Sons, Ltd. Published 2011 by John Wiley & Sons, Ltd.
This chapter is based on Chapter 78 (B. Timothy Walsh) of *Psychiatry, Third Edition*

Table 16-1	Medical problems associated with anorexia nervosa
Skin	**Lanugo**
Cardiovascular	Hypotension
	Bradycardia
	Arrhythmias
Hemopoietic system	Normochromic normocytic anemia
	Leukopenia
Fluid and electrolyte balance	Elevated urea nitrogen and creatinine
	Hypokalemia
	Hyponatremia
	Hypochloremia
	Alkalosis
Gastrointestinal system	Elevated liver enzymes
	Delayed gastric emptying
	Constipation
Endocrine system	Diminished thyroxine level with normal thyroid stimulating hormone level
	Elevated plasma cortisol
	Diminished secretion of luteinizing hormone, follicle stimulating hormone, estrogen, or testosterone
Bone	Osteoporosis

- **Binge eating/purging type:** The person self-induces vomiting or misuses laxatives, diuretics, or enemas.

16.2.1 Physiological disturbances

An impressive array of physical disturbances has been documented in anorexia nervosa (Table 16.1). Most of these appear to be secondary consequences of starvation, and it is not clear whether or how the physiological disturbances listed contribute to the development and maintenance of the psychological and behavioral abnormalities characteristic of the illness.

Common laboratory findings are a mild-to-moderate normochromic, normocytic anemia and leukopenia, with a deficit in polymorphonuclear leukocytes leading to a relative lymphocytosis. Elevations of blood urea nitrogen and serum creatinine concentrations may occur because of dehydration, which can also artificially elevate the hemoglobin and hematocrit. A variety of electrolyte abnormalities may be observed, reflecting the state of hydration and the history of vomiting and diuretic and laxative abuse. Serum levels of liver enzymes are usually normal but may transiently increase during refeeding.

Cholesterol levels may be elevated. The electrocardiogram typically shows sinus bradycardia and, occasionally, low QRS voltage and a prolonged QT interval. A variety of arrhythmias have also been described in the literature.

16.2.2 Epidemiology

Anorexia nervosa is a relatively rare illness. The point prevalence of strictly defined AN is only about 0.5%. The prevalence rates of partial syndromes (those not meeting the complete criteria) are substantially higher. Some studies suggest that its incidence has increased significantly during the last 50 years, and that the increase is due to changes in cultural norms regarding desirable body shape and weight. Anorexia nervosa mostly affects women, the ratio of men to women being between 1 : 10 and 1 : 20. It occurs primarily in industrialized and affluent countries, with data suggesting that the condition is more common among the higher socioeconomic classes. Some occupations, such as ballet dancing and fashion modeling, appear to confer a particularly high risk for the development of anorexia nervosa.

16.2.3 Course

The course of the illness is fairly typical across cases. An adolescent girl or young woman who is of normal weight or, perhaps, a few pounds overweight decides to diet. This decision may be prompted by an important but not extraordinary life event, such as attending a new school. Initially the dieting seems moderate but it intensifies as weight falls. Dietary restrictions become broader and more rigid. The person begins to avoid meals with others. The individual has idiosyncratic rules about eating and exercise. Food avoidance and weight loss are accompanied by a sense of accomplishment, and weight gain is viewed as a failure and a sign of weakness. Physical activity, such as running or aerobic exercise, often increases as the dieting and weight loss develop. Inactivity and complaints of weakness usually occur only when emaciation has become extreme. The person's life becomes centered around food and exercise. The person may become depressed and emotionally labile, withdrawn and secretive. She or he may lie about weight and eating behavior. Despite the profound disturbances in the way the person views her or his weight and calorie needs, reality testing is otherwise intact, and the person may continue to function well in school or at work. Symptoms usually persist for months or years until, typically at the insistence of friends or family, the person reluctantly agrees to see a professional. When the illness occurs in males the course is very similar to that in females.

Patients with this illness exhibit significant impairment in their lives as a result of their eating rituals and chronic states of semi-starvation. There is also an associated mortality. Data suggest that 10–20% of patients who have been hospitalized for AN will, in the next 10–30 years, die as a result of their illness. Much of the mortality is due to severe and chronic starvation, which eventually terminates in sudden death. A significant proportion of patients commit suicide.

16.2.4 Etiology

Anorexia nervosa occurs most frequently in biological relatives of patients who present with the disorder. However, conclusive data for genetic transmission of the disorder are not yet available.

Because anorexia nervosa typically begins during adolescence, developmental issues are thought to play an important etiological role. These include the critical challenges of establishing independence, defining a personal identity, family struggles, and conflicts regarding sexuality. However, it is not clear that difficulties over these issues are more salient for individuals who will develop anorexia nervosa than for other adolescents.

Family traits, such as over-protective mothers and passive fathers, have been identified in the literature as typical of parents of suffers. But few empirical studies have been conducted to date, particularly studies that also examine psychiatrically or medically ill comparison groups. Hence, despite theorizing, the precise role of the family in the development and course of anorexia nervosa has not been clearly delineated.

Cognitive–behavioral theories emphasize the distortions and dysfunctional thoughts (e.g., dichotomous thinking) that may stem from various causal factors, all of which eventually focus on the belief that it is essential to be thin. Certain personality traits have commonly been reported among women with the illness. These include high degrees of self-discipline, conscientiousness, and emotional caution. Depression has been implicated as a nonspecific risk factor.

Social psychologists suggest that an increased prevalence of anorexia nervosa is related to the emphasis in contemporary Western society on an unrealistically thin appearance in women which has increased significantly during the past several decades. Other authors have noted that the core features of the illness have been described in other cultural settings, indicating that the current societal emphasis on thinness is not a necessary precondition for the development of this syndrome.

16.2.5 Differential diagnosis

Anorexia nervosa is not difficult to recognize. Although depression, schizophrenia, and obsessive–compulsive disorder may be associated with disturbed eating and weight loss, it is rarely difficult to differentiate these disorders from anorexia nervosa. Individuals with major depression may lose significant weight but do not exhibit the relentless drive for thinness characteristic of anorexia nervosa. In schizophrenia, starvation may occur because of delusions about food.

Individuals with obsessive–compulsive disorder may describe irrational concerns about food and develop rituals related to meal preparation and eating but do not describe the intense fear of gaining weight and the pervasive wish to be thin that characterize anorexia nervosa. A wide variety of medical problems cause serious weight loss in young people and may at times be confused with anorexia nervosa. Examples of such problems include gastric outlet obstruction, Crohn's disease, and a brain tumor. Individuals whose weight loss is due to a general medical illness generally do not show the drive for thinness, the fear of gaining weight, and the increased physical activity characteristic of anorexia nervosa.

16.2.6 Comorbidities

Symptoms of mood and anxiety disturbances, especially obsessive–compulsive disorder, are commonly observed among individuals with anorexia nervosa. These symptoms improve substantially with weight gain but often do not resolve completely. Some individuals, especially those with the binge/purge subtype, may also have problems with substance abuse.

16.2.7 Treatment

Treatment of anorexia nervosa is challenging because of denial and the myriad of associated conditions and need for intervention beyond that which can normally be provided by a single clinician. A team approach, whether in an inpatient or partial hospitalization program, is optimal. There are six goals of treatment:

- Engagement of the patient and family in treatment

- Assessment of and addressing acute medical problems, such as fluid and electrolyte disturbances and cardiac arrhythmias (this may require the involvement of a general medical physician)

- Restoration of a more normal body weight

- Normalization of eating (this and the preceding may require the services of a professional dietician)

- Resolution of the associated psychological disturbances

- Prevention of relapse.

Despite the multiple physiological disturbances associated with anorexia nervosa, there is no clearly established role for medication. There is, at present, no general agreement about the most useful type of psychotherapy or the specific topics that need to be addressed. Most eating disorder programs employ a variety of psychotherapeutic interventions. There is good evidence supporting the involvement of the family in the treatment of younger patients with anorexia nervosa.

A large percentage of patients remain chronically ill; 30–50% of those successfully treated in hospital require rehospitalization within a year of discharge. Therefore, post-hospitalization outpatient treatments are recommended to prevent relapse and improve overall short- and long-term functioning.

Some patients with anorexia nervosa refuse to accept treatment and thereby can raise difficult ethical issues. If weight is extremely low or there are acute medical problems, it may be appropriate to consider involuntary commitment.

16.3 Bulimia nervosa

The salient behavioral disturbance of bulimia nervosa (BN) is the occurrence of episodes of binge-eating. During these episodes, the individual consumes an amount of food that is unusually large, considering the circumstances under which it was eaten. Episodes of binge-eating are associated with a sense of loss of control. Once the eating has begun, the individual feels unable to stop until an excessive amount has been consumed. After overeating, individuals engage in some form of inappropriate behavior in an attempt to avoid weight gain. This can include self-induced vomiting, abuse of laxatives, misusing diuretics, fasting for long periods, and exercising extensively after binges.

The DSM-IV-TR criteria require that the overeating episodes and the compensatory behaviors both occur at least twice a week for 3 months to merit a diagnosis of bulimia nervosa. Criterion D in the DSM-IV-TR definition requires that individuals exhibit an over-concern with body shape and weight. Also, in the DSM-IV-TR nomenclature, the diagnosis of bulimia nervosa is not given to individuals with anorexia nervosa. Individuals with the latter illness who recurrently engage in binge-eating or purging behavior should be given the diagnosis of anorexia nervosa (binge-eating/purging subtype) rather than an additional diagnosis of bulimia nervosa.

There are two principal types of bulimia nervosa. In the purging type, the person regularly engages in self-induced vomiting or the misuse of laxatives, diuretics, or enemas. In the non-purging type, the individual uses fasting or excessive exercise to control weight, but does not regularly purge.

16.3.1 Physiological disturbances

In a small proportion of individuals, bulimia nervosa is associated with the development of fluid and electrolyte abnormalities that result from the self-induced vomiting or the misuse of laxatives or diuretics. The most common electrolyte disturbances are hypokalemia, hyponatremia, and hypochloremia. Patients who lose substantial amounts of stomach acid through vomiting may become slightly alkalotic; those who abuse laxatives may become slightly acidotic.

There is an increased frequency of menstrual disturbances such as oligomenorrhea among women with bulimia nervosa. Patients who induce vomiting for many years may develop dental erosion, especially of the upper front teeth. Some patients develop painless salivary gland enlargement, which is thought to represent hypertrophy resulting from the repeated episodes of binge-eating and vomiting. The serum level of amylase is sometimes mildly elevated because of increased amounts of salivary amylase. Potentially life-threatening complications such as an esophageal tear or gastric rupture occur rarely. The longstanding use of syrup of ipecac to induce vomiting can lead to permanent damage to nerves and muscles, including clinically significant cardiomyopathy. Routine laboratory testing reveals an abnormality of fluid and electrolyte balance such as those described above in 5–10% of patients with bulimia nervosa.

16.3.2 Epidemiology

Although binge-eating is frequent, the full-blown disorder of bulimia nervosa is much less common, with a lifetime prevalence of 1–2% among women in the United States. Data suggest a significant increase in the incidence of bulimia nervosa in the last several decades.

16.3.3 Course

Bulimia nervosa typically starts after a young woman who sees herself as somewhat overweight diets and, after some initial success, begins to overeat. Distressed by her lack of control and fear of gaining weight, she turns to compensatory mechanisms, such as inducing vomiting or taking laxatives. The episodes of binge-eating usually increase in intensity and frequency, occuring after a variety of stimuli such as transient depression or anxiety. Patients describe themselves as "numb" during a binge-eating episode and are intensely ashamed of their condition. Once established, binges tends to occur in the late afternoon or evening and almost always while the person is alone. The typical patient presenting to an eating disorders clinic has been binge-eating and inducing vomiting five to ten times weekly for 3–10 years. Binges tend to contain 1000 or more calories and to consist of sweet, high-fat foods.

Over time the symptoms of bulimia nervosa tend to improve, although a substantial proportion of individuals continue to engage in binge-eating and purging.

16.3.4 Comorbidity patterns

Among patients with bulimia nervosa who are seen at eating disorders clinics, there is an increased frequency of anxiety and mood disorders, especially major depressive disorder and dysthymic disorder, drug and/or alcohol abuse, and personality disorders. It is not certain whether this comorbidity is also observed in community samples or whether it is acharacteristic of individuals who seek treatment.

16.3.5 Differential diagnosis

Bulimia nervosa is not difficult to recognize if a full history is available. The binge-eating/purging type of anorexia nervosa has much in common with bulimia nervosa but is distinguished by the characteristic low body weight and, in women, amenorrhea. Some individuals with atypical forms of depression overeat when depressed; but unless there is a pattern of binging and purging, an additional diagnosis of bulimia nervosa is not warranted.

Many individuals who believe they have bulimia nervosa have a symptom pattern that fails to meet the full diagnostic criteria. Individuals with these characteristics fall into the broad and heterogeneous category of "atypical eating disorders." Binge-eating disorder (discussed later), a category currently included in the DSM-IV-TR appendix B for categories that need additional research, is characterized by recurrent binge-eating similar to that seen in bulimia nervosa but without the regular occurrence of inappropriate compensatory behavior.

16.3.6 Etiology

The etiology of bulimia nervosa is uncertain. Predisposing factors include being an adolescent girl or young adult woman and having a personal or family history of obesity and of mood disturbance. Twins studies suggest that there may be inheritance factors that contribute to bulimia nervosa, but what these are is unclear.

Many of the same psychosocial factors related to the development of anorexia nervosa are also applicable to bulimia nervosa, including the influence of cultural esthetic ideals of thinness and physical fitness. Similarly, bulimia nervosa primarily affects women; the ratio of men to women is approximately 1 : 10. It also occurs more frequently in certain occupations (e.g., modeling) and sports (e.g., wrestling, running).

Cognitive–behavioral theories emphasize the role of rigid rules regarding food and eating, and the distorted and dysfunctional thoughts that are similar to those seen in anorexia nervosa. Interpersonal theories also implicate interpersonal stressors as a primary factor in triggering binge-eating. There is no evidence to suggest that a particular personality structure is characteristic of women with bulimia nervosa.

Compared with women without psychiatric illness, women with bulimia nervosa report increased frequencies of sexual abuse. However, the rates of abuse are similar to those found in other psychiatric disorders and occur in a minority of women with bulimia nervosa. Thus, while early abuse may predispose an individual to psychiatric problems generally, it does not appear to lead specifically to an eating disorder, and most patients with bulimia nervosa do not have histories of sexual abuse.

16.3.7 Treatment

The goals of the treatment of bulimia nervosa include stopping the binge-eating and inappropriate compensatory behaviors, and refocusing on factors other than shape and weight as a basis for self-esteem. The power struggles that often complicate the treatment process in anorexia nervosa occur much less frequently in the treatment of patients with bulimia nervosa, largely because the critical behavioral disturbances are less ego-syntonic and are more distressing. Most bulimia nervosa patients who pursue treatment agree with the primary treatment goals and wish to give up the core behavioral features of their illness.

The form of psychotherapy that has been examined most intensively is highly structured cognitive–behavioral therapy (CBT) concentrating on the distorted ideas about weight and shape, on the rigid rules regarding food consumption and the pressure to diet, and on the events that trigger episodes of binge-eating. Therapy can be individual or in a group. Up to 50% of patients with bulimia nervosa achieve abstinence from binge-eating and purging during a course of CBT, and in most, this improvement appears to be sustained.

Although antidepressant medication is clearly superior to placebo in the treatment of bulimia nervosa, several studies suggest that a course of a single antidepressant medication is generally inferior to a course of CBT. However, patients who fail to respond adequately to, or who relapse following, a trial of psychotherapy may respond to antidepressant medication.

Although psychotherapy and antidepressant medication are effective interventions for many patients with bulimia nervosa, some individuals have little or no response. There is no clearly established algorithm for the treatment of such refractory patients.

A major factor influencing the treatment of bulimia nervosa is the presence of other significant psychiatric or medical illness. For example, it can be difficult for individuals who are currently abusing drugs or alcohol to use the treatment methods described, and many experts suggest that the substance abuse needs to be addressed before the eating disorder can be effectively treated.

16.4 Binge-eating disorder

Binge-eating disorder (BED) is a proposed diagnostic category related to, but quite distinct from, bulimia nervosa. Suggested diagnostic criteria for BED are included in an appendix of DSM-IV-TR, which provides criteria sets for further study. These criteria require recurrent episodes of binge-eating, which are defined just as for bulimia nervosa. The major difference is that individuals with BED do not regularly use inappropriate compensatory behavior, although the precise meaning of "regularly" is not specified. Other differences from the definition of bulimia nervosa relate to the frequency of binge-eating: individuals with bulimia nervosa must have binged, on average, at least two times per week over the last 3 months, whereas individuals with binge- eating disorder must have binged at least 2 days per week over the last 6 months.

Individuals who describe binge-eating disorder are likely to be obese, and it is important to obtain a history of changes in weight and of efforts to lose weight. It is important to obtain a clear understanding of daily food intake and of what the individual considers to be a binge. The use of purging and other inappropriate weight-control methods and symptoms of mood disturbance and anxiety should be assessed.

16.4.1 Physical examination and laboratory findings

The salient general medical issue is that of obesity. Individuals with binge-eating disorder who are obese should be followed by a primary-care physician for assessment and treatment of the complications of obesity.

16.4.2 Epidemiology

The prevalence of binge-eating disorder is much greater than that of anorexia nervosa or bulimia nervosa. A recent study reports a lifetime prevalence of 3.5% among women and 2% among men. The prevalence among obese individuals who attend weight-loss clinics is substantially higher, and the frequency of binge-eating disorder increases with the degree of obesity. In contrast to anorexia nervosa and bulimia nervosa, individuals with BED are more likely to be from minority ethnic groups, and middle-aged.

16.4.3 Comorbidity patterns

Binge-eating disorder is frequently associated with symptoms of mood and anxiety disorder.

16.4.4 Course

As the recognition of binge-eating disorder is relatively recent, there is little definitive information about the natural history of this disorder. However, recent data suggest that the symptoms tend to be stable over time.

16.4.5 Differential diagnosis

Individuals who meet the proposed definition of binge eating disorder clearly have increased complaints of depression and anxiety, compared to individuals of similar weight without binge-eating disorder. The most difficult issue in the diagnostic assessment of binge-eating disorder is determining whether the eating pattern of concern to the individual meets the proposed definition of binge-eating. There are numerous varieties of unhealthy eating, such as the consumption of high-fat foods, and the nosology of these patterns of eating is not well worked out. Some individuals with atypical depression binge-eat when depressed; if the individual meets criteria for both a binge-eating disorder and an atypical depression, both diagnoses should be made.

16.4.6 Etiology and pathophysiology

Little is known about the etiology of binge-eating disorder. It is clearly associated with obesity, but it is uncertain to what degree the binge-eating is a contributor to, or a consequence of, the obesity.

16.4.7 Treatment

For most individuals with binge-eating disorder, there are three related goals. One is behavioral, to cease binge-eating. A second focuses on improving symptoms of mood and anxiety disturbance, which frequently are associated. The third is weight loss for individuals who are also obese.

Treatment approaches to binge-eating disorder are currently under active study. Definitive information about the best treatment algorithm has not yet been developed.

Clinical Vignette

When Ms A, a 24-year-old single white woman, was first evaluated for admission to an inpatient eating disorders program she had been restricting her food intake for about 5 years and had been amenorrheic for 4 years. At the time of her admission she weighed 71 pounds at a height of 61.5 inches.

In twelfth grade, Ms A menstruated for the first time and also developed "very large" breasts. She had a difficult first year at college, where she increased to her maximum weight of 120 pounds. The following year she transferred to a smaller college, became a vegetarian "for ethical reasons," and began to significantly restrict her food intake. She limited herself to a total of 700–800 calories a day, with a maximum of 200 calories per meal, and gradually lost weight in the next 5 years. She did not binge, vomit, abuse laxatives, or engage in excessive exercise. She considered herself to be "obsessed with calories" and observed a variety of rituals regarding food and its preparation (e.g., obsessively weighing her food).

Although Ms A excelled academically, she had no close friends and had never been involved in a romantic relationship. She was quite close to her mother and sister and had always been dependent on her parents. After graduating (with honors) from college, she worked at a series of temporary jobs but was unemployed and living at home with her mother at the time of admission. She had been in outpatient psychotherapy with two different therapists during the previous 2 years. The first therapist did not address her eating disorder, and Ms A continued to lose weight, from 90 to 80 pounds. Although her second therapist confronted her about her anorexia nervosa and started her on desipramine at 20 mg/day for depressive symptoms, Ms A continued to lose weight.

During her first 5-month hospitalization, Ms A was treated with a multimodal program (behavioral weight gain protocol, individual and family therapy, fluoxetine at 60–80 mg/day for obsessive–compulsive traits, and depressive symptoms) and gained up to a weight of 98 pounds. At discharge, she was maintaining her weight on food but remained concerned about her weight and was particularly frightened of reaching "the triple digits" (100 pounds). After leaving the hospital, Ms A continued with outpatient psychotherapy and fluoxetine for several months. She was then seriously injured in a car accident and, during a prolonged convalescent period, discontinued treatment for her eating disorder. She remained unemployed, eventually moved in with her sister and her sister's family, and gradually lost weight.

About 3.5 years after discharge, at the age of 27 years, Ms A again sought inpatient treatment. At admission she weighed 83 pounds but still felt "fat." During hospitalization she steadily gained weight and was prescribed sertraline at 100 mg/day for feelings of low self-esteem, anxiety, and obsessional thinking. When she was discharged 5 months later, at a weight of 108 pounds, she noted menstrual bleeding for the first time in more than 7 years. After leaving the hospital, Ms A continued taking medication and began outpatient cognitive–behavioral psychotherapy. For the next year she continued to struggle with eating and weight issues but managed to maintain her weight and successfully expand other aspects of her life by independently supporting herself with a full-time job, making new friends, and becoming involved in her first romantic relationship.

KEY POINTS

- Anorexia nervosa and bulimia nervosa are eating disorders that share many etiologic factors and can be viewed as existing along a single spectrum of eating disorders.

- Binge-eating disorder is a proposed diagnostic category related to, but quite distinct from, bulimia nervosa.

- The etiology of these disorders develop from a complex interaction of individual, family, sociocultural, and physiological factors.

- Patients with eating disorders exhibit disturbances in many or all the functional health patterns.

- Treatment of eating disorders happens in community-based and inpatient settings and is a complex and often lengthy process.

- Treatment outcomes include normalization of weight and eating patterns, improved self-esteem, and development of more realistic thought processes, adaptive coping mechanisms, and constructive family processes.

Further Reading

Mehler, P.S. and Andersen, A.E. (2010) *Eating Disorders: A Guide to Medical Care and Complications*, Johns Hopkins University Press, Baltimore, MD.

17.1 Introduction

In most cognitive disorders, the brain is organically compromised. This state may be temporary or permanent. In either case, it causes the affected person to exhibit cognitively disturbed behavior.

Cognitive disorders are a group characterized by a disruption of, or deficit in, cognitive functioning. The specific categories within this disorder, as delineated by DSM-IV-TR, include the following:

1. Delirium, dementia, amnestic, and other cognitive disorders

2. Mental disorders resulting from a general medical condition

3. Substance-related disorders.

Their hallmarks are pathologically driven changes in cognition that can be recognized clinically as notable deficits or impairments. Delirium, dementia, and amnestic disorders are classified as cognitive because they feature impairment in such parameters as memory, language, or attention as a cardinal symptom. Each of these three major cognitive disorders is subdivided into categories that ascribe the etiology of the disorder to a general medical condition, the persisting effects of a substance, or multiple etiologies. A "not otherwise specified" category is included for each disorder.

In the case of delirium, the primary disturbance is in the level of consciousness with associated impairments in orientation, memory, judgment, and attention. Dementia features cognitive deficits in memory, language, and intellect. The amnestic disorder is characterized by impairment in memory in the absence of clouded consciousness or other noteworthy cognitive dysfunction. In general, the cognitive disorders should represent a decline from a previous higher level of functioning, of either acute (delirium) or insidious (dementia) onset, and should interfere with the patient's social or occupational functioning.

Delirium is discussed in Chapter 38. Mental disorders resulting from a general medical condition are discussed in Chapter 23. This chapter specifically discusses the dementias.

The prognosis for individuals with progressive dementia is very poor. Currently, no *cures* are available for the dementias; however, certain interventions appear to *delay* or *slow* the progression of some of the disorders.

17.2 The dementias

"Dementia" is defined in DSM-IV-TR as a group of disorders characterized by the development of multiple cognitive deficits (including memory impairment) that are due to the direct physiologic effects of a general medical condition, the persisting effects of a substance, or multiple etiologies (e.g., the

Fundamentals of Psychiatry, First Edition. Allan Tasman and Wanda K. Mohr.
© 2011 John Wiley & Sons, Ltd. Published 2011 by John Wiley & Sons, Ltd.
This chapter is based on Chapter 51 (Robert L. Frierson) of *Psychiatry, Third Edition*

combined effects of a metabolic and a degenerative disorder). The disorders constituting the dementias share a common symptom presentation and are identified and classified on the basis of etiology.

The cognitive deficits exhibited in these disorders must be of sufficient severity to interfere with either occupational functioning or the individual's usual social activities or relationships. In addition, the observed deficits must represent a decline from a higher level of functioning and not be the consequence of a delirium. A delirium can, however, be superimposed on a dementia, and both can be diagnosed if the dementia is observed when the delirium is not in evidence. Dementia is typically chronic and occurs in the presence of a clear sensorium. If clouding of consciousness occurs, the diagnosis of delirium should be considered. Classifications of dementia are considered in Box 17.1.

17.2.1 Prevalence

The prevalence of dementias is not precisely known. Estimates vary depending on the age range of the population studied and whether the individuals sampled were in the general community, acute care facilities, or long-term nursing institutions.

17.2.2 Symptoms

Essential to the diagnosis of dementia is the presence of cognitive deficits that include memory impairment and at least one of the following abnormalities of cognition: aphasia, agnosia, apraxia, or a disturbance in executive function. In addition to defects in memory, patients with dementia often exhibit impairments in language, recognition, object naming, and motor skills. *Aphasia* is an abnormality of language that often occurs in vascular dementias involving the dominant hemisphere. Because this hemisphere controls verbal, written, and sign language, these individuals may have significant problems interacting with people in their environment. People with dementia and aphasia

---

Box 17.1 Classifications of Dementia.

Dementia of the Alzheimer type

- Early-onset versus late-onset
- Uncomplicated
- With delirium
- With delusions
- With depressed mood

Vascular dementia

- Uncomplicated
- With delirium
- With delusions
- With depressed mood

Dementia due to head trauma
Dementia due to Parkinson's disease
Dementia due to HIV disease
Dementia due to Huntington's disease
Dementia due to Pick's disease
Dementia due to Creutzfeldt–Jakob disease
Dementia due to other general medical conditions (e.g., neurosyphilis, normal-pressure hydrocephalus)
Substance-induced persisting dementia
Dementia due to multiple etiologies
Dementia not otherwise specified

may exhibit paucity of speech, poor articulation, and a telegraphic pattern of speech (nonfluent, Broca's aphasia). Despite faulty communication skills, patients with dementia with nonfluent aphasia have normal comprehension and awareness of their language impairment. As a result, such individuals often present with significant depression, anxiety, and frustration.

By contrast, patients with dementia with fluent (Wernicke's) aphasia may be quite verbose and articulate, but much of the language is nonsensical and rife with such paraphasias as neologisms and clang (rhyming) associations. Whereas nonfluent aphasias are usually associated with discrete lesions, fluent aphasia can result from such diffuse conditions as dementia of the Alzheimer type. More commonly, fluent aphasias occur in conjunction with vascular dementia secondary to a temporal-lobe or parietal-lobe cerebrovascular accident (CVA). Because the demented patients with fluent aphasia have impaired comprehension, they may seem apathetic and unconcerned with their language deficits, if they are in fact aware of them at all. They do not generally display the emotional distress of patients with dementia and nonfluent aphasia.

Patients with dementia may also lose their ability to recognize. *Agnosia* is a feature of a dominant hemisphere lesion and involves altered perception in which, despite normal sensations, intellect, and language, the patient cannot recognize objects. This is in contrast to aphasia in which the patient with dementia may not be able to name objects, but can recognize them. The type of agnosia depends on the area of the sensory cortex that is involved. Some demented patients with severe visual agnosia cannot name objects presented, match them to samples, or point to objects named by the examiner. Other patients may present with auditory agnosia and be unable to localize or distinguish such sounds as the ringing of a telephone. A minority of demented patients may exhibit astereognosis, the inability to identify an object by palpation.

Demented patients may also lose their ability to carry out selected motor activities despite intact motor abilities, sensory function, and comprehension of the assigned task (*apraxia*). Affected patients cannot perform such activities as brushing their teeth, chewing food, or waving goodbye when asked to do so.

The two most common forms of apraxia in demented individuals are ideational and gait apraxia. Ideational apraxia is the inability to perform motor activities that require sequential steps and results from a lesion involving both frontal lobes or the complete cerebrum. Gait apraxia, often seen in such conditions as normal-pressure hydrocephalus, is the inability to perform various motions of ambulation. It also results from conditions that diffusely affect the cerebrum.

Impairment of executive function is the inability to think abstractly, plan, initiate, and end complex behavior. On Mental Status Examination (MSE), patients with dementia display problems coping with new tasks. Such activities as subtracting serial sevens may be impaired.

Clearly, aphasia, agnosia, apraxia, and impairment of executive function can seriously impede the demented individual's ability to interact with his or her environment. An appropriate MSE of the patient with suspected dementia should include screening for the presence of these abnormalities.

Patients with dementia display other identifying features that often prove problematic. Poor insight and poor judgment are common in dementia and often cause individuals to engage in potentially dangerous activities or make unrealistic and grandiose plans for the future. Visual–spatial functioning may be impaired, and if patients have the ability to construct a plan and carry it out, suicide attempts can occur. More common is unintentional self-harm resulting from carelessness, undue familiarity with strangers, and disregard for the accepted rules of conduct.

Emotional lability, as seen in pseudobulbar palsy after cerebral injury, can be particularly frustrating for caregivers, as are occasional psychotic features such as delusions and hallucinations. Changes in their environment and daily routine can be particularly distressing for demented patients, and their frustration can be manifested by violent behavior.

17.2.3 Course

The course of a particular dementia is influenced by its etiology. Although historically the dementias have been considered progressive and irreversible, there is, in fact, significant variation in the course of individual dementias. The disorder can be progressive, static, or remitting. In addition to the etiology, factors that influence the course of the dementia include: the time span between the onset and the initiation of prescribed treatment; the degree of reversibility of the particular dementia; the presence of comorbid psychiatric disorders; and the level of psychosocial support.

The earlier distinction between "treatable" and "untreatable" dementias has been replaced by the concepts of "reversible," "irreversible," and "arrestable." Most reversible cases of dementia are associated with shorter duration of symptoms, mild cognitive impairment, and superimposed delirium. Specifically, the dementias caused by drugs, depression, and metabolic disorders are most likely to be reversible. Other conditions such as normal-pressure hydrocephalus, subdural hematoma, and tertiary syphilis are more commonly arrestable.

Although potentially reversible dementias should be aggressively investigated, in reality only 8% of dementias are partially reversible and about 3% fully reversible. There is some evidence to suggest that early treatment of demented patients, particularly those with Alzheimer type, with agents such as donepezil (which acts as an inhibitor of acetylcholinesterase) and galanthamine may slow the rate of progression of the dementia – although some investigators doubt the ability of these agents to slow the rate of progression.

17.2.4 Differential diagnosis

Memory impairment occurs in a variety of conditions including delirium, amnestic disorders, and depression. In delirium, the onset of altered memory is acute and the pattern typically fluctuates (waxing and waning) with increased proclivity for confusion during the night. Delirium is more likely to feature autonomic hyperactivity and alterations in level of consciousness. In some cases a dementia can have a superimposed delirium.

Patients with major depression often complain of lapses in memory and judgment, poor concentration, and seemingly diminished intellectual capacity. Often these symptoms are mistakenly diagnosed as dementia, especially in elderly populations. A thorough medical history and MSE focusing on symptoms of hopelessness, crying episodes, and unrealistic guilt in conjunction with a family history can be diagnostically beneficial.

The term *pseudodementia* has been used to denote cognitive impairment secondary to a psychiatric disorder, most commonly depression. In comparison with demented patients, those with depressive pseudodementia exhibit better insight regarding their cognitive dysfunction, are more likely to give "I don't know" answers and may exhibit neuro-vegetative signs of depression. Pharmacologic treatment of the depression should improve the cognitive dysfunction as well.

An amnestic disorder also presents with a significant memory deficit, but without the other associated features such as aphasia, agnosia, and apraxia. If cognitive impairment occurs only in the context of drug use, substance intoxication or substance withdrawal is the appropriate diagnosis. Although mental retardation implies below-average intellect and subsequent impairment in other areas of function, the onset is before 18 years of age and abnormalities of memory do not always occur. Mental retardation must be considered in the differential diagnosis of dementias of childhood and adolescence along with such disorders as Wilson's disease (hepatolenticular degeneration), lead intoxication, subacute sclerosing panencephalitis, HIV spectrum disorders, and substance abuse (particularly abuse of inhalants).

Patients with schizophrenia may also exhibit a variety of cognitive abnormalities, but this condition also has an early onset and a distinctive constellation of symptoms, and it does not result from a medical condition or the persisting effects of a substance.

Factitious disorder must be distinguished from dementia. Unlike dementia, this condition presents with inconsistent symptoms that, although similar in some respects, are not totally consistent with those of a dementia. For example, a patient with factitious disorder with psychological symptoms (in this case dementia) might have equal impairment in all phases of memory, while patients with dementia usually have better remote than recent memory.

Dementia must also be distinguished from benign senescence (normal aging). Only when such changes exceed the level of altered function to be expected for the patient's age is the diagnosis of dementia warranted.

17.3 Dementia due to alzheimer's disease

Alzheimer's disease is the most common cause of dementia, accounting for 55–65% of all cases. The etiology and pathogenesis of Alzheimer's disease are unknown.

17.3.1 Biological features

The brains of patients with Alzheimer's disease contain many senile plaques, neurofibrillary tangles, and Hirano's bodies. There is degeneration of nerve cells, but the significant atrophy seen on neurodiagnostic examination may be more the result of shrinkage of neurons and loss of dendritic spines than of actual neuronal loss. The atrophy is most apparent in the associational cortex areas, and early on the primary motor and sensory areas are relatively spared. Significant degenerative changes in neurons are seen in the hippocampus, locus ceruleus, and nucleus basalis of Mynert. With advancing disease these changes, in effect, separate the hippocampus from the remainder of the brain. Initially, the parietal and temporal regions are most affected by plaques and tangles, accounting for the memory impairment and syndromes sometimes associated with the parietal lobe and Alzheimer's disease (some apraxias, hemi-attention, anosognosia, Gerstmann's syndrome).

Neurofibrillary tangles do not correlate with the severity of the dementia; however, the concentration of neuritic plaques is directly associated with the severity of the disease. Neurochemically, the brains of patients with Alzheimer's disease exhibit significant cholinergic abnormalities. There is a profound decrease in acetylcholine in almost all patients, as well as decreased immunologic activity of somatostatin- and corticotropin-releasing factors. The enzyme required for ACh synthesis, choline acetyltransferase, is also greatly reduced. Other studies suggest involvement of noradrenergic and serotoninergic systems in later-onset disease and diminished gamma-aminobutyric acid. Specifically, the noradrenergic deficiencies seen in younger patients may be connected to changes in the locus ceruleus, and abnormalities of serotonin to effects on the raphe nuclei.

The role of genetic factors in the development of Alzheimer's disease has received increased attention as the role of the apolipoprotein E4 allele as a major genetic susceptibility risk factor has been confirmed by numerous studies.

Finally, several studies suggest that changes in membrane function, metabolism, and morphology are involved in the pathology of Alzheimer's disease. Nonetheless, the basic molecular defect responsible for the associated dementia has not been defined.

17.3.2 Clinical features

The course and clinical features of Alzheimer's disease parallel those discussed earlier in this chapter for the dementias in general.

17.3.3 Pharmacologic treatment

The two principles of management of Alzheimer's disease are to treat what is treatable without aggravating existing symptoms, and to support the caregivers who are also victims of this disease. Despite the significant decrease in ACh and choline acetyltransferase in Alzheimer's disease, treatments based on the cholinergic hypothesis have been unsuccessful.

Because vasopressin levels are slightly decreased in the hippocampus of patients with Alzheimer's disease, and somatostatin is adversely affected as well, attempts were made to replace these agents but with little effect. In the belief that improving blood flow might be of benefit, such agents as the metabolic enhancer and vasodilator ergoloid mesylates (hydergine, an ergot alkaloid) were tried. Hydergine did seem to have some benefit, but the effects may have been related to its mild antidepressant action. Onset of action of any beneficial effects of hydergine was quite long.

Despite lackluster effects of physostigmine, a second cholinesterase inhibitor had shown promise. Tetrahydroaminoacridine (tacrine) produced significant cognitive improvement in 16 of 17 patients with Alzheimer's disease in an early study. Subsequent studies have been less impressive, but significant improvement in a number of scales measuring cognitive performance illustrated the benefit of this agent for some patients (see Chapter 33). Donepezil and rivastigmine, inhibitors of acetylcholinesterase, have also been employed in an attempt to enhance cholinergic function by inhibiting its breakdown. These agents must be given early in the course of the dementia. Memantine can be used in patients with more advanced dementia and is often used in combination with donepezil. Donepezil has been approved for mild to moderate dementia, while memantine is approved for moderate to severe dementia. In those instances where improvement is not demonstrated after an adequate trial of donezepil, the addition of memantine has been beneficial for some patients. Many clinicians, when treating patients with severe dementia will start with donezepil and memantine simultaneously.

Depression is often associated with Alzheimer's disease. If antidepressant medication is to be used, low doses (about one-third to one-half of the usual initial dose) are advised, and only agents with minimal anticholinergic activity should be employed. An appropriate choice would be a selective serotonin-reuptake inhibitor such as paroxetine, fluoxetine, or sertraline, but even these have the potential to increase confusion. Agents such as trazodone and mirtazapine have occasionally been employed because of their sedating properties.

Anxiety and psychosis, particularly paranoid delusions, are common. Benzodiazepines can be disinhibiting in these patients and may exacerbate confusion, so they should be avoided if possible. If they are required, agents with a shorter duration of action (e.g., lorazepam, oxazepam) are preferred. Antipsychotic medications with high anticholinergic potential (thioridazine, chlorpromazine) may also affect memory adversely. While these agents have been favored in the past because of their tendency to produce sedation, second-generation antipsychotics have been reported to have lower incidences of neuroleptic-related side-effects. Haloperidol has less anticholinergic activity but has a greater tendency toward extrapyramidal effects. Some studies have associated the use of atypical antipsychotics to treat agitation and aggressiveness in Alzheimer patients, with a higher incidence of sudden deaths in rare cases. Therefore, these agents should be reserved in most cases for those demented patients with both agitation and psychosis. If they are used, cardiac parameters such as QTc interval length should be monitored, and the lowest possible effective dose should be employed. In such patients, where agitation (and not psychosis) is a major factor, the use of low-dose valproic acid has been helpful.

In summary, the psychopharmacologic management of Alzheimer's disease is designed to ameliorate cognitive deficits if possible, to control agitated, psychotic, and dangerous behavior, and to treat any underlying psychiatric disorder (e.g., major depression) that might be comorbid with dementia.

17.4 Vascular dementia

After Alzheimer's disease, this is the second most common form of dementia. Although its incidence is thought to be considerably less, some researchers suggest that it may be the most common dementia in men and in those aged 85 years of older.

Risk factors for vascular dementia parallel those for cerebrovascular accident and include hypertension, smoking, hyperlipidemia, atrial fibrillation, and diabetes. Computed tomography scan and magnetic resonance imaging often verify the brain disease in this particular dementia. Cognitive deficits arise from the multiple infarcts in the cortex and the white matter of the brain after the hemorrhage or ischemia inherent in a CVA. Historically, the patient experiences a more abrupt onset, and a stepwise or fluctuating pattern of progression rather than a steady and gradual deterioration. The patient exhibits focal neurologic signs. The specific symptomatology seen with this dementia depends on the sectors of the brain infarcted and the extent to which they are damaged. Frequently, there is accompanying neurologic evidence of cerebrovascular disease, such as paresis or paralysis of a limb or headaches. The patient with vascular dementia also will experience impaired memory aphasia, apraxia, agnosia, and difficulties with executive functioning. Mixed dementias of both vascular and Alzheimer's type are common.

17.5 Dementia due to Huntington's disease

Huntington's disease is a hereditary disorder associated with the development of dementia. It is an autosomal dominant trait. Unfortunately, this condition does not become apparent until age 35–45 years, usually after childbearing has occurred. Fifty percent of offspring are affected. There is also a juvenile form of the disease. Huntington's disease affects about 4 in 100 000 people, making it a significant cause of dementia in middle-aged adults.

The pathology of Huntington's disease involves selective destruction in the caudate and putamen. Men and women are affected equall. The course of the disease from onset to death is approximately 15 years. A genetic marker for Huntington's chorea makes presymptomatic and prenatal testing possible; however, the test is not always available. Moreover, when the test is available, it produces a high anxiety quotient for the at-risk person.

The person with Huntington's disease experiences chorea or involuntary, jerky, arrhythmic movements that intensify during times of stress (the illness was formerly referred to as Huntington's chorea). Clumsiness, muscle weakness, and gait disturbance are also present. The jerking movements usually peak 10 years after onset and then stabilize or decrease. This particular dementia causes no aphasia, agnosia, or apraxia, but memory deficits, slowed thinking, problems with sustained attention span, and deficiency in judgment occur. Cognitive symptoms often begin with mild emotional manifestations such as irritability and progress to anxiety and depression. As the frontal lobe begins to deteriorate, the person becomes labile, impulsive, easily frustrated, irritable, hostile, and aggressive. The illness becomes more relentless with time, and the affected patient often exhibits affective or intermittent explosive disorders.

17.6 Dementia due to Lewy-body disease

A dementia sometimes mistaken for Alzheimer's disease because of the clinical similarity, Lewy-body disease is characterized by earlier and more prominent visual hallucinations, parkinsonian features, and behavioral disturbances. The exact incidence is unknown. The presence of Lewy inclusion bodies in the cerebral cortex on autopsy confirms the diagnosis. A distinguishing characteristic is that patients have significant adverse effects when given antipsychotic drugs.

17.7 Dementia due to Pick's disease

Pick's disease is a rare form of progressive dementia clinically indistinguishable from Alzheimer's disease but is about one-fifth as common. Pick's disease occurs in middle adult life and has a duration that varies from 2 to 15 years. It has a strong familial tendency, but definite genetic pattern has not been established. ACh levels are reduced.

17.8 Dementia due to Parkinson's disease

Parkinson's disease is a neurodegenerative illness that progresses slowly and has no known cure. It is characterized by a decreasing number of brain cells in the substantia nigra, resulting in a depletion of the neurotransmitter, dopamine.

The clinical features of Parkinson's disease are well described, with the cardinal triad being tremor, rigidity, and bradykinesia. Associated features include postural instability, a festinating gait, micrographia, seborrhea, urinary changes, constipation, hypophonia, and an expressionless facial countenance. The tremor in Parkinson's disease has a regular rate and is most prominent when the patient is sitting with arms supported; it has therefore been described as "intention tremor." Paranoid delusions and visual hallucinations may occur, but auditory hallucinations are rare. Antipsychotics with low incidence of extrapyramidal symptoms are recommended (e.g., quetiapine).

The pharmacologic treatment of Parkinson's disease involves the use of a number of categories of medication. These include selegiline, a selective monoamine oxidase inhibitor, levodopa, other dopamine agonists, bromocriptine, pergolide mesylate, and various anticholinergic agents (e.g., benztropine). Selegiline should not be given to patients on antidepressant medication, and there is a risk that dopaminergic agents may produce/activate psychosis or mania and anticholinergic drugs may increase confusion.

Several researchers are looking into the possibility of using embryonic stem-cell implants as treatment for Parkinson's disease and several other conditions. Deep brain stimulation (DBS) is a surgical procedure used to treat Parkinson's disease in patients whose symptoms cannot be adequately controlled with medication. DBS uses a surgically implanted, battery-operated medical device called a neurostimulator to deliver electrical stimulation to targeted areas of the brain that control movement, blocking the abnormal nerve signals that cause tremor and other Parkinson's disease symptoms.

17.9 Dementia associated with Human Immunodeficiency Virus

This dementia is seen more frequently in a younger population than the other dementias because HIV is more prevalent in the younger population. Although HIV dementia is found in up to 75% of those with HIV, other causes of dementia such as infections, tumors, and adverse response to drugs need to be considered. Magnetic resonance imaging of the brain often reveals a type of pathologic change, and the patient usually manifests the other symptoms accompanying an incidence of AIDS. The clinician should be alert for mild cognitive decline or neurological symptoms such as headaches, vision changes, and neuropathies that might signal central nervous system involvement in the patient with AIDS.

The patient with HIV dementia has the typical dementia signs of memory loss, poor judgment, and decreased executive functions such as planning and reasoning. At times, patients have slowed motor movements. The progression of this dementia differs from other dementias that have a predictably steady mental deterioration. Some patients with HIV dementia have daily episodes of memory loss and confusion alternating with mental clarity. The dementia also can stabilize for months or even years before its downward progression resumes.

HIV dementia is best treated by identifying the associated medical condition, instituting appropriate therapy, and managing behavior in the interim.

17.10 Dementia associated with Creutzfeldt–Jakob disease

Creutzfeldt–Jakob disease is a rare condition that causes a cognitive disorder by targeting the central nervous system. With a worldwide incidence of about one new case per 1 million people per year, this rapidly progressive and ultimately fatal disease is caused by a protein-like agent called a prion. The disease generally affects people aged 65 years or older, with a life expectancy of 1 month to 6 years after onset and an average lifespan of 15 months.

The disease is thought to be spread through contact with contaminated human brain tissue, pituitary growth hormone, organ transplantation or from improperly sterilized neurosurgical tools. The ingestion of certain neurologic parts of cows that have been infected with a prion similar to the one of Creutzfeldt–Jakob disease has been implicated in its transmission (so called "mad cow disease"), as well as cannibalism.

The patient with Creutzfeldt–Jakob disease passes through three distinct stages. Initially, mental abnormalities progress into a rapidly deteriorating dementia. Later, a jerking, seizure-like activity appears. Many patients exhibit ataxia, dysarthria, and other cerebellar signs. Extrapyramidal signs, disruption in many of the senses, and seizures are other manifestations during the middle phase of this disease. The final phase is usually marked by coma, with the patient dying from infections and respiratory problems.

17.11 Dementia due to head trauma

Head trauma is the leading cause of brain injury for children and young adults. It is estimated that more than 7 million head injuries and 500 000 related hospital admissions occur in the US annually. Traumatic head injuries result in concussions, contusions, or open head injuries, and the physical examination often reveals such features as blood behind the tympanic membranes (Battle's sign), infraorbital ecchymosis, and pupillary abnormalities.

The psychiatric manifestations of an acute brain injury are generally classified as a delirium or amnestic disorder. However, head trauma-induced delirious states often merge into a chronic dementia. Episodes of repeated head trauma, as in dementia pugilistica (punchdrunk syndrome), can lead to permanent changes in cognition and thus are appropriately classified as demented states. The punchdrunk syndrome is seen in aging boxers and includes dysarthric speech, emotional lability, slowed thought, and impulsivity. A single head injury may result in a postconcussional syndrome with resultant memory impairment, alterations in mood and personality, hyperacusis, headaches, easy fatiguability, anxiety, belligerent behavior, and dizziness. Alcohol abuse, postural hypotension, and gait disturbances are often associated with head injuries that result in dementia.

17.12 Substance-induced persisting dementia

In instances in which the features of dementia result from central nervous system effects of a medication, toxin, or drug of abuse (including alcohol), the diagnosis of dementia due to the persisting effects of a substance should be made. The most common dementias in this category are those associated with alcohol abuse, accounting for about 10% of all dementias.

The diagnosis of alcohol-abuse dementia requires that the cognitive changes persist after the cessation of alcohol use and are not the result of changes in mentation associated with early abstinence, amnestic episodes (blackouts), or Wernicke–Korsakoff syndrome. In addition to various nutritional deficiencies and the toxic effects of alcohol itself, alcohol abusers are more prone to develop dementia as a result of head trauma and chronic hepatic encephalopathy.

Chronic alcohol abuse is the third leading cause of dementia. It affects a higher proportion of women than men, and alcohol-induced dementia is a relatively late occurrence, generally following 15–20 years of heavy drinking. Dementia is more common in individuals with alcoholism who are malnourished. The CT scan shows cortical atrophy and ventricular dilatation after about 10 years, with neuronal loss, pigmentary degeneration, and glial proliferation. The frontal lobes are the most affected, followed by parietal and temporal areas. The amount of deterioration is related to age, number of episodes of heavy drinking, and total amount of alcohol consumed over time.

Alcohol-induced dementia secondary to the toxic effects of alcohol develops insidiously and often presents initially with changes in personality. Increasing memory loss, worsening cognitive processing, and concrete thinking follow. The presence of a dementia due to alcohol abuse dictates an alcohol treatment program that is behavior-based, structured, supportive, and repetitive. Some medications such as acamprosate and naltrexone have been shown to decrease craving in alcoholics and may be of some benefit as part of an overall rehabilitation program.

Many other agents can produce dementia as a result of their persisting effects. Exposure to such heavy metals as mercury and bromide, chronic contact with various insecticides, and use of various classes of drugs of abuse may produce dementia. In particular, the abuse of organic solvents (inhalants) has been associated with neurological changes.

17.13 Dementia due to other general medical conditions

Normal-pressure hydrocephalus is generally considered the fifth leading cause of dementia after Alzheimer's, vascular, alcohol-related, and AIDS dementias. Long considered irreversible but often merely arrestable, normal-pressure hydrocephalus is a syndrome consisting of dementia, urinary incontinence, and gait apraxia. It results from subarachnoid hemorrhage, meningitis, or trauma that impedes cerebrospinal fluid absorption.

Unlike other dementias, the dementia caused by normal-pressure hydrocephalus has physical effects that often overshadow the mental effects. Psychomotor retardation, marked gait disturbances, and, in severe cases, complete incontinence of urine occur. The hydrocephalus can be relieved by insertion of a shunt into the lateral ventricle to drain CSF into the chest or abdominal cavity, where it is absorbed. Clinical improvement with shunting approaches 50% with a neurosurgical complication rate of 13–25%. Infection remains the most common complication.

Hepatolenticular degeneration (Wilson's disease) is an inherited autosomal recessive condition associated with dementia, hepatic dysfunction, and a movement disorder. Localized to chromosome 13, this disorder features copper deposits in the liver, brain, and cornea. Symptoms begin in adolescence to the early twenties, but cases are often seen in younger children. Wilson's disease should be considered along with Huntington's disease, HIV/AIDS dementia, substance-abuse dementia, head trauma, and subacute sclerosing panencephalitis in the differential diagnosis of dementia that presents in adolescence and early adulthood. Personality, mood, and thought disorders are common, and physical findings include a wing-beating tremor, rigidity, dystonia, and the pathognomonic Kayser–Fleischer ring around the cornea. Wilson's disease can mimic other conditions including Huntington's disease, Parkinson's disease, atypical psychosis, and neuroleptic-induced dystonia. Chelating agents such as penicillamine, if administered early, can reverse central nervous system and non-neurological findings in about 50% of cases.

In addition to the conditions mentioned above, *other medical illnesses* can be associated with dementia. These include endocrine disorders (hypothyroidism, hypoparathyroidism), chronic metabolic conditions (hypocalcemia, hypoglycemia), nutritional deficiencies (thiamine, niacin, vitamin B_{12}), structural lesions (brain tumors, subdural hematomas), and multiple sclerosis.

Dementia may have more than one cause in a particular patient. Certain types of dementia tend to occur together, including alcohol-induced persisting dementia and dementia caused by head trauma, vascular dementia, and dementia of the Alzheimer type, and alcohol-abuse dementia and a nutritional dementia.

17.14 Management of the dementias

Box 17.2 gives a summary of the management approach to dementias.

The ability of patients to care for themselves decreases as the severity of the cognitive order increases. The goals of care for people with dementia are to enhance function and prevent further decline. Preservation of function requires the nurse to encourage the patient to perform his or her own activities of daily living, rather than to do these tasks for the patient.

The healthcare team and the family caregivers need to continually re-evaluate the patient's ability to meet self-care needs. Caregivers can help by enhancing the patient's environment to facilitate his or her limited ability to perform activities of daily living and by fulfilling unmet patient needs themselves. Written daily reminders can be helpful in the performance of daily activities. Prominent clocks, calendars, and windows are important, and an effort should be made to minimize changes in the patient's daily activities. Repeated demonstrations of how to lock doors and windows and operate appliances are helpful, and arranging for rapid dialing of essential telephone numbers can be important. Maintaining adequate hydration, nutrition, exercise, and cleanliness is essential.

Family members must watch the gradual deterioration of the patient and accept that a significant part of their own lives must be devoted to the care of the individual. Difficult decisions about institutionalization and termination of life support are distinct possibilities, and the patients often turn their anger and paranoia toward the caregiver.

Education is a valuable treatment tool for families. Information about the disease and peer support is available through Alzheimer's associations, and many such agencies provide family members with a companion for the patient to allow the family some time away. Many studies suggest that the primary reason for institutionalization of these patients is the tremendous burden of care they pose for their families.

Aimless wandering seems to be a particularly disturbing behavior. Unfortunately, the unfamiliar surroundings of a nursing home often increase the patient's level of confusion and anxiety. For these reasons, family members are at risk for depression, anxiety syndromes, insomnia, and a variety of other psychological manifestations. When these occur, they should be promptly treated. In the United States, the National Alzheimer's Education and Referral Service can be accessed by calling 1-800-621-0379.

Box 17.2 Summary of the Management of Dementia.

- Identify and, if possible, correct the underlying cause.
- Manipulate the environment to reorient the patient.
- Intervene with the family by means of education, peer support, providing access to community organizations, discussing powers of attorney, living wills, and institutionalization if appropriate, and arranging therapy if indicated.
- Institute pharmacologic management of psychiatric symptoms and behavior.

Teaching families and ancillary caregivers about the behavior of people with dementia is important. For example, sometimes patients display aberrant behavior because of unmet needs. An underlying medical problem may have gone undetected, or they may be experiencing pain. As the ability to communicate decreases, the caregivers and the healthcare team may need to carefully observe the patient to try to discern the meaning behind the individual's actions. Problem behavior can be driven by something as basic as the discomfort of constipation. Problematic behavior may subside after a basic need has been met.

17.15 Amnestic disorders

Amnestic disorders include conditions characterized by *short-term memory loss*. The deterioration of memory is so great that it prevents patients from functioning at previous levels of social and occupational performance and seriously deters them from learning new information. Patients typically cannot recollect any events as recent as 2 minutes before. They may have some difficulty recalling events or knowledge that they formerly knew to be fact. The acuity of remote memory recall varies, and patients become adept at confabulation to hide memory deficits.

The brain damage that causes the condition is oriented as to person, but leaves the patient disoriented to time and place to some degree. Patients have a superficiality of emotions that precludes deep emotional ties with others. They frequently adopt an emotional blandness in their affect. The progression of the symptomatology depends on the underlying etiology and its severity. Like the dementias, the symptomatology shares a commonality; the etiology is the differentiating factor. The two most common reasons for amnestic disorders are alcohol abuse and head trauma.

Wernicke–Korsakoff syndrome, one of the substance-induced persisting amnestic disorders, has been known for years as Korsakoff syndrome. The two occur so frequently together that they present a classic picture and thus often are combined and referred to as the Wernicke–Korsakoff syndrome. By itself, Wernicke syndrome produces physical symptoms of ataxia, confusion, and paralysis of some of the motor muscles of the eye. Both syndromes are caused by the patient's compulsion for ingestion of alcohol, which supersedes the need for nutritional intake. Indeed, this syndrome usually is found in the 40- to 70-year-old patient with alcoholism and a history of steady and progressive alcohol intake. In time, this person develops a vitamin B_1 (thiamin) deficiency that directly interferes with the production of the brain's main nutrient, glucose, resulting in the symptomatology of this syndrome.

A patient with this disorder has great difficulty with recent memory, and specifically the ability to learn new information. Because of the inability to recall recent events, the individual fills in memory gaps with fabricated or imagined data (confabulation). This is truly a case of anterograde amnesia, and patients have no idea that there is not a memory defect.

The prognosis for an individual experiencing an amnestic disorder varies greatly. As with the other cognitive disorders, the etiology of an amnestic disorder determines the duration and the severity of the course of illness. In the case of the amnestic disorder "type" presented here (Wernicke–Korsakoff syndrome), the administration of the B vitamin, thiamin, can help alleviate some of the ataxic symptomatology. For the most part, however, the memory impairment remains. The primary goal in the amnestic disorders is to discover and treat the underlying cause.

Because some of these conditions are associated with serious psychological states (e.g., suicide attempts by hanging, carbon monoxide poisoning, deliberate motor vehicle accidents, self-inflicted gunshot wounds to the head), some form of psychiatric involvement is often necessary. In the hospital, continuous reorientation by means of verbal redirection, clocks, and calendars can allay the patient's fears. Supportive individual psychotherapy and family counseling are beneficial.

Clinical Vignette

Ms X, a 75-year-old woman, presented to the emergency room with complaints of memory loss and inability to "think straight." For the past month, she and her family had noted a marked change in her mental state that "seemed to happen overnight." She would forget the names of her grandchildren and showed little interest in activities she had previously enjoyed. Apparently, she had been hospitalized twice in the past for depression, but had never exhibited cognitive impairments. On the Mental Status Examination, she exhibited marked psychomotor retardation and a blunted affect. She was oriented only to person and all three spheres of memory were significantly impaired. In fact, she responded to most questions with a shrug of her shoulders and the comment "I don't know." As the interview continued she became more frustrated with her inability to perform, and asked the physician to "stop asking all these questions." She was hospitalized and a complete work-up was initiated.

The evaluation for dementia revealed negative results on drug and heavy-metal screening, the absence of any potentially offending medications, normal CT and MRI scans, and a normal EEG. Chemistry assays, hematology, thyroid functions, vitamin studies, serological tests for syphilis, chest radiography, and urinalysis were normal. Psychological testing revealed inconsistent cognitive deficits.

A psychiatric consultation was obtained, and it was recommended that a trial of psychostimulants be undertaken to rule out the possibility of depression as the cause of her cognitive impairment. The following day Ms X received methylphenidate 2.5 mg at 7 a.m. and 2.5 mg at noon before lunch. She tolerated the medication well, and her dose was increased to 7.5 mg on the second day. By the third day, she demonstrated improvement in her affect, concentration, and attention span, and in subsequent days her cognition improved significantly. Eventually, she had a complete recovery and the methylphenidate was discontinued after 2 months without relapse.

This case illustrates the difficulty in distinguishing dementia from cognitive impairment in depression. Features suggestive of depression included the relatively rapid onset, the patient's insight into the cognitive deficits, the presence of some vegetative signs of depression, absence of an identified medical condition judged to be responsible, pervasive yet inconsistent cognitive deficits, a past history of treatment for depression, and a positive response to a psychostimulant trial. The psychostimulant was chosen because the onset of action is faster than that of the other antidepressant agents. The principal problems encountered in treating a patient such as this are the tendency of physicians to underdiagnose depression in the elderly and the hesitancy of many caregivers to use psychostimulants for the treatment of depression.

KEY POINTS

- Cognitive disorders appear in the aging population as well as the general population.

- The possible etiologies of cognitive disorders include primary brain disease, systemic disturbances, influences of exogenous substances, and withdrawal and residual effects of exogenous substances.

- Aberrant behaviors associated with these disorders may include deficits in the sensorium, attention span, orientation, perception, and memory.

- Symptoms of cognitive disorders may be approached in terms of acute onset and chronic progression.

- Gathering and analyzing assessment data for a patient with a cognitive disorder requires participation of family members or friends who have been in close contact.

- Continuum of care involves the collaborative efforts of the entire interdisciplinary health-care team, including the family.

- Goal-setting for the client with an organic disorder focuses on eliminating the organic etiology, preventing acceleration of symptoms, and preserving dignity.

- Preserving optimal levels of functioning and preventing further decline are key goals. Psychosocial interventions strive to maintain the client's optimal physical health, structure the environment, promote socialization and independent functioning, and preserve the family unit.

Further Reading

Cohen-Mansfield, J. (2003) Non-pharmacologic interventions for psychotic symptoms in dementia. *Journal of Geriatric Psychiatry and Neurology*, **16** (4), 219–224.

Coon, D.W., Thompson, L., Steffan, A. *et al.* (2003) Anger and depression management: psychoeducation skill training interventions for women caregivers of a relative with dementia. *Gerontologist*, **43** (5), 678–689.

Hepburn, K.W., Lewis, M., and Sherman, C.W. (2003) The savvy caregiver program: developing and testing a transportable dementia family caregiver training program. *Gerontologist*, **43** (6), 908–915.

National Institute on Aging, Alzheimer's Disease Education and Referral Center (2003) *Alzheimer's Disease Genetics Fact Sheet* (NIH Publication 03-4012). US Government Printing Office.

National Institute of Neurological Disorders (2004) *The Dementias: Hope Through Research*. Available at: http://www.ninds.nih.gov/disorders/dementias/detail_dementia.htm.

18   Substance Use, Abuse, and Dependence

18.1 Introduction

This chapter discusses patients who abuse substances that affect the central nervous system (CNS). It examines systems of substance classification, concepts related to the etiology and dynamics of substance abuse and dependency, physical and behavioral changes that occur in people who abuse and become dependent on substances, and interdisciplinary treatment interventions.

These disorders are seen across many educational, treatment, and counseling settings. They are often, but not always, seen in conjunction with another major mental health problem. Problems occur on a spectrum from use to dependence, and it is important to understand the entire spectrum to properly diagnose, prevent progression of, and treat these disorders. The treatment of these disorders is a complex specialty area of mental health.

18.2 Terminology of substance abuse and dependence

Substance *abuse* is a maladaptive pattern of substance use leading to impairment, distress, and recurrent significant negative consequences. These adverse consequences can occur in medical, psychosocial, or legal domains. Individuals who abuse licit or illicit substances often engage in situations that are physically hazardous.

Substance *dependence* is the compulsive use of a substance, accompanied by tolerance and withdrawal. A diagnosis of substance dependence (once called "addiction") pre-empts a diagnosis of abuse, as tolerance, compulsive use and withdrawal are generally not present in substance abuse. In both instances, DSM specifies that the behaviors will have occurred in the past year. The major differences are outlined in Table 18.1. Since tolerance and withdrawal require a sustained period of use, and these manifestations of substance dependence may not typically begin until the individual is in the twenties or thirties. However, some older adolescents may meet the criteria for substance dependence by age 18.

Prolonged heavy ingestion of a substance results in *physical tolerance* and more of the drug is needed to achieve the desired effect. When physical tolerance develops, the person may experience withdrawal or an abstinence syndrome after cessation or a decrease in consumption.

All drugs of abuse and dependency share certain factors, while some factors are specific to each drug. The commonalities underlying these disorders is that the core problem is the abuse of, or dependency on, a substance, although the manifestations or functional disturbances resulting from the problem may differ. The words "addiction" and "dependence" are frequently confused. There is little consensus on what addiction actually means and it is not a DSM term. Addiction usually refers to a behavioral pattern of drug abuse characterized by overwhelming involvement with use of a drug

Fundamentals of Psychiatry, First Edition. Allan Tasman and Wanda K. Mohr.
© 2011 John Wiley & Sons, Ltd. Published 2011 by John Wiley & Sons, Ltd.

Table 18-1 Substance abuse versus substance dependence	
Abuse (1 out of 4 in past year)	**Dependence (3 out of 7 in past year)**
Recurrent use resulting in failure to fulfill major roles	Tolerance
Recurrent use in situations that are physically hazardous	Withdrawal
Recurrent substance-related legal problems	Substance taken in larger amounts and/or for a longer period than was intended
Continued use despite having persistent and social problems due to use	Unsuccessful attempts to cut down or control use
	Great deal of time spent in activities necessary to obtain substance or recover from its effects
	Important social, occupational, or recreational activities given up because of use
	Substance use continues despite knowledge that medical or psychological problems are due to use

(compulsive use) and with the securing of its supply, and by a high tendency to relapse after discontinuation. Addiction is often used when dependence is what is meant.

The use and abuse of substances happen in fads, but the most commonly abused substances include alcohol, opioids the stimulants, such as cocaine and the amphetamines, and the cannabinoids. Prescription sedative abuse and dependence have become problematic among psychiatric and other patients.

Owing to the sheer volume of material available on scores of drugs of abuse, this chapter will highlight those that are most commonly encountered in clinical practice. The remainder are presented in a table with their intoxication manifestations, health effects, and withdrawal symptoms.

18.3 Recreational use of substances

Recreational use of drugs and alcohol has become an increasingly part of Western culture. Only the use of tobacco and alcohol is endorsed legally, but (with some exceptions) recreational use of other substances is overlooked by authorities. Some users are apparently unharmed, using substances episodically and in small doses and avoiding toxicity and tolerance. Recreational drugs and substances are taken orally or inhaled, their use is often accompanied by rituals, and they are rarely ingested alone. It is important for the clinician to be aware of recreational drug and alcohol use and patterns in that such use can interfere with therapeutics and has the potential to turn into more serious use.

An estimated 20% of people in the United States have used prescription drugs for nonmedical reasons. This is called "prescription drug abuse" and is a growing problem. Prescription drugs that are abused or used for nonmedical reasons can lead to dependence. Commonly abused classes of prescription drugs include opioids, CNS depressants, and stimulants.

A study in 2007 showed that 2.7% of eighth-graders, 7.2% of tenth-graders, and 9.6% of twelfth-graders had abused hydrocodone, and 1.8% of eighth-graders, 3.9% of tenth-graders, and 5.2% of twelfth-graders had abused oxycodone, for nonmedical purposes at least once in the year prior to being surveyed.

18.4 Epidemiology

Approximately 22% of US adults have a substance abuse disorder. In 2008, an estimated 20.1 million of the population aged 12 years or older were current (past month) illicit drug users, meaning they had used an illicit drug during the month prior to the survey interview. This estimate represents 8.0% of the population aged 12 years or older. Illicit drug use is higher among males than females. Further statistics on substance abuse and dependence can be found on the SAMHSA website at http://www.oas.samhsa.gov/nhsda.htm.

18.5 Etiology of drug and alcohol dependence

Commonly used psychoactive drugs vary in their potential for creating dependence. Drug dependence develops in a way that is both complex and unclear. The process is influenced by the properties of the psychoactive drugs, genetic predispoisition, cultural and social settings.

Heritability or genetic vulnerability may be important in the development of drug and alcohol dependence. Epidemiological studies of twins suggest that, while both genetic and environmental factors play a role in twin concordance of drug use, concordance of abuse and dependence are more influenced by genetic factors. While no single gene has been definitively linked to any substance use disorder, certain alleles may play a role in their development and/or clinical manifestations.

Research has focused on the effects of illicit drugs on reward pathways in the brain. The most prevalent reward pathway involves several sequential parts of the brain: the ventral tegmental area, the nucleus accumbens, and the prefrontal cortex. When the brain perceives a pleasure stimulus, the neurotransmitter dopamine normally sends the stimulus along this pathway. Drugs of abuse interfere with this normal neurotransmission by binding themselves to dopamine receptors sites, thus replacing the normal effect of dopamine with the drug's effect. The result is the stimulation of receiving neurons by the substance, resulting in the initial mood-altering effect of the drug (depression or euphoria). With continued presence of the addictive drug, dopamine levels either drop or the pleasure pathway is destroyed, reducing normal neurotransmission of pleasure experiences. The physiologic dependence and addiction to a substance is characterized when the person experiences cravings for stimulation of the pleasure pathway, often leading to engagement in compulsive behavior to obtain the chemicals of stimulation. The craving for the stimulus eventually becomes stronger than the reward.

Environment and the presence and availability are also critical factors in the development of substance use. Experimentation can only occur when substances of abuse are accessible. The development of substance use and dependence disorders depends on a myriad of risk factors, which are listed in Table 18.2.

The "gateway" drug use hypothesis, in which experimentation with drugs evolves into more serious drug use, was described over three decades ago. The natural history of substance abuse and dependence typically follows a chronic relapsing pattern, although many youths experiment with drugs and never progress to dependence.

18.6 Comorbidity and dual diagnoses

One of the emerging issues from the Healthy People 2010 midcourse review was co-occurring mental health and substance abuse disorders and the outcomes resulting from this combination. About 50% of adults who have a diagnosable mental disorder will also have a substance abuse disorder at some point during their lifetime. Co-occurring disorders tend to be more chronic and disabling than either disorder alone. Individuals with co-occurring disorders are more likely to experience a chronic course or to require more services than people with either type of disorder alone.

The terms *comorbidity* and *dual diagnosis* describe a patient with coexisting substance abuse or dependency and a major psychiatric disorder. The disorders are unrelated and meet the DSM-IV-TR criteria.

Table 18-2 Risk factors for substance use disorders	
Genetic factors	Studies have found rates of substance dependence 3–4 times higher in identical twins than in dizygotic twins
Psychologic factors	High rates of depressive disorders and sensation seeking
Social and environmental factors	Peer and family influences
Biologic factors	Repeated exposure to the substance results in neural adaptation that perpetuates the dependence cycle

Reports estimate that dual diagnoses in chronically mentally ill patients range from 30% to 40% of outpatients and from 60% to 80% of inpatients. Traditional methods of treatment for major psychiatric disorders and substance dependency (i.e., substance dependency programs) have not been successful in treating patients with dual diagnoses. Ongoing research on the identification, treatment, and rehabilitation of patients with dual diagnoses is needed.

18.7 Alcohol use and dependence

18.7.1 Pharmacology and effects

Alcohol (ethanol) is a legal chemical having pharmacologic properties that produce mind- and mood-altering effects. It is a CNS depressant. Alcohol-containing beverages include beer, wine, and distilled spirits. In contrast to some other drugs that produce their effects from small quantities, alcohol usually requires large quantities used over a period of time to cause physical dependence.

As the dose of alcohol increases, a pattern of effects emerge: sedation, impaired mental and motor functioning, deepening stupor with a decrease in stimulation response (including painful stimulus response), coma, and eventually death from respiratory and circulatory collapse. The physical and behavioral manifestations of the effects of alcohol on the CNS are related directly to the level of alcohol in the blood and the concentration of alcohol in the brain. The blood's alcohol level is expressed as milligrams of alcohol per milliliter of blood (mg/mL). Alcohol concentration in the blood depends on the rate of absorption, transportation to the CNS, redistribution to other parts of the body, metabolism, and elimination. Alcohol is absorbed through the mouth, stomach, and small intestine. It is absorbed unchanged into the blood and circulates throughout the body, including the brain. It also crosses the placenta into fetal circulation. Intoxication occurs when the circulating alcohol interferes with the normal functioning of brain nerve cells.

The rate of absorption of alcohol into the blood varies and depends on the rate of ingestion, substances in the beverage (e.g., carbonation can increase absorption), food in the stomach, and the drinker's physical or emotional state.

Body size affects the concentration of alcohol in the blood. The same amount of alcohol ingested by a small person results in greater blood alcohol concentration than in a big person, because the latter has more blood volume in which the alcohol is diluted. A person's body chemistry and cultural influences also may alter the behavioral effects of alcohol.

Oxidation, which occurs mainly in the liver, eliminates 90% of the alcohol absorbed by the body. The other 10% is eliminated unchanged through body fluids such as breath, sweat, and urine. The rate of drinking may vary, but the excretion of alcohol from the body remains at a fixed rate. A healthy liver metabolizes about one ounce of alcohol per hour.

18.7.2 Tolerance

Alcohol-tolerant individuals may also be cross-tolerant to other CNS depressants. The drinking history of alcoholics often reveals the ability to increase tolerance and to maintain this increase for long periods. Frequently, an irreversible drop in tolerance follows this increased tolerance; the person becomes intoxicated with smaller amounts of alcohol.

18.7.3 Intoxication

Intoxication occurs after drinking excessive amounts of alcohol and is evidenced in maladaptive behavior such as fighting, impaired judgment, or interference with social or occupational functioning. Physiologic signs such as slurred speech, incoordination, unsteady gait, and flushed face may accompany intoxication. Psychologic signs may be observed, such as mood change, irritability, talkativeness, or impaired attention.

18.7.4 Abuse and dependence

Alcohol *abuse* refers to a maladaptive pattern of episodic drinking resulting in failure ot fulfill obligations, exposure to physically hazardous situations, legal problems or social and interpersonal problems without evidence of dependence. Alcohol *dependence* refers to frequent consumption of large amounts of alcohol over time, resulting in tolerance, physical and psychologic dependence, and withdrawal syndrome. People who abuse or who are dependent on alcohol often experience serious social consequences from their drinking. They can also experience serious medical and neurological conditions. These are briefly described below.

18.7.4.1 Alcoholic hallucinosis
Alcoholic hallucinosis usually occurs within 48 hours after cessation of, or a reduction in, drinking. Vivid, perhaps threatening, auditory hallucinations may develop, but clouding of consciousness does not occur.

18.7.4.2 Alcoholic amnestic disorder
The alcoholic amnestic disorder results from heavy, prolonged drinking and is thought to be related to poor nutrition. Amnesia consists of impairment in the ability to learn new information (short-term memory) and to recall remote information (long-term memory). Other neurologic signs, such as neuropathy, unsteady gait, or myopathy, may be present.

Amnestic disorders related to thiamine deficiency include Wernicke's encephalopathy, a mild to severe decrease in mental functioning characterized by ataxia, nystagmus, ophthalmoplegia, and mental status changes. These symptoms improve with thiamine replacement. Korsakoff's psychosis also results from thiamine deficiency and involves gait disturbance, short-term memory loss, disorientation, delirium, confabulation, and neuropathy. Korsakoff's psychosis is not reversed by thiamine replacement therapy. Wernicke–Korsakoff syndrome is the coexistence of Wernicke's encephalopathy and Korsakoff's psychosis.

18.7.4.3 Alcoholic dementia
Alcoholic dementia is associated with prolonged, chronic alcohol dependence. Signs of dementia include loss of intellectual ability that is severe enough to interfere with social or occupational functioning and impairment in memory, abstract thinking, and judgment. The degree of impairment may range from mild to severe.

18.7.5 Associated medical conditions

Heavy consumption of alcohol adversely affects most body systems. Gastrointestinal problems occur as a result of the irritating effects of alcohol on the GI tract, resulting in gastritis or gastric ulcers. Acute or chronic pancreatitis may occur. Esophagitis may result from the direct toxic effects of alcohol on the esophageal mucosa, increased acid production in the stomach, or frequent vomiting. Cardiovascular problems such as mild to moderate hypertension, cardiomyopathy, or arrhythmias result from the direct toxic effects of the substance and malnutrition.

The liver is highly susceptible to the damaging effects of alcohol because it is the primary organ that metabolizes the substance. Alcohol is toxic to the liver, regardless of the person's nutritional status. *Alcoholic hepatitis* is a serious condition involving inflammation and necrosis of the liver cells and sometimes is reversible. *Cirrhosis* of the liver, in which the liver cells are destroyed and replaced by scar tissue, is the most serious condition and is irreversible. A high risk of *cancer*, especially of the mouth, pharynx, larynx, esophagus, pancreas, stomach, and colon, is associated with alcoholism.

Hematopoietic complications include decreased white blood cell production, decreased granulocyte adherence, and thrombocytopenia, leading to compromised immune function. Nonspecific indicators of regular alcohol use include elevated levels of mean corpuscular volume, gammaglutamyltransferase, and carbohydrate-deficient transferrin. While other conditions such as nonalcoholic liver disease, hyperthyroidism, and use of anticonvulsants also can elevate the gammaglutamyltransferase level, this combination of findings should raise suspicion of regular alcohol consumption of 6–8 ounces a day.

18.7.6 Other complications of alcohol consumption

Among pregnant women aged 15–44, an estimated 10.6% reported current alcohol use, 4.5% reported binge-drinking, and 0.8% reported heavy drinking. This is a troubling statistic in that such activity can lead to *fetal alcohol syndrome*. FAS is a serious syndrome characterized by a group of congenital birth defects caused by chronic drinking while pregnant. These include prenatal and postnatal growth deficiency, facial malformations (small head circumference, flattened and elongated groove between nose and upper lip, flattened midface, sunken nasal bridge), CNS dysfunction, and varying degrees of major organ system malfunction. FAS is associated with poor academic performance and behavioral difficulties in children and it is the leading cause of mental retardation.

18.7.7 Alcohol withdrawal

Alcohol withdrawal, also referred to as "abstinence syndrome," occurs after a reduction in, or a cessation of, prolonged heavy drinking. Earliest signs of withdrawal include irritability and impatient behavior. A coarse tremor of hand, tongue, and eyelids may follow, as may nausea and vomiting, general malaise or weakness, autonomic nervous system hyperactivity (e.g., increased blood pressure and pulse), headache, paroxysmal sweats, anxiety, a depressed or irritable mood, and orthostatic hypotension. Sleep disturbances, insomnia, nightmares, or hallucinations also may occur during withdrawal. Alcohol withdrawal is often assessed using the Clinical Institute Withdrawal Assessment of Alcohol Scale – Revised (CIWA-AR).

Alcohol withdrawal delirium (delirium tremens, or DTs), is the most serious form of withdrawal syndrome. It occurs within 48 hours after cessation of, or reduction in, prolonged heavy drinking and can occur as long as 1 week after cessation of drinking. Symptoms involve increased agitation, confusion, anxiety, hallucinations, delusions, course tremors, fever, diaphoresis, increased heart rate, and precordial pain. Prompt and adequate sedation at the onset of withdrawal symptoms can prevent the occurrence of DTs.

18.7.8 Treatment for alcohol misuse

When a patient presents with acute intoxication, the clinician's priority is to stop any further ingestion that might lead to unconsciousness or death. The second priority is to maintain the person's safety (and the safety of others) by preventing him or her from engaging in any behavior that might result in injury or death to self or others. It should be noted that, if a patient is somnolent while intoxicated, he or she may become combative when the blood alcohol level (BAL) decreases.

In chronic use, treatment involved detoxification and medical evaluation for illnesses that might complicate withdrawal. Withdrawal symptoms should be identified and treated. Most patients can be detoxified from alcohol in 3–5 days. The withdrawal time frame should be considered in the context of when they will need the most support; for alcoholics, this is the second day after the last ingestion of alcohol. Other factors influencing the length of the detoxification period include the severity of the dependency and the person's overall heath status. Patients who are medically debilitated detoxify more slowly. Withdrawal should be carefully managed. Detoxification protocols have been developed through the Center for Substance Abuse Treatment (CSAT) as a Treatment Improvement Protocol (see suggested readings at the end of the chapter). Benzodiazepines are recommended as first-line agents for alcohol withdrawal. All of the benzodiazepines are equally efficacious in reducing withdrawal signs and symptoms.

The rehabilitation program usually involves detoxification, restoration of physical and emotional stability, intervention methods to increase motivation to continue in treatment, confronting pathologic defenses, facilitation of insight into problem areas, planning for discharge, and follow-up care.

18.8 Hypnotic or anxiolytic use or dependence

Most people do not find the subjective effects of sedative–hypnotics pleasant or appealing beyond their therapeutic effects (e.g., relief of anxiety or facilitation of sleep). Many sedative–hypnotic abusers have a subjectively different response. Addict's qualitative difference in subjective responses to medications is an important reason why medications that are safe and efficacious for non-addicts cannot be safely prescribed for addicts. In addition, addicts may take doses of medications above recommended dosages, take them by injection or means other than prescribed (e.g., dissolving tablets and injecting them, crushing tablets and snorting them), or take them in combination with other prescription medications or street drugs such as heroin or cocaine, that put them at risk for adverse consequences.

Most individuals with sedative–hypnotic dependence are patients whose dependence evolved during a course of medical treatment, drug abusers (including alcohol) who use sedative–hypnotics in addition to other drugs, or drug abusers who use sedative–hypnotics to self-medicate adverse effects of other drugs of abuse such as cocaine or methamphetamine.

18.8.1 Intoxication

Acute intoxication with sedative–hypnotics produces slurred speech, incoordination, ataxia, sustained nystagmus, impaired judgment, and mood lability. When taken in large amounts, they produce progressive respiratory depression and coma. The amount of respiratory depression produced by the benzodiazepines is much less than that produced by the barbiturates and other sedative–hypnotics.

18.8.2 Dependence

Sedative–hypnotics can produce tolerance and physiologic dependence. Physiologic dependence can be induced within several days with continuous infusion of anesthetic doses.

18.8.3 Withdrawal syndrome

The withdrawal syndrome arising from the discontinuation of short-acting sedative–hypnotics is similar to that from stopping or cutting down on the use of alcohol. Signs and symptoms include anxiety, tremors, nightmares, insomnia, anorexia, nausea, vomiting, postural hypotension, seizures, delirium, and hyperpyrexia. The syndrome is qualitatively similar for all sedative–hypnotics, but the time course of symptoms depends on the particular drug. With short-acting sedative–hypnotics, withdrawal symptoms typically begin 12–24 hours after the last dose and peak in intensity at between 24 and 72 hours.

With long-acting drugs, withdrawal signs and symptoms peak on the fifth to eighth day. During untreated sedative–hypnotic withdrawal, the EEG may show paroxysmal bursts of high-voltage, low-frequency activity that precedes the development of seizures. The withdrawal delirium may include confusion, visual and auditory hallucinations. The delirium generally follows a period of insomnia. Some patients may have only delirium, others have only seizures, and some may have both delirium and convulsions.

Benzodiazepines, may also produce a severe, protracted withdrawal syndrome, and withdrawal symptoms may be produced in some patients after cessation of long-term therapeutic dosing.

18.8.4 Treatment for sedative–hypnotic misuse

Once a diagnosis of dependence is manifested it is unlikely that a patient will be able to return to controlled, therapeutic use of sedative–hypnotics. All these substances, including alcohol, are cross-tolerant, and physical dependence and tolerance are quickly reestablished if a patient resumes use.

If after sedative–hypnotic withdrawal the patient has another primarily psychiatric disorder, such as generalized anxiety disorder (GAD), panic attacks, or insomnia, alternate treatment strategies other than sedative–hypnotics should be used if possible. Treatment of sedative–hypnotic dependence that has developed as a result of treatment of an underlying psychiatric disorder is usually a lengthy undertaking.

Three general strategies are used for withdrawing patients from sedative–hypnotics, including benzodiazepines. The first is to use decreasing doses of the agent of dependence. The second is to substitute phenobarbital or some other long-acting barbiturate for the addicting agent, and gradually withdraw the substitute medication. The third, used for patients with a dependence on both alcohol and a benzodiazepine, is to substitute a long-acting benzodiazepine, such as chlordiazepoxide, and taper it over 1–2 weeks.

The preferred withdrawal strategy depends on the particular benzodiazepine, the involvement of other drugs of dependence, and the clinical setting in which the detoxification program takes place. The gradual reduction of the benzodiazepine of dependence is used primarily in medical settings for dependence arising from treatment of an underlying condition. The patient must be cooperative, must be able to adhere to dosing regimens, and must not be abusing alcohol or other drugs.

18.9 Cocaine abuse and dependence

Cocaine is a CNS stimulant produced from the coca plant. Cocaine is consumed in several preparations. Cocaine hydrochloride powder is usually snorted through the nostrils, or it may be mixed in water and injected intravenously. Cocaine hydrochloride powder is also commonly heated (cooked up) with ammonia or baking soda and water to remove the hydrochloride, thus forming a gel-like substance that can be smoked (freebasing). "Crack" cocaine is a precooked form of cocaine alkaloid that became popular in the 1980s.

18.9.1 Cocaine abuse

Episodes of cocaine abuse may occur around paydays, days off from work or weekends, holidays or special occasions, and may be characterized by brief periods (hours to days) of high-dose binging use followed by longer periods of abstinence or unproblematic use.

18.9.2 Cocaine dependence

Cocaine dependence can develop quickly after initiation of use because of the potent euphoria produced by the drug. The route of administration is related to the development of cocaine dependence; smoked and intravenous routes are more highly correlated with dependence than the intranasal route of administration. Cocaine has a short half-life requiring frequent dosing to maintain the "high" (binge use). Individuals with cocaine dependence often spend large amounts of money for the drug and may be involved in illegal activities to obtain it. Binges may be separated by several days while the individual recovers or attempts to obtain more money for drug purchase. Illegal activities such as theft and prostitution are often engaged in to obtain cash for cocaine. Obligations such as employment and childcare are often neglected.

Tolerance to cocaine effects develops quickly, resulting in larger amounts of drug use with time. This is often associated with mental or physical complications of use including paranoia, aggressive behavior, anxiety and agitation, depression, and weight loss.

18.9.3 Intoxication

The clinical effects of cocaine intoxication are characterized initially by euphoria (referred to as a "high") and also include agitation, anxiety, irritability or affective lability, grandiosity, impaired judgment, increased psychomotor activity, hypervigilance or paranoia, and sometimes hallucinations (visual, auditory, or tactile) may occur. Physical symptoms that can accompany cocaine intoxication include hypertension, tachycardia, hyperthermia, mydriasis, nausea, vomiting, tremor, diaphoresis, chest pain, arrhythmia, confusion, seizures, dyskinetic movements, dystonia, and, in severe cases, coma. These effects are more frequently seen in high-dose binge users of cocaine. Cardiovascular effects are probably a result of sympathomimetic properties of cocaine (i.e., release of norepinephrine and blockade of norepinephrine reuptake).

18.9.4 Withdrawal syndrome

unease/dissatisfaction w/ life

Cocaine withdrawal develops within a few hours to a few days after stopping or reducing cocaine use that has been heavy and prolonged. The syndrome is characterized by dysphoria and two or more physiologic changes including fatigue, vivid and unpleasant dreams, insomnia or hypersomnia, hyperphagia, and psychomotor agitation or retardation. Anhedonia and craving for cocaine can be part of the withdrawal syndrome. Depression and suicidal ideation are the most serious complications and require individualized assessment and treatment. The syndrome may last up to several days but generally resolves without treatment.

18.9.5 Associated medical complications

Cardiac toxicity is one of the leading causes of morbidity and mortality associated with cocaine use. The risk of myocardial infarct is well established and is not related to dose, route, or frequency of administration. About one-half of patients with cocaine-related myocardial infarction have no evidence of atherosclerotic coronary artery disease.

Cocaine use is associated with a wide range of cardiac arrhythmias including sinus tachycardia, sinus bradycardia, supraventricular and ventricular tachycardia, ventricular premature contractions, ventricular tachycardia and fibrillation, torsades de pointes, and asystole. Several cases of cardiomyopathy and left ventricular hypertrophy attributed to cocaine use have been reported. The condition is often associated with chronic cocaine use and cocaine-related myocardial ischemia and infarction.

Intranasal abuse of cocaine has been associated with a number of medical complications including chronic sinusitis, septal perforation, subperiosteal abscess, pneumomediastinum, pneumothorax, and pulmonary edema. Cerebrovascular accidents related to cocaine use have been well documented. Cerebral infarct, subarachnoid hemorrhage, intraparenchymal hemorrhage, and intraventricular hemorrhage have been observed as acute complications of cocaine use.

Seizures may occur as a primary effect of cocaine owing to its ability to lower the seizure threshold or may be secondary to other CNS or cardiac events precipitated by cocaine use.

Recently, acute renal failure as a result of rhabdomyolysis has been recognized as an important complication of cocaine abuse. Pregnancy may increase the risk of rhabdomyolysis and renal failure. Renal failure may progress rapidly in the context of cocaine-induced rhabdomyolysis, and dialysis may be necessary for some patients.

18.9.6 Treatment for cocaine misuse

The majority of patients with cocaine-related disorders are most appropriately treated in an outpatient setting. Treatment may vary by provider but generally includes multiple weekly contacts for the initial months of treatment because less frequent contact is not effective in the initiation or maintenance of abstinence. These sessions consist of some combination of individual drug counseling, peer support groups, family or couples therapy, urine toxicology monitoring, education sessions, psychotherapy, and psychiatric treatment that may include pharmacotherapy for cocaine addiction and/or comorbid psychiatric disorders.

Inpatient treatment is reserved for those who have been refractory to outpatient treatment, whose compulsive use of cocaine represents an imminent danger (e.g., suicidality associated with cocaine toxicity or acute abstinence), who have other comorbid psychiatric or medical disorders complicating their treatment, or who are dependent on more than one substance and require monitored detoxification.

18.10 Amphetamine abuse and dependence

The illicit abuse of substances such as methamphetamine and of prescribed substances such as methylphenidate represent a growing health concern. While the major abused psychostimulant in the US is cocaine, this is not the case in several Western US cities, nor in the state of Hawaii. Worldwide abuse or regular use of amphetamines is more than double that of cocaine. Amphetamine-type stimulants (ATSs) include the phenylisopropylamines amphetamine (AMPH), methamphetamine (METH), and phenylpropanolamine (PPA), the natural substances ephedrine and pseudoephedrine, and phenylethylamines including methylphenidate and pemoline. While METH and AMPH cause the vast majority of abuse and dependence, use of any of these substances has been associated with abuse and dependence.

By far the most widely abused amphetamine-type substance is METH, which is commonly known as meth, speed, crank, CR, wire, and jib, and in its re-crystallized smoked form, ice, crystal, or glass. Legitimate forms of METH prescribed for attention-deficit hyperactivity disorder and weight control undoubtedly represent a miniscule source of the total amount abused each year.

AMPH, most prevalent in Western Europe, is commonly known as amp, bennies, dex, or black beauties, and is prescribed in the treatment of attention-deficit hyperactivity disorder, narcolepsy, weight control, and depression.

The socially acceptable and very desirable effects of prescribed ATSs – weight loss and productivity enhancement – make their widespread use, and thus the potential for abuse, unavoidable. Students and athletes appear particularly at risk for development of stimulant abuse, given that both exposure to licit and illicit sources and the pressures to use are high. Those whose jobs require sleep-cycle reversal, long hours and so on, such as truck drivers, also appear at high risk. Amphetamine-type substances are commonly injected or smoked by heavy users, or they may be snorted.

Designer amphetamines (analogues, the best-known of which is Ecstasy or 3,4-methylenedioxymethamphetamine, MDMA) are used recreationally with increasing popularity despite animal studies showing neurotoxic effects to serotonin (5-HT) and/or dopamine neurones. Ecstasy use leads to symptoms of classic amphetamine use. Users report a sense of feeling unusual closeness with other people and enhanced personal comfort. They describe seeing an increased luminescence of objects in the environment, although these hallucinogenic effects are less than those caused by other hallucinogens, such as LSD.

18.10.1 Intoxication

Acute amphetamine intoxication begins with a "high" feeling which may be followed by feelings of euphoria. The user experiences enhanced energy, becoming more outgoing and talkative, and more alert. Other symptoms include anxiety, tension, grandiosity, repetitive behavior, anger, fighting, and impaired judgment.

18.10.2 Amphetamine dependence

As with any addiction process, abuse and dependence are characterized by continued use in the face of negative consequences. These consequences may include physical and psychologic health, occupational functioning, legal problems, interpersonal relationships, and financial affairs. Amphetamine dependence occurs when an individual uses one or more of the amphetamine substances in a maladaptive way resulting in at least three of the following symptoms: a need for increased amounts of amphetamines to achieve the desired subjective effect (tolerance); the presence of withdrawal symptoms such as depression, fatigue, insomnia or hypersomnia, increased appetite, or agitation; using amphetamines in larger amounts or for longer duration; a persistent, unsuccessful attempt to control use of the substance; increased amount of time spent using or obtaining amphetamines; giving up important activities in deference to the use of amphetamines; and continued amphetamine use despite related physical, emotional, occupational, legal, or relational difficulties.

18.10.3 Withdrawal syndrome

ATS withdrawal states occur in some 87% of users. Following amphetamine intoxication, a "crash" occurs with symptoms of anxiety, shakiness, depressed mood, lethargy, fatigue, nightmares, headache, perspiring, muscle cramps, stomach cramps, and increased appetite. Withdrawal symptoms usually peak in 2–5 days and are gone within a week. The most serious withdrawal symptom is depression, possibly very severe and leading to suicidal thoughts. Resurgence of craving when exposed to drug-associated environmental cues probably persists for years, as is the case with other substance-dependence disorders. A protracted state of depression and low energy often persists for weeks. The occurrence of ATS withdrawal usually occurs in those who have progressed from the diagnosis of abuse to dependence.

18.10.4 Associated medical complications

For heavy users, a number of general consequences of ATS dependence include malnutrition and cachexia from sleep deprivation, exposure to the elements, and so on. Skin disorders, including infections and lesions from "picking" are common. More serious are ATS-related deaths due to cardiac arrhythmias, stroke, and rhabdomyolysis that have been documented since the 1950s. These problems were similar to those reported for cocaine (see earlier). ATS users are at high risk for contraction of HIV, and likely hepatitis B and C, secondary to sharing needles. Some of the medical complications can also result from exposure to contaminants during ATS use.

18.10.5 Treatment for amphetamine misuse

Management of acute intoxication is guided by the presenting medical and psychiatric symptoms. Anxiety and agitation are first treated by an environment that reduces stimulation and provides orientation, with staff providing reassurance and talk-downs. Physical restraints should be avoided as these may worsen rhabdomyolysis or hyperthermia. When nonpharmacological means are insufficient, benzodiazepines, typically lorazepam or diazepam, are first-line treatments since they protect against imminent seizures. Antipsychotics for agitation should be avoided because of the risk of worsening hyperthermia or rhabdomyolysis if neuroleptic malignant syndrome were to occur, and their ability to lower seizure threshold. However, since benzodiazepines run the risk of disinhibiting some individuals, typical antipsychotics, such as haloperidol, are often the preferred choice.

Emergency considerations in the withdrawal phase of ATS intoxication are principally psychiatric. Medical complications of ATS withdrawal, such as myalgias, involuntary motor movements and so on can be treated symptomatically and should spontaneously remit.

The use of antidepressants for 3–4 weeks following cessation of ATS use is suggested, because depression is a hallmark of ATS withdrawal. Often, allowing the individual increased time to sleep and re-establishment of normal nutrition is quite helpful. Where needed, the use of trazodone for sleep or short-term benzodiazepines for anxiety is needed along with antidepressant therapy.

Cognitive–behavioral therapy forms the basis of many treatments for psychostimulant dependence. Contingency incentives, skills training, and family member participation are helpful for maintaining abstinence. The community-reinforcement-plus-vouchers approach is described in the Treatment Improvement Protocol Series (TIPS) (see http://csat.samhsa.gov/faqs.aspx). This approach combines couples counseling, vocational training and skills training, and contingency management through rewards for negative urine testing. This combined approach for treatment of cocaine dependence is shown to improve treatment retention and decrease drug use.. Further, the approach has been manualized to improve consistency among clinicians (see Budney and Higgins in the further reading section).

18.11 Opioid abuse and dependence

In the US there has been a marked increase in prescription opioid abuse and dependence such that it now has surpassed heroin. For example, the US National Survey on Drug Use and Health found in

2005 that abuse or dependence on unprescribed pain relievers was almost seven times more prevalent among persons aged 12 years or older than abuse and dependence on heroin. The overall number of persons meeting criteria for abuse or dependence on pain relievers was estimated at 1.55 million, compared with 227 000 abusing or dependent on heroin.

Oxycodone and hydrocodone products have traditionally been the main prescription opioids of abuse. Much attention has focused on Oxycontin R, a long-acting formulation of oxycodone that contains doses up to 80 mg per tablet. Though the slow absorption of this medication is unlikely to result in abuse when taken as prescribed, substance abusers have discovered that the tablets can be crushed, freeing much of the oxycodone that can then be inhaled or injected to produce a potent euphoria.

Opioid-related disorders, as in the case of other substance-related disorders, are felt to arise from a variety of social, psychologic, and biologic factors. Among those identified as especially important are opioid use within the individual's immediate social environment and peer group, availability of opioids, a history of childhood conduct disorder or adult antisocial personality disorder, and a family history of one or more substance-use disorders. The families of persons with opioid dependence are likely to have higher levels of psychopathology, especially an increased incidence of alcohol and drug-use disorders, and antisocial personality disorder. These findings suggest that there is a genetic susceptibility. The exact mechanism or mix of factors that produce opioid dependence or abuse are unknown, as are the factors that contribute to the chronic relapsing pattern that is typically seen in many of these patients.

18.11.1 Intoxication

Opioid intoxication is characterized by maladaptive and clinically significant behavioral changes developing within minutes to a few hours. Symptoms include an initial euphoria sometimes followed by dysphoria or apathy. Psychomotor retardation or agitation, impaired judgment, and impaired social or occupational functioning are commonly seen. Intoxication is accompanied by papillary constriction unless there has been a severe overdose with consequent anoxia and pupillary dilatation. Individuals with intoxication are often drowsy (described as being "on the nod") or even obtunded, have slurred speech, impaired memory, and demonstrate inattention to the environment to the point of ignoring potentially harmful events. Dryness of secretions in the mouth and nose, slowing of gastrointestinal activity, and constipation are associated with both acute and chronic opioid use. Visual acuity may be impaired as a result of pupillary constriction. The magnitude of the behavioral and physiologic changes depends on the dose as well as individual characteristics of the user, such as rate of absorption, chronicity of use, and tolerance.

Symptoms of intoxication usually last for several hours, but are dependent on the half-life of the particular opioid that has been used. Severe intoxication following an opioid overdose can lead to coma, respiratory depression, pupillary dilatation, unconsciousness, and death.

18.11.2 Opioid abuse

Opioid abuse is a maladaptive pattern of intermittent use in hazardous situations (driving under the influence, being intoxicated while using heavy machinery, working in dangerous places, and so on), or periodic use resulting in adverse social, legal, or interpersonal problems. All of these signs and symptoms can also be seen in people who are dependent; abuse is characterized by less regular use than dependence (i.e., compulsive use not present) and by the absence of significant tolerance or withdrawal. As with other substance use disorders, opioid abuse and dependence are hierarchical and thus people diagnosed as having opioid abuse must never have met criteria for opioid dependence

18.11.3 Opiod dependence

Opioid dependence is diagnosed by the signs and symptoms associated with compulsive, prolonged self-administration of opioids that are used for no legitimate medical purpose; or, if a medical condition exists that requires opioid treatment, are used in doses that greatly exceed the amount needed for pain relief. Persons with opioid dependence typically demonstrate continued use in spite of adverse physical, behavioral, and psychologic consequences. Almost all individuals meeting criteria for opioid dependence have significant levels of tolerance and will experience withdrawal upon abrupt discontinuation of opioid drugs. Those with opioid dependence tend to develop such regular patterns of compulsive use that daily activities are typically planned around obtaining and administering drugs.

Opioids are usually purchased on the illicit market, but they can also be obtained by forging prescriptions, faking or exaggerating medical problems, or by receiving simultaneous prescriptions from several physicians. Physicians and other healthcare professionals who are dependent will often obtain opioids by writing prescriptions or by diverting opioids that have been prescribed for patients.

18.11.4 Course and natural history of dependence

Opioid dependence can begin at any age, but problems associated with opioid use are most commonly first observed in the late teens or early 20s. Once dependence occurs it is usually continuous over a period of many years even though periods of abstinence are frequent. Reoccurrence is common even after many years of forced abstinence, such as occurs during incarceration. Increasing age appears to be associated with a decrease in prevalence. This tendency for dependence to remit generally begins after age 40 and has been called "maturing out." However, others remain opioid dependent into their fifties and beyond. Thus, though spontaneous remission can and does occur, most cases of untreated opioid dependence follow a chronic, relapsing course for many years.

18.11.5 Withdrawal syndrome

Opioid withdrawal is a clinically significant, maladaptive behavioral and physiological syndrome associated with cessation or reduction of opioid use that has been heavy and prolonged. It can also be precipitated by administration of an opioid antagonist such as naloxone or naltrexone.

Patients in opioid withdrawal typically demonstrate a pattern of signs and symptoms that are opposite the acute agonist effects. The first of these are subjective and consist of complaints of anxiety, restlessness, and an "achy feeling" that is often located in the back and legs. These symptoms are accompanied by a craving to obtain opioids, drug-seeking behavior, along with irritability and increased sensitivity to pain. Additionally, patients typically demonstrate three or more of the following: dysphoric or depressed mood; nausea or vomiting; diarrhea; muscle aches; lacrimation or rhinorrhea; increased sweating; yawning; fever; insomnia; pupillary dilatation; fever; and piloerection. Piloerection and withdrawal-related fever are rarely seen in clinical settings (other than prison) as they are signs of advanced withdrawal in persons with a very significant degree of physiologic dependence; opioid-dependent persons with "habits" of that magnitude usually manage to obtain drugs before withdrawal becomes so far advanced.

For short-acting drugs such as heroin, withdrawal symptoms occur within 6–24 hours after the last dose in most dependent individuals, peak within 1–3 days, and gradually subside over a period of 5–7 days. Symptoms may take 2–4 days to emerge in the case of longer-acting drugs such as methadone. Less acute withdrawal symptoms are sometimes present and can last for weeks to months. These more persistent symptoms can include anxiety, dysphoria, anhedonia, insomnia, and drug craving.

Table 18-3 Commonly abused substances

Category	Example	Effects of Intoxication	Health Consequences	Withdrawal Symptoms
Cannabinoids	Marijuana Hashish	Euphoria, slowed thinking and reaction time, confusion, impaired balance and coordination	Cough, respiratory infections, impaired memory and concentration, tolerance, dependence	Appear within 24 hours with pronounced symptoms for the first 10 days Include irritability, anxiety, physical tension, decreased appetite and mood
Dissociative anesthetics	Ketamine	Increased heart rate and blood pressure Impaired motor function	Memory loss	Mental instability
	PCP and analogs	Decrease in blood pressure and heart rate, panic, aggression and violence	Delirium at high doses, depression Loss of appetite, depression	Mental instability
Hallucinogens	LSD Mescaline Psilocybin	Altered states of perception and feeling, increased body temperature, blood pressure and heart rate, tremors, numbness, weakness, nervousness, paranoia	Persisting perception disorder (flashbacks)	Psychotic-like episodes persisting long after use
Inhalants	Solvents Gases Nitrites	Stimulation, loss of inhibition, headache, slurred speech, loss of motor coordination	Wheezing, memory impairment, depression, damage to cardio-vascular systems, sudden death	Mild withdrawal syndrome
Opioids	Codeine Heroin Morphine Fentanyl (and derivatives) Oxycodone Hydrocodone	Euphoria, sedation, relief of pain, staggering gait	Nausea, constipation, respiratory depression, tolerance, addiction, coma death	Runny nose, twitching, diaphoresis, nausea and vomiting, high blood pressure, fever, muscle aches, stomach cramps, insomnia, weakness Symptoms pass within a few days (5–7) but cravings may persist and it may take many months to feel "normal"
Anabolic steroids	–	No intoxication effects	Hypertension, blood clotting and cholesterol changes, reduced sperm production, shrunken testicles, breast enlargement; in females and development of masculine characteristics	Mood swings, insomnia, fatigue, loss of appetite, depression, suicide attempts
Dextromethorphan	–	Dissociative effects, distorted visual perceptions	Similar to dissociative anesthetics at high doses	As for anabolic steroids

18.11.6 Treatment for opioid misuse

There are currently a number of effective pharmacologic and behavioral therapies for the treatment of opioid dependence, with these two approaches often combined to optimize outcome. There are also some newer options, which may take various forms. For example, methadone maintenance is an established treatment, while the use of buprenorphine and buprenorphine/naloxone in a clinic-based setting represents a relatively new variation on that theme. Clonidine has been used extensively to treat opioid withdrawal while lofexidine is a structural analog that appears to have fewer hypotensive and sedating effects. The depot dosage form of naltrexone, available in the US currently for the treatment of alcohol dependence and under development for opioid dependence treatment, may increase compliance with a medication that is a highly effective opioid antagonist but which has been underutilized because of poor acceptance by patients. In almost every treatment episode using pharmacotherapy, it is combined with some type of psychosocial or behavioral treatment.

18.12 Other substances of abuse and dependence

Owing to the sheer number of potential substances that can result in abuse or dependence, this chapter has discussed only those most commonly encountered by clinicians. Table 18.3 provides an overview of some other drugs of abuse, the effects of intoxication, health consequences, and withdrawal symptoms. Readers are encouraged to avail themselves of the websites and readings suggested at the end of the chapter for further study.

Clinical Vignette 1

Mr A first sought psychiatric help at the age of 19 years. During his first year of college he had a difficult adjustment. He had never had close friends, but at school he felt isolated from his family. Although he had always been a good student, averaging As and Bs in high school, he was unable to achieve the same level of academic performance. He became increasingly distressed by his sense of isolation and his inability to maintain an adequate grade point average. Around the middle of his first year of college he saw a psychiatrist, who thought he was having an adjustment reaction to his new surroundings. He was not given medication at the time but was referred for supportive psychotherapy. After two appointments with his therapist, he decided it was not helpful.

Shortly thereafter, he began to feel that the other students were staring at him and laughing at him behind his back. Then he began to feel as if they were playing tricks on him, sending secret messages to him over the radio to torment him. This experience lasted over 6 months. He also began hearing two voices, which he did not recognize. These voices would comment on his behavior and criticize his actions. They began to tell him to stay out of his dormitory room at night. The voices also warned him that the dormitory food was poisoned. One night, he was picked up by police for loitering and was brought to an emergency department.

The emergency department psychiatrist saw him as a disheveled, unshaven man who was agitated during the interview, pacing across the examining room. He was wearing dark sunglasses, although it was the middle of the night, and he said he did not want the examiner to read his mind by looking into his eyes, so he kept the sunglasses on throughout the interview. His speech was of normal rate and prosody, although there were long pauses in some of his responses. He was able to respond to questions clearly, and his thought processes were logical, although he repeatedly spoke angrily as if responding to voices. He did say that the voices had been telling him to kill himself for the past two nights, although he said he was trying not to listen to them. The patient showed only some difficulty in concentration on a cognitive examination. His judgment was fair in that he recognized his need for some help, but he showed no insight into his symptoms.

The psychiatrist felt that the patient was potentially a risk of harm to himself because of the command auditory hallucinations and required hospitalization. Mr A did not agree to come into the hospital, and the psychiatrist sought involuntary hospitalization through appropriate procedures. In the hospital, the patient was initially quite agitated, requiring intramuscular haloperidol and lorazepam. Almost immediately his behavior calmed, and he was able to agree to hospitalization and treatment. He was treated with risperidone, and the dose was titrated up to 3 mg/day by mouth at bedtime. After 1 week with this medication regimen, he began to experience a decrease in his auditory hallucinations and paranoid ideation. He was sleeping better and was no longer concerned about the foods he was eating.

Clinical Vignette 2

Mr Z, a 42-year-old male, presented for treatment of opioid dependence; this was his sixth episode of methadone maintenance. He had a long history of alcoholism that interfered with treatment in the past and had begun using cocaine regularly.

Mr Z had done fairly well in the past on methadone as far as illicit opioid use was concerned, but clinic attendance and his ability to comply with clinic rules, especially regarding take-home doses, had been severely compromised by alcohol abuse. He would typically remain in treatment for about a year, then become angry over his inability to obtain take-home doses due to ongoing positive breathalyzer readings, and drop-out of treatment; relapse to opioid use always immediately followed. During previous treatment episodes, he had frequently been offered inpatient detoxification for alcoholism but always refused because "alcohol was not his problem, heroin was the problem," and he could not take time off work.

When Mr Z presented for treatment this time, he had severe social stressors. He was unemployed (secondary to his alcohol problems) and living with his parents, who were threatening to put him out because of drug use. He was told that, this time, methadone would not be offered unless he first entered the hospital. After some discussion he agreed that as part of his treatment plan he would first enter the hospital for 21–28 days of treatment including alcohol detoxification and stabilization on methadone and then be discharged to maintenance therapy.

This approach worked. After inpatient discharge, the patient kept regular counseling appointments, continued to attend self-help meetings to which he had been introduced while on the inpatient unit, "requested" daily breathalyzer testing, and turned down an offer to return to his job in the liquor store. Over the following three years his liver function tests returned to normal levels. He was stable on 65 mg of methadone per day with urine tests negative for opioids, although occasionally his urine was positive for cocaine.

Clinical Vignette 3

Mrs W, a 33-year-old woman, was referred by her internist for treatment of alcohol dependence after an overdose of alprazolam (Xanax) and alcohol. She had ingested about 30 tablets of alprazolam 2 mg and a bottle of wine after an argument with her husband. She and her husband were in the process of an acrimonious separation, and during the 3 months before her hospitalization she had increased her alcohol consumption from one or two glasses of wine with the evening meal to 1.5 bottles of wine each night.

Mrs W stated that she had wanted to die and that she had heard that the combination of alprazolam and alcohol was lethal. She had not previously made a suicide attempt. However, she was under the ongoing care of a psychiatrist because of panic attacks. A previous psychiatrist had started the patient with alprazolam about 6 years before the overdose. Before treatment with alprazolam, her panic attacks had become disabling. While she was taking 4 mg/day of alprazolam, the panic attacks became infrequent, and much attenuated in intensity. She had resumed employment as a travel agent. As her alcohol use increased, the frequency and intensity of her panic attacks increased. Until the overdose, she took alprazolam exactly as prescribed, 2 mg twice a day at the same time each day. Her psychiatrist verified that her refills were consistent with her history.

Mrs W was frightened by having overdosed and acknowledged that her alcohol use was excessive and that she needed treatment. However, she did not want to discontinue alprazolam because she feared worsening of the panic attacks.

Mrs W presented a challenging clinical situation, often referred to in the chemical dependence treatment field as "dual diagnosis: a major psychiatric disorder and chemical dependence." Alcohol and drug treatment programs generally want patients to discontinue all mood-altering medications, particularly those with abuse potential, when they enter treatment. Chemical dependence treatment staffs often observe that alcohol-abusing patients increase their use of prescription medication when they stop drinking.

Because Mrs W's panic attacks had been disabling, and because the alcohol abuse seemed a response to an acute situational stress, the patient began outpatient chemical dependence treatment, four nights per week. She and her husband began couples therapy, and Mrs W increased the frequency of visits with her psychiatrist. With the increased support, she completed the separation from her husband, remained abstinent from alcohol, and remained on a carefully monitored dose of alprazolam.

KEY POINTS

- Substance abuse occurs when a person uses alcohol or other drugs repeatedly to the extent that functional problems occur. However, it does not include compulsive use or addiction.

- Substance dependency is diagnosed when the individual continues using alcohol or other drugs in spite of negative consequences such as significant functional problems in daily living. An individual with dependency is likely to experience tolerance as the use of the substance escalates, and a withdrawal syndrome when the drug of abuse is stopped.

- Substance abuse disorders can be classified into 12 categories of substances: alcohol, amphetamines, caffeine, cannabis, cocaine, hallucinogens, inhalants, nicotine, opioids, phencyclidines, sedative–hypnotics, and polysubstance abuse.

- All of the disorders may be associated with any of the four common subdiagnoses of dependence, abuse, intoxication, and withdrawal.

- Substance abuse disorders are multidimensional and related strongly to neurophysiologic processes as well as to psychosocial and behavioral processes.

- People with drug or alcohol dependence or abuse are impaired in multiple areas (physically, socially, and psychologically) at some time during their disorder.

- Signs and symptoms of abuse and dependence are specific to which drug is being used. However, functional impairment in several areas is a requisite for diagnosis.

- Many patients have coexistence of a substance abuse disorder and a major psychiatric disorder (comorbidity).

- Interdisciplinary treatment includes detoxification programs and facilities, inpatient rehabilitation, outpatient programs, and private practice physician treatment. There is a wide network of 12-step treatment programs throughout the world, led by lay people and paraprofessionals.

This chapter contains material from the following chapters in *Psychiatry, Third Edition*: Chapter 53 (Thomas R. Kosten); Chapter 54 (Thomas F. Babor, Carlos A. Hernandez-Avila, Jane A. Ungemack); Chapter 55 (Kevin A. Sevarino); Chapter 57 (Benjamin R. Nordstrom, Frances R. Levin); Chapter 58 (Jennifer R. Baker, Charles Y. Jin, Elinore F. McCance-Katz); Chapter 60 (Rif S. El-Mallakh, John H. Halpern, Henry D. Abraham); Chapter 61 (Charles W. Sharp, Neil Rosenberg, Fred Beauvais); and Chapter 63 (George E. Woody, Paul J. Fudala).

Further Reading

Budney, A.J. and Higgins, S.T. (1998) A community reinforcement plus vouchers approach: treating cocaine addiction. Therapy Manuals for Drug Addiction, Manual 2, DHHS Publication (ADM) 98-4309, National Institute on Drug Abuse, Rockville, MD. Available at: http://165.112.78.61/TXManuals/CRA/CRA1.html.

Kandel, D. (2002) *Stages and Pathways of Drug Involvement: Examining the Gateway Hypothesis*, Cambridge University Press, Cambridge, UK.

National Institute on Drug Abuse (NIDA): http://www.nida.nih.gov.

Reis, R.K. (2009) *Principles of Addiction Medicine*, 4th edn, Lippincott, Williams & Wilkins, Philadelphia, PA.

University of Michigan: *Monitoring the Future*. Available at: http://www.monitoringthefuture.org/.

NIDA Research Report (2002) Methamphetamine Abuse and Addiction, NIH Publication 02-4210, printed April 1998, reprinted January 2002.

19 ● Personality Disorders

19.1 Introduction

Personality traits have long been the focus of considerable scientific research. Their heritability, childhood antecedents, temporal stability, universality and functional relevance to work, well-being, marital stability, and even physical health have been well established across many studies. Every human has a personality or a characteristic manner of thinking, feeling, behaving, and relating to others, and each person has a constellation of traits that makes him or her unique. When these traits become inflexible or maladaptive and are the cause of functional impairment or subjective distress, they comprise personality disorders. This chapter outlines what is known about the personality disorders delineated in DSM-IV-TR, their etiologies and approaches to treatment.

Personality disorders are a collection of personality traits that have become fixed and rigid to the point that the person experiences inner distress and behavioral dysfunction. They are lifelong patterns of behavior that adversely affect many areas of the person's life and functioning and are not produced by another disorder or illness. "Personality disorder" is the only class of mental disorders in DSM-IV-TR for which an explicit definition and criterion set are provided.

DSM defines a personallity disorder as "an enduring pattern of inner experience and behavior that deviates markedly from the expectations of the individual's culture, is pervasive and inflexible, has an onset in adolescence or early adulthood, is stable over time, and leads to distress or impairment."

Personality disorders are considered serious psychiatric conditions because of their associated symptoms. Their seriousness is underscored by the fact that they increase the risk of developing comorbid psychiatric disorders such as major depression, anxiety disorder, and substance abuse.

19.2 The categorical–dimensional debate

In DSM-IV-TR, personality disorders are polythetic categories that have defined criteria and for which a certain number must be present to meet the diagnostic threshold. They are defined within a categorical, hierarchical taxonomic system, clustering into three groupings that are based on severity. The categorical approach is practical insofar as it is relatively easy to use for purposes of communication and conceptualization. Much information can be conveyed using a single diagnostic label regarding features, associated conditions, and possible treatment options.

Unfortunately, there are a number of serious problems with the categorical system of personality disorder diagnosis presented in DSM-IV-TR. Personality disorder categories are quite heterogeneous with regard to symptoms and traits (e.g., there are 256 combinations of symptoms that can result in the diagnosis of borderline personality disorder), comorbidity among personality disorder diagnoses is common, and diagnoses do not appear to be very stable over time. Hence, the idea that

Fundamentals of Psychiatry, First Edition. Allan Tasman and Wanda K. Mohr.
© 2011 John Wiley & Sons, Ltd. Published 2011 by John Wiley & Sons, Ltd.
This chapter is based on Chapter 82 (Thomas A. Widiger, Stephanie N. Mullins-Sweatt) of *Psychiatry, Third Edition*

personality disorders represent distinct diagnostic entities may not be valid and their categorical classification may not be optimal.

An alternative to representing personality pathology and disorder categorically is a *dimensional model* of classification. Dimensional models provide more reliable scores (e.g., across raters and across time); help to explain symptom heterogeneity and the lack of clear boundaries between categorical diagnoses through the lens of underlying personality traits or dimensions; retain important information about sub-threshold traits and symptoms that may be of clinical interest; and allow for integration of scientific findings concerning the distribution of personality traits and associated maladaptivity into a classification system.

It is possible that a dimensional model of personality disorders will be adopted in future editions of DSM. However, much work will need to be done before the dimensional model is accepted by researchers who study these disorders and clinicians who treat them. Barriers that must be overcome include the perception that dimensional models are more cumbersome and less user-friendly than the cleanly delineated categorical ones. A second concern is determining how appropriate cutoffs would be established for distress or maladaptation and impairment, such that pathology can be established and treated. A final practical issue that must be addressed is that of insurance coverage: third-party payers are not likely to reimburse for treatment unless they know concretely what they are funding and how interventions are tied to diagnosis.

19.3 Epidemiology

Information is limited about the incidence and prevalence of personality disorders because people with them often do not seek help from professionals. Estimates of their prevalence within clinical settings are typically above 50%. As many as 60% of inpatients within some clinical settings would be diagnosed with borderline personality disorder (BPD), and as many as 50% of inmates within a correctional setting could be diagnosed with antisocial personality disorder (ASPD). Although the comorbid presence of a personality disorder is likely to have an important impact on the course and treatment of an Axis I disorder, the prevalence of personality disorder is generally underestimated in clinical practice, due in part to the failure to provide systematic or comprehensive assessments of personality disorder symptomatology and perhaps as well to the lack of funding for the treatment of personality disorders.

Approximately 10–15% of the general population would be diagnosed with one of the DSM-IV-TR personality disorders.

19.4 Course

The requirement that a personality disorder be evident since late adolescence and be relatively chronic thereafter has been a traditional means with which to distinguish a personality disorder from an Axis I disorder. Mood, anxiety, psychotic, sexual, and other mental disorders have traditionally been conceptualized as conditions that arise at some point during a person's life and that are relatively limited or circumscribed in their expression and duration. Personality disorders, in contrast, are conditions that are evident as early as late adolescence (and in some instances prior to that time), are evident in everyday functioning, and are stable throughout adulthood.

19.5 Etiology

Little information is available or verifiable about what actually causes personality disorders despite several theories regarding personality development. Some scholars suggest that they actually represent variants of normal personality structure rather than disease processes. Most likely, the DSM-IV-TR personality disorders might be, for the most part, constellations of maladaptive personality traits that are the result of multiple genetic dispositions interacting with a variety of detrimental environmental experiences.

19.6 The three clusters of personality disorder

DSM-IV-TR includes ten individual personality disorder diagnoses that are organized into three clusters: (A) paranoid, schizoid, and schizotypal (placed within an odd–eccentric cluster); (B) antisocial, borderline, histrionic, and narcissistic (dramatic–emotional–erratic cluster); and (C) avoidant, dependent, and obsessive–compulsive (anxious– fearful cluster). Two others are included in the appendix to DSM-IV-TR for disorders needing further study (passive–aggressive and depressive). Readers of this text are referred to DSM-IV-TR for specific diagnostic criteria for each.

19.6.1 Cluster A disorders

People with a Cluster A personality disorder manifest signs and symptoms sometimes associated with the schizophrenic spectrum. In addition to appearing odd or eccentric, those affected often seem cold, withdrawn, suspicious, and irrational.

19.6.1.1 Paranoid personality disorder

People with paranoid personality disorder (PPD) are suspicious, quick to take offense, and usually cannot acknowledge their own negative feelings toward others. However, they often project these negative feelings onto others. They have few friends and may project hidden meaning into innocent remarks. They may be litigious and guarded, and they may bear grudges for imagined insults or slights. Marital or sexual difficulties are common and often involve issues related to fidelity. People with PPD are quick to react with anger and counterattack in response to imagined character or reputation attacks. Despite their tendency to interpret the actions of others as deliberately threatening or demeaning, these people do not lose contact with reality.

As children, these individuals may appear odd and peculiar to their peers and they may not have achieved to their capacity in school. Their adjustment as adults will be particularly poor with respect to interpersonal relationships. They may become socially isolated or fanatic members of groups that encourage or at least accept their paranoid ideation. They might maintain a steady employment but will be difficult coworkers, as they will tend to be rigid, controlling, critical, blaming, and prejudicial. They are likely to become involved in lengthy, acrimonious, and litigious disputes that are difficult, if not impossible, to resolve.

There are no systematic studies on the treatment of PPD. Individuals rarely seek treatment for their feelings of suspiciousness and distrust. They will experience these traits as simply accurate perceptions of a malevolent and dangerous world (i.e., ego-syntonic). They may not consider the paranoid attributions to be at all problematic, disruptive, or maladaptive. They will not be delusional, but they will fail to be reflective, insightful, or self-critical. They may recognize only that they have difficulty controlling their anger and getting along with others. They might be in treatment for an anxiety, mood, or substance-related disorder or for various marital, familial, occupational, or social (or legal) conflicts that are secondary to their personality disorder; but they will also externalize the responsibility for their problems and will have substantial difficulty recognizing their own contribution to their internal dysphoria and external conflicts. They will consider their problems to be due to what others are doing *to them*, not to how they perceive, react, or relate to others.

These individuals are exceedingly difficult to engage in treatment. They are not good candidates for individual or group therapy. People with PPD may perceive the use of a medication to represent an effort to simply suppress or control their accusations and suspicions. However, they may be receptive and responsive to the benefits of a medication to help control feelings of anxiousness or depression that are secondary to their personality disorder.

19.6.1.2 Schizoid personality disorder

Schizoid personality disorder (SZPD) is a pervasive pattern of social detachment and restricted emotional expression. Individuals are lifelong loners. They exhibit indifference to social relationships, a flattened affectivity, and a cold, unsociable, reclusive demeanor. They take pleasure in few, if any, activities. People with this disorder usually never marry, have little interest in exploring their sexuality, and frequently live as adult children with their parents or other first-degree relatives.

There are few systematic studies on the childhood antecedents of and adult course of SZPD. Individuals are likely to have been socially isolated and withdrawn as children. They may not have been accepted well by their peers and may have even been the brunt of some peer ostracism. Psychosocial models for the etiology of SZPD are lacking. It is possible that a sustained history of isolation during infancy and childhood, with an encouragement and modeling by parental figures of interpersonal withdrawal, indifference, and detachment, could contribute to the development of schizoid personality traits.

Prototypic cases of SZPD would rarely present for treatment, whether it is for their schizoid traits or a concomitant Axis I disorder. They would feel little need for treatment, as their isolation will often be ego-syntonic. Their social isolation will be of more concern to their relatives, colleagues, or friends than to themselves. Their disinterest in, and withdrawal from, intimate or intense interpersonal contact will also be a substantial barrier to treatment. They will at times appear depressed but one must be careful not to confuse their anhedonic detachment, withdrawal, and flat affect with symptoms of depression.

If a person with SZPD is seen for treatment for a concomitant Axis I disorder (e.g., a sexual arousal disorder or substance dependence), it is advisable to work within the confines and limitations of the schizoid personality traits. Charismatic, engaging, emotional, or intimate therapists can be very uncomfortable, foreign, and even threatening to people with SZPD. A more businesslike approach can be more successful. Patients are perhaps best treated with a supportive psychotherapy that emphasizes education and feedback concerning interpersonal skills and communication.

19.6.1.3 Schizotypal personality disorder

People with schizotypal personality disorder (STPD) display an enduring and pervasive pattern of social and interpersonal deficits marked by extreme discomfort with, and intolerance for, close relationships. The symptomatology of STPD has been differentiated into components of positive symptoms (cognitive–perceptual aberrations) and negative symptoms (social aversion and withdrawal) comparable to the distinctions made for schizophrenia.

These individuals may have disturbed thought patterns and manifest odd behavior, speech, and appearance. They may be suspicious and display ideas of reference without delusions of reference. They may be superstitious and believe that they are capable of unusual forms of communication such as telepathy and clairvoyance. Patients with STP have a constricted or otherwise inappropriate affect and lack friends or confidantes other than first-degree relatives. They experience great social anxiety that does not diminish with familiarity and that seems to be associated with paranoid fearfulness rather than issues of low self-esteem.

There is insufficient research to describe the childhood precursors of adult STPD. Persons with STPD would be expected to appear peculiar and odd to their peers during adolescence, and may have been teased or ostracized. Achievement in school might be impaired, and they may have been heavily involved in esoteric fantasies and peculiar interests. As adults, they may drift toward esoteric fringe groups that support their magical thinking and aberrant beliefs. These activities can provide structure for some people with STPD, but they can also contribute to a further loosening and deterioration if there is an encouragement of aberrant experiences.

The symptomatology of STPD does not appear to remit with age. The course appears to be relatively stable, with some proportion of schizotypal persons remaining marginally employed, withdrawn, and transient throughout their lives. There is compelling empirical support for a genetic association of STPD with schizophrenia. Some patients meeting DSM-IV-TR criteria for STPD do eventually go on to develop schizophrenia but the vast majority do not.

Individuals with STPD may seek treatment for their feelings of anxiousness, perceptual disturbances, or depression. Treatment should be cognitive, behavioral, supportive, and/or pharmacologic, as they will often find the intimacy and emotionality of reflective, exploratory psychotherapy to be too stressful and they have the potential for psychotic decompensation.

Most of the systematic empirical research on the treatment of STPD has been confined to pharmacologic interventions. Low doses of antipsychotic medications have shown some effectiveness in the treatment of schizotypal symptoms, particularly the perceptual aberrations and social anxiousness. Group therapy has also been recommended for persons with STPD but only when the group is highly structured and supportive.

19.6.2 Cluster B disorders

A patient with a Cluster B disorder displays dramatic, emotional, and attention-seeking behaviors. He or she might also display labile and shallow moods and tend to become involved in all kinds of intense interpersonal conflicts.

19.6.2.1 Antisocial personality disorder

People with antisocial personality disorder (ASPD) display aggressive, irresponsible behavior that often leads to conflicts with society and involvement in the criminal justice system. People with this disorder commonly display behaviors such as fighting, lying, stealing, abusing children and spouses, abusing substances, and participating in confidence schemes. These people, while often superficially charming, lack genuine warmth.

While the diagnosis of antisocial personality disorder is limited to patients older than 18 years, the person also must have had a history of conduct disorder before 17 years of age.

ASPD will at times be difficult to differentiate from a substance-dependence disorder in young adults because many individuals with ASPD develop a substance-related disorder and many with a substance dependence engage in antisocial acts.

The US National Institute of Mental Health Epidemiologic Catchment Area Study indicated that approximately 3% of males and 1% of females have ASPD. There is considerable support from twin, family, and adoption studies for a genetic contribution to the etiology of ASPD. Exactly what is inherited in ASPD, however, is not known. It could be impulsivity, an antagonistic callousness, or an abnormally low anxiousness, or all of these dispositions combined. Numerous environmental factors have also been implicated in the etiology of antisocial behavior. Shared, or common, environmental influences account for 15–20% of variation in criminality or delinquency. Shared environmental factors such as low family income, inner-city residence, poor parental supervision, single-parent household, rearing by antisocial parents, delinquent siblings, parental conflict, harsh discipline, neglect, large family size, and young mother have all been implicated as risk factors for antisocial behavior.

ASPD is one personality disorder for which much is known about childhood antecedents, as it is well documented that people diagnosed with childhood-onset conduct disorder have a considerable risk of meeting the DSM-IV-TR criteria for ASPD as an adult. There are also compelling data to indicate that ASPD is a relatively chronic disorder, although, as the person reaches middle to older age, research suggests that the frequency of criminal acts appears to decrease. Nevertheless, the core personality traits may remain largely stable.

As adults, people with ASPD are unlikely to maintain steady employment, and they may even become impoverished, homeless, or spend years within penal institutions. However, some individuals with ASPD may express their psychopathic tendencies within a socially acceptable or at least legitimate profession, and they may in fact be quite successful as long as their tendency to bend or violate the norms or rules of their profession and exploit, deceive, and manipulate others contribute to a career advancement. Their success may at some point unravel when their psychopathic behaviors become problematic or evident to others. The same pattern may also occur within sexual and marital relationships.

ASPD is considered to be the most difficult personality disorder to treat. Individuals with ASPD can be seductively charming and declare a commitment to change, but they often lack sufficient motivation. They often fail to see the costs associated with antisocial acts (e.g., imprisonment, eventual impoverishment, and lack of meaningful interpersonal relationships) and may stay in treatment only as required by an external source, such as a parole. Residential programs that provide a carefully controlled environment of structure and supervision, combined with peer confrontation, have been recommended. However, it is unknown what benefits may be sustained after the ASPD individual leaves this environment.

Rather than attempt to develop a sense of conscience in these individuals, therapeutic techniques should perhaps be focused on rational and utilitarian arguments against repeating past mistakes. These approaches would focus on the tangible, material value of prosocial behavior.

19.6.2.2 Borderline personality disorder

Borderline personality disorder (BPD) is the most frequently diagnosed and studied of the personality disorders. By early adulthood, patients with BPD evidence instability in mood, impulse control, and interpersonal relationships. pervasive pattern of impulsivity and instability in interpersonal relationships, affect, and self-image. The primary diagnostic criteria include frantic efforts to avoid abandonment, unstable and intense relationships, impulsivity (e.g., substance abuse, binge-eating, sexual promiscuity), recurrent suicidal thoughts and gestures, self-mutilation, and episodes of rage and anger. Moreover, most people with BPD develop quite a number of Axis I mental disorders, including mood, dissociative, eating, substance-use, and anxiety disorders. It can be difficult to differentiate BPD from these disorders if assessment is confined to current symptomatology and the context and history of patient dysfunction is not taken into account.

Approximately 1–2% of the general population would meet the DSM-IV-TR criteria for BPD. It is the most prevalent personality disorder within most clinical settings. Approximately 15% of all inpatients (51% of inpatients with a personality disorder) and 8% of all outpatients (27% of outpatients with a personality disorder) will have borderline personality disorder. Approximately 75% of people with BPD will be female.

Individuals with BPD are likely to have been emotionally unstable, impulsive, and hostile as children, but there is little longitudinal research on the childhood antecedents of BPD. As adolescents, their intense affectivity and impulsivity may contribute to involvement with rebellious groups. BPD has been diagnosed in children and adolescents, but considerable caution should be used when doing so, as some of the symptoms of BPD could be confused with a normal adolescent rebellion or identity crisis.

As adults, people with BPD may be repeatedly hospitalized, due to their affect and impulse dyscontrol, psychotic-like and dissociative symptomatology, and suicide attempts. The risk of suicide is increased with a comorbid mood disorder and substance-related disorder. It is estimated that 3–10% of people with BPD will have committed suicide by the age of 30.

Intimate relationships tend to be very unstable and explosive, and employment history is generally poor. As the person reaches the age of 30, affective lability and impulsivity may begin to diminish. These symptoms may lessen earlier if the person becomes involved with a supportive and patient sexual partner. Occurrence of a severe stressor can easily disrupt the lessening of symptomatology, resulting in a brief psychotic, dissociative, or mood-disorder episode.

Patients with BPD form relationships with therapists that are similar to their other significant relationships; that is, the therapeutic relationship can often be tremendously unstable, intense, and volatile. Ongoing consultation with colleagues is recommended to address the therapist's reactions toward the patient that might interfere with the therapeutic relationship. Sessions should emphasize the building of a strong therapeutic alliance, monitoring of self-destructive and suicidal behaviors, validation of suffering and abusive experience (but also helping the patient take responsibility for actions), promotion of self-reflection rather than impulsive action, and setting of limits on self-destructive behavior.

Dialectical behavior therapy (DBT) has been shown empirically to be a particularly effective treatment of BPD. The therapist attempts to assist the person to overcome debilitating experiences with an "invalidating environment" by achieving goals of stabilization, behavioral control, emotional calmness, effectiveness, joy, and wholeness. The therapist uses a dialectical approach of acceptance, validation, and problem-solving to assist the patient to synthesize inner contradictions and conflicts. The American Psychiatric Association also concluded that psychodynamic psychotherapy has obtained empirical support for the treatment of borderline personality disorder that is equal to DBT, although this conclusion has been disputed.

Pharmacologic treatment of patients with BPD is varied, as it depends primarily on the predominant Axis I symptomatology. As mentioned, individuals with BPD can display a wide variety of Axis I symptoms, including anxiety, depression, hallucinations, delusions, and dissociations. It is important in their pharmacologic treatment for clinicians not to be unduly influenced by transient symptoms or by symptoms that are readily addressed through exploratory or supportive techniques, but to be flexible and not be unduly resistant to their use. Relying solely upon one's own psychotherapeutic skills can be unnecessary and even irresponsible, and clinicians are urged to have a consulting and supportive supervisory system in place when treating these individuals.

19.6.2.3 Histrionic personality disorder

Patients with histrionic personality disorder (HPD) have a longstanding pattern of excessive emotionality and attention-seeking behaviors. Histrionic individuals tend to be emotionally manipulative and intolerant of delayed gratification.

Approximately 1–3% of the general population may be diagnosed with HPD. It has typically been found that at least two-thirds of those with HPD are female.

Little is known about the premorbid behavior pattern. During adolescence the person with HPD is likely to have been flamboyant, flirtatious, and attention-seeking. Adults with HPD will readily form new relationships but will have difficulty sustaining them. They strive to be at center stage by focusing exclusively on their own desires and interests during conversations with others. They often express themselves in dramatic and highly emotional ways, but, despite their theatricality, their speech style is superficial and lacking in detail.

People with this disorder often engage in seductive behaviors to gain approval. Their extreme dependence on the favor of others may result in their moods appearing shallow or excessively reactive to their surroundings. Additionally, they can be naive, gullible, and easily influenced, and may be given to emotional outbursts as a result of low frustration tolerance. Hence, people with this disorder often appear inconsistent and unpredictable. They usually blame failure or disappointment on others.

There is little research on the etiology of HPD. There is a suggestion that HPD may share with ASPD a genetic disposition toward impulsivity or sensation-seeking. The tendency of a family to emphasize, value, or reinforce attention-seeking in a person with a genetic disposition toward emotionality may represent a general pathway toward HPD.

People with HPD will readily develop rapport but it will often be superficial and unreliable. A key task in treating the patient with HPD is countering his or her global and diffuse cognitive style by insisting on attending to structure and detail within sessions and to the practical, immediate problems within daily life. It is also important to explore within treatment the historical source for the individual's need for attention and involvement.

The intense affectivity of people with HPD may also be responsive to antidepressant treatment, particularly those patients with substantial mood reactivity, hypersomnia, and rejection sensitivity.

19.6.2.4 Narcissistic personality disorder

This diagnostic category is considered to be an American concept, as it does not appear in the World Health Organization International Classification of Diseases. Patients with narcissistic personality disorder (NPD) have a lifelong pattern of self-centeredness, self-absorption, inability to empathize with others, grandiosity, and extreme desire for the admiration of others. They feel that they are unusually special and often exaggerate their accomplishments to appear more important than they actually are. Despite their grandiose ideas, these patients have fragile self-esteem and are overly sensitive to what others think or say about them. As sensitive as they are to the opinions of others, they are particularly insensitive to the needs or feelings of others and lack empathy. In fact, they often feel entitled to special treatment from others; when it is denied, these patients can become demanding, angry, and offended. People with NPD can be haughty, arrogant, and capable of taking advantage of others to achieve their own ends. They also are often intensely envious of others and believe others are envious of them.

NPD overlaps substantially with ASPD and may lie along a common continuum of psychopathology. Both disorders include a disposition to dominate, humiliate, and manipulate others. NPD is among the least frequently diagnosed personality disorders within clinical settings, with estimates of prevalence as low as 2%. Those with NPD are considered to be prone to mood disorders, as well as anorexia and substance-related disorders, especially involving cocaine.

Little is known empirically about the course of narcissism. Clinical experience suggests that this disorder does not abate with age and may even become more evident into middle or older age. People with this disorder might be seemingly well adjusted and even successful as a young adult, having experienced substantial achievements in education, career, and perhaps even within relationships. However, their relationships with their colleagues, peers, and intimates might become strained over time as their lack of consideration for, and even exploitative use of, others becomes cumulatively evident.

There has been little systematic research on the etiology of narcissism. Two twin studies have supported heritability for narcissistic personality traits, although given the complexity of narcissism it is not entirely clear what precisely is being inherited.

The predominant models for the etiology of narcissism have been largely social learning or psychodynamic. One model proposes that narcissism develops through an excessive idealization by parental figures, which is then incorporated by the child into his or her self-image. Narcissism may also develop through unempathic, neglectful, inconsistent, or even devaluing parental figures who have failed to adequately mirror a child's natural need for idealization.

People rarely seek treatment for their narcissism. Individuals with NPD enter treatment-seeking assistance for another mental disorder, such as substance abuse (secondary to career stress), mood disorder (secondary to career setback), or even something quite specific, such as test anxiety.

Once an individual with NPD is in treatment, he or she will have difficulty perceiving the relationship as collaborative and will likely attempt to dominate, impress, or devalue the therapist. Cognitive–behavioral approaches to NPD emphasize increasing awareness of the impact of narcissistic behaviors and statements on interpersonal relationships. Group therapy can be useful for increasing awareness of the grandiosity, lack of empathy, and devaluation of others. However, these traits not only interfere with the narcissistic person's ability to sustain membership within groups (and within individual therapy), they may also become quite harmful and destructive to the rapport of the entire group. There is no accepted pharmacologic approach to the treatment of narcissism.

19.6.3 Cluster C disorders

A patient with a Cluster C personality disorder is often anxious, tense, and overcontrolled. These disorders may occur with Axis I anxiety disorders and require effort to distinguish between the two axes.

19.6.3.1 Avoidant personality disorder

Avoidant personality disorder (AVPD) is a pervasive pattern of timidity, inhibition, inadequacy, and social hypersensitivity. People with AVPD may have a strong desire to develop close, personal relationships but feel too insecure to approach others or to express their feelings. People with avoidant personality disorder have a pattern of social discomfort and fear of negative evaluation beginning in early adulthood. They are preoccupied with what they perceive as their own short-comings and will risk forming relationships with others only if they believe acceptance is guaranteed.

People with this disorder often view themselves as unattractive and inferior to others and are often socially inept. Consequently, they usually avoid occupations that have social demands. They are reluctant to take risks or try new activities for fear of being embarrassed, shamed, or ridiculed.

Timidity, shyness, and social insecurity are not uncommon problems, and AVPD is one of the more prevalent personality disorders within clinical settings, occurring in 5–25% of all patients. However, AVPD may be diagnosed in only 1–2% of the general population. It appears to occur equally among males and females, with some studies reporting more males and others reporting more females. People with AVPD are likely to have symptoms that meet the DSM-IV-TR criteria for a generalized social phobia, and others may have a mood disorder. While most patients with avoidant personality also may be diagnosed with social phobia, most patients with social phobia do not qualify for the diagnosis of avoidant personality disorder. That is, avoidant personality disorder pervades all social situations, while social phobia is confined to specific situations (e.g., speaking or eating in public).

Adolescence will have been a particularly difficult developmental period, due to the importance at this time of attractiveness, dating, and popularity. Occupational success may not be significantly impaired, as long as there is little demand for public performance. Avoidance of social situations will impair the ability to develop adequate social skills, and this will then further handicap any eventual efforts to develop relationships. As a parent, the person may be very responsible, empathic, and affectionate, but may unwittingly impart feelings of social anxiousness and awkwardness. Severity of the AVPD symptomatology diminishes as the person becomes older.

There is limited research on the etiology or pathology of AVPD. It may involve elevated peripheral sympathetic activity and adrenocortical responsiveness, resulting in excessive autonomic arousal, fearfulness, and inhibition. The pathology of AVPD, however, may be as much psychologic as neurochemical, with the timidity, shyness, and insecurity being a natural result of a cumulative history of denigrating, embarrassing, and devaluing experiences.

People with AVPD will seek treatment for their avoidant personality traits, although many will initially seek treatment for symptoms of anxiety, particularly social phobia. Social skills training, systematic desensitization, and a graded hierarchy of *in vivo* exposure to feared social situations have been shown to be useful in the treatment of AVPD. Persons with AVPD will often find group therapies to be helpful. Exploratory and supportive groups can provide them with an understanding environment in which to discuss their social insecurities, to explore and practice more assertive behaviors, and to develop an increased self-confidence to approach others and to develop relationships outside of the group.

19.6.3.2 Dependent personality disorder

Patients with dependent personality disorder (DPD) have a pervasive and excessive need to be taken care of, leading to submissive and clinging behavior and fears of separation. They need the approval of others to such an extent that they have tremendous difficulty making independent decisions or starting projects. People with dependent personality disorder fear abandonment and feel helpless when alone. Consequently, they urgently seek another relationship to provide them with care and support if a relationship ends. People with DPD will also have low self-esteem, and will often be self-critical and self-denigrating. They may go to great lengths, even suffering abuse, to stay in a relationship. As a result of their intense need for reassurance, they often have occupational difficulties.

Excessive dependency will often be seen in people who have developed debilitating mental and general medical disorders, such as agoraphobia, schizophrenia, mental retardation, severe injuries, and dementia. However, a diagnosis of DPD requires the presence of the dependent traits since late childhood or adolescence.

Deference, politeness, and passivity will also vary substantially across cultural groups. It is important not to confuse differences in personality that are due to different cultural norms with the presence of a personality disorder.

DPD is among the most prevalent of the personality disorders, occurring in 5–30% of patients and 2–4% of the general community. It is more commonly diagnosed in females.

People with DPD are likely to have been excessively submissive as children and adolescents, and some may have had a chronic physical illness or a separation anxiety disorder during childhood, but there is actually little systematic research on the etiology of excessive dependency. Central to its etiology and pathology is considered to be an insecure interpersonal attachment. Individuals with DPD are prone to mood disorders throughout life, particularly major depression and dysthymia, and to anxiety disorders, particularly agoraphobia, social phobia, and panic disorder.

There are no empirically validated treatments for DPD. Treatment recommendations are essentially based on anecdotal clinical experience. People with DPD will often be in treatment for one or more Axis I disorders, particularly a mood (depressive) or an anxiety disorder. These individuals will tend to be very agreeable, compliant, and grateful, at times to excess.

Therapists should be careful not to unwittingly encourage this submissiveness, nor to reject the client in order to be rid of their clinging dependency. An important component of treatment will often be a thorough exploration of the need for support and its root causes. Cognitive–behavioral techniques can be useful to address feelings of inadequacy and helplessness, and to provide training in assertiveness and problem-solving techniques. People with DPD may also benefit from group therapy. A supportive group is useful in diffusing the feelings of dependency onto a variety of persons, in providing feedback regarding their manner of relating to others, and in providing practice and role models for more assertive and autonomous interpersonal functioning. There is no known pharmacologic treatment for DPD.

19.6.3.3 Obsessive–compulsive personality disorder

Obsessive–compulsive personality disorder (OCPD) is characterized by a preoccupation with orderliness, perfectionism, and mental and interpersonal control. These lifelong traits exist at the expense of the person's efficiency and flexibility. The individual's rigid perfectionism often results in indecisiveness, preoccupation with detail, and an insistence that others should do things their way. Thus, they may have difficulty being effective in their occupational and social roles. Additionally, people with obsessive–compulsive personality disorder may have difficulty expressing affection and may appear depressed.

OCPD resembles, to some extent, obsessive–compulsive anxiety disorder (OCAD). However, many people with OCPD fail to develop OCAD, and vice versa. There is in fact little empirical support for a close relationship of OCAD with OCPD. Unlike Axis I obsessive–compulsive disorder (see Chapter 15), patients with OCPD do not have actual obsessions or compulsions. OCPD, in contrast, involves rigid, inhibited, and authoritarian behavior patterns that are more ego-syntonic.

Only 1–2% of the general community may meet the diagnostic criteria for the disorder but this could be an under-estimation. It appears to be more common in men.

There is little systematic research on the childhood antecedents or adult course of OCPD. As children, some with OCPD may have appeared to be relatively well behaved, responsible, and conscientious. However, they may have also been overly serious, rigid, and constrained. As adults, it is expected that many will obtain good to excellent success within a job or career. They can be excellent workers to the point of excess, sacrificing their social and leisure activities, marriage, and family for their job. Relationships with spouse and children are likely to be strained owing to their tendency to be detached and uninvolved, and yet authoritarian and domineering with respect to decisions. A spouse may complain of a lack of affection, tenderness, and warmth. Relationships with colleagues at work may be equally strained by the excessive perfectionism, domination, indecision, worrying, and anger.

A variety of studies have indicated heritability for the trait of obsessionality, and there is considerable empirical support for the heritability of conscientiousness. OCPD includes personality traits that are highly valued within most cultures, and some instances of OCPD may reflect exaggerated or excessive responses to the expectations of, or pressures by, parental figures.

People with OCPD may fail to seek treatment for the symptomatology. They may seek treatment instead for disorders and problems that are secondary to their OCPD traits, including anxiety disorders, health problems, and problems within various relationships (e.g., marital, familial, occupational). Treatment will be complicated by their inability to appreciate the contribution of their personality to these problems and disorders.

Cognitive–behavioral techniques that address the irrationality of excessive conscientiousness, moralism, perfectionism, devotion to work, and stubbornness can be effective. People with OCPD can be problematic in groups because they will tend to be domineering, constricted, and judgmental. There is no accepted pharmacologic treatment. Some will benefit from anxiolytic or antidepressant medications, but this will typically reflect the presence of associated features or comorbid disorders. The core traits of OCPD might not be affected by pharmacologic interventions.

19.6.4 Personality disorder not otherwise specified

DSM-IV-TR includes a diagnostic category for patients with a personality disorder who do not meet the diagnostic criteria for any of the ten officially recognized diagnoses considered above. In fact, "personality disorder not otherwise specified" (PDNOS) is one of the more commonly used personality disorder diagnoses in clinical practice.

It is not possible to discuss the etiology, pathology, course, or treatment of PDNOS since the diagnosis refers to a wide variety of personality types. However, one usage of PDNOS is for the two personality disorders presented in the appendix to DSM-IV-TR for criterion sets provided for further study, the passive–aggressive and the depressive.

19.6.4.1 Passive–aggressive personality disorder

Passive–aggressive personality disorder (PAPD) is a pervasive pattern of negativistic attitudes and passive resistance to authority, demands, responsibilities, or obligations. There have been no longitudinal studies to address this concern. It was shifted to the appendix of DSM-IV-TR because there had been little research to support its validity. A primary concern about PADP has been whether it is a situational reaction to authoritative control or in fact a temporally stable personality trait.

19.6.4.2 Depressive personality disorder

Depressive personality disorder (DPPD) was proposed for inclusion in DSM-III and DSM-III-R, but there were concerns that it may not be adequately distinguished from the mood disorder of dysthymia. It was decided that the DSM-IV-TR diagnostic criteria for DPPD lacked sufficient empirical support to warrant full recognition.

DPPD is defined as a pervasive pattern of depressive cognitions and behaviors that have been evident since adolescence and characteristic of everyday functioning. These are people who characteristically display a gloominess, cheerlessness, pessimism, brooding, rumination, and dejection.

Clinical Vignette 1

Ms C, a 36-year-old, was referred to a day-hospital program for borderline personality disorders after her fourth hospitalization for depression and suicidality.

Ms C had not known her father. She was raised by her mother who had a polysubstance dependence. Her relationship with her mother was described as negligent and distant. She had two brothers. The oldest brother abused her sexually for three years since she was 13 years old, the abuse ending when he was drafted into the army. She denied any feelings of anger or bitterness toward him, and in fact described substantial feelings of fondness and affection. He died while serving in Vietnam.

Ms C obtained good to excellent grades in school but had a history of indiscriminant sexual behavior, substance abuse, and bulimia. Her common method for purging was to attempt to swallow a belt, thereby inducing vomiting. Her first treatment was at the age of 19. She became significantly depressed when she discovered that her fiancé was sexually involved with her best friend. Her hospitalization was precipitated by the ingestion of a lethal amount of drugs. Subsequent to this hospitalization she began to mutilate herself by scratching or cutting her arms with broken plates, dinner knives, or metal. The self-mutilation was usually precipitated by episodes of severe loneliness and feelings of emptiness.

Ms C had a very active social life and a large network of friends. However, her relationships were unstable. She could be quite supportive, engaging, and personable, but would overreact to common conflicts, disagreements, and difficulties. She would feel intensely hurt, depressed, angry, or enraged, and would hope that her friends would relieve her pain through some gesture. However, they would typically feel frustrated, annoyed, or overwhelmed by the intensity of her affect and her reactions.

Her sexual relationships were even more problematic. She would quickly develop intense feelings of attraction, involvement, and dependency. However, she would soon experience her lovers as disappointing and neglectful, which at times had more than a kernel of truth. Many were neglectful, unempathic, or abusive, but all of them found the intensity of the inevitable conflicts and her anger to be intolerable.

She was also questioning her sexual orientation. She had never been sexually involved with a woman, but she did have fantasies of an involvement with various women she had known. It was conceivable that she might find a relationship with a woman to be more stable and satisfying, but it was likely that as much conflict would occur with women as had occurred with men.

Ms C attended the day-hospital BPD program for two years. Treatment included group therapy, individual psychotherapy (using both cognitive–behavioral and insight), and antidepressant medication. The CBT focused on daily management of problems, exploring alternate perceptions of, and means for, addressing conflicts with others, and gradually developing more effective coping strategies. The irrationality of her reactions became more apparent to her as their source within her past relationships was better understood.

Treatment was successful in ending her reliance on self-mutilation and in decreasing the intensity of her interpersonal conficts. She continues to have unstable relationships, but she was much more successful in acknowledging and resolving conflicts in ways that were more realistic and appropriate.

Clinical Vignette 2

Ms L, a 21-year-old college sophomore, unexpectedly returned home in the middle of the first semester proclaiming that she could no longer suffer the anxiety and depression she felt at college. Neither she nor her parents felt they had a clear understanding of what was making her feel so distraught. She was doing fine in her classes and was actively involved in a number of college organizations. Her mother called her academic advisor at college for advice, and Ms L was referred to a clinician for consultation and treatment.

Ms L indicated at the initial session that she had been intensely ambivalent about attending college and had in fact delayed enrollment for two years in the hope that she could convince her parents that she would not have to leave home. She indicated that she felt overwhelmingly frightened and tearful away from home. She had been calling her parents three to five times each week, seeking their advice and reassurance but also simply to maintain regular contact. Her level of anxiety decreased substantially when she returned home but quickly emerged at the thought of leaving home again.

Ms L's parents were concerned that she was returning home to be close to a boy that she had once dated. She, however, denied this motivation, indicating that she had long abandoned any hope of a future in that particular relationship. She was a popular young woman, generally considered to be quite amicable, modest, friendly, warm, attractive, bright, and engaging. However, she acknowledged that she often felt very insecure in her relationships, requiring reassurances from her girlfriends and boyfriends that she was not a burden to them, as she in fact grew increasingly burdensome in part from her need for their reassurance. She indicated that she had often fallen in love but had repeatedly felt crushed and devastated when the object of her love failed to become as attached. She said that one boyfriend broke up with her explicitly because he experienced her as being too "needy" and "clinging." She admitted that this was "not far from the truth" but had pleaded to him that she would no longer be so needy if only he would not leave her.

Ms L described her relationship with parents, particularly her mother, as being very close, supportive, and dependable. Her childhood history, however, included many examples of failures to develop an independent self-confidence. For example, she felt unable to attend a summer camp attended by her best friends because of fears of separation from her parents. She did attend the following summer but taxed the patience of the camp counselors with her demands for attention and support. Her parents verbally encouraged her to develop greater independence and self-confidence but they also would repeatedly give in to her requests for protection and support. Her mother in fact often appeared to be somewhat reluctant to be separate from her.

Ms L was seen in twice-weekly individual psychotherapy. Pharmacotherapy was provided for her anxious and depressive symptoms but was discontinued after 2 months after to complaints of side-effects. Cognitive therapy focused on her self-denigrating beliefs of helplessness, behavioral therapy included a gradual shaping of independence from her parents, and insight therapy explored the relationship of her self-image with her relationships with her parents. Treatment was successful in developing sufficient independence and self-esteem for her to feel comfortable and confident enough to return the following year to college. She successfully completed college although abandoned aspirations to pursue a social work career after she became married and had children of her own.

KEY POINTS

- A personality disorder may be defined as an enduring collection of personality character-istics that have become fixed and rigid to the point that the patient experiences distress and behavioral dysfunction.

- Personality disorders can occur singularly or with other serious psychiatric disorders such as major depression, anxiety disorder, and substance abuse.

- The cause or causes of personality disorders are unknown. Scholars speculate that personality disorders may actually represent variants of normal personality rather than disease processes. Some also speculate that personality disorders are caused by psycho-social factors, while others point to growing evidence that personality disorders have a genetic component. It is likely that a combination of biologic and psychosocial factors is responsible for the formation of personality itself and personality disorders.

- Some patients with personality disorders worsen over time, while others improve. Some patients drop out of treatment, preventing further follow-up; others refuse treatment, creating unknown variables in studies.

- Ten types of personality disorder are organized into three clusters: A, B, and C. Patients with type A typically are described as cold, withdrawn, suspicious, and irrational. Those with type B display dramatic, emotional, and attention-seeking behaviors. Those with type C are often anxious, tense, and overcontrolled.

- Two personality disorders are included in the DSM appendix for which there is insufficient evidence or consensus and which require further study. These are passive–aggressive and depressive types.

- Patients may benefit from individual psychotherapy using supportive, insight-oriented, and cognitive–behavioral approaches. Group and family therapy may even benefit some patients.

- Clinicians should develop skills in assessing, forming trust, setting limits, and using therapeutic confrontation to provide effective care.

- Clinicians are also advised that they should have a supportive supervisor or mentor, as these patients may cause negative feelings and progress in treating personality disorders is usually slow and requires patience and maturity.

Further Reading

Lilienfeld, S.O., O'Donohue, W.T., and Fowler, K.A. (2007) *Personality Disorders: Toward the DSM-V,* Sage, New York.

Reich, J. (2001) *Personality Disorders: Current Research and Treatments,* Taylor & Francis, New York.

20 Stereotyped Movement Disorder and Reactive Attachment Disorder

20.1 Introduction

This chapter discusses stereotyped movement disorder, which involves abnormal motor behaviors and reactive attachment disorder (RAD), which involves abnormal social behaviors. Both tend to occur in association with socially deprived environments, most often occurring in individuals who have developmental delays or mental retardation.

20.2 Stereotypic movement disorder

Stereotypic movement disorder is characterized by repetitive, seemingly driven, nonfunctional movements including hand-waving, head-banging, body-rocking, fiddling with fingers, self-biting, or hitting various parts of one's own body. These behaviors can be problematic for a number of reasons because they may result in self-injury, affect general health, result in significant social stigmatization, interfere with acquisition of new skills, and interfere with performance of existing skills.

20.2.1 Diagnostic features

Stereotypies are repetitive, driven, and nonfunctional motor behavior. They are voluntary, lack variability, persist over time, are immutable even when the environment changes, and are inconsistent with the person's expected development. Stereotypic movements are problematic when they interfere with a person's overall functioning, become socially stigmatizing, or result in self-injury.

20.2.2 Epidemiology

Stereotypic movements are relatively common. For example, as many as 90% of typically developing children engage in body-rocking as a normal part of motor development, and 10% of normally developing 2-year-olds engage in head-banging while having tantrums.

Stereotypic movements are present but rare in populations of adults with average intelligence. These behaviors are predictably longer-lived and more impairing in developmentally delayed

Fundamentals of Psychiatry, First Edition. Allan Tasman and Wanda K. Mohr.
© 2011 John Wiley & Sons, Ltd. Published 2011 by John Wiley & Sons, Ltd.
This chapter is based on Chapter 50 (Morgan Feibelman, Charles H. Zeanah) of *Psychiatry, Third Edition*

populations. In fact, the more severe the level of retardation, the more likely the person is to exhibit stereotypic movements, and the more likely these will be self-injurious.

20.2.3 Comorbidity

Stereotypic movement disorder occurs most frequently in people with mental retardation, or pervasive developmental disorders. Because they are both related to conditions of neglect, stereotypic movement disorder may co-occur with RAD. Several other conditions are also associated with stereotypic movements. Some genetic syndromes associated with it are Lesh–Nyhan syndrome (self-biting of the forearms), Prader–Willi syndrome (picking skin of the back of the hands), and Fragile X syndrome.

20.2.4 Differential diagnosis

The stereotypic behaviors must be distinguished from a variety of other movements. Like most other DSM-IV-TR diagnoses, the behaviors must be severe enough to cause impairment in functioning. Stereotypic movement disorder is often diagnosed in people with mental retardation. However, stereotypic movements are considered a feature of pervasive developmental disorders and therefore would not be given a separate diagnosis when they occur in such individuals.

Stereotypic movement disorder must also be distinguished from a variety of different behaviors. For example, compulsions associated with obsessive–compulsive disorder (see Chapter 15) can look like stereotypic movements. Likewise, movements from the effects of certain medications, such as the antipsychotic group, should be taken into consideration and ruled out.

Developmentally appropriate self-stimulatory behaviors such as thumb-sucking can be differentiated by the appropriateness of the behavior to the child's developmental level, changes in the behavior in response to the environment, and extinction of the behavior as the child develops.

Trichotillomania is another condition that must be distinguished from stereotypic movement disorder. Factitious disorder with predominantly physical signs and symptoms, and self-mutilation associated with personality disorders, mood disorders, and psychotic disorders, should also be differentiated from stereotypic movement disorder.

20.2.5 Etiology

Stereotypic movement disorder has a multifactorial pathophysiology involving a complex interaction between several neurological pathways, psychological factors, and social factors. Considerable research had addressed the neurobiology of stereotypies. Dopaminergic, serotinergic, and endogenous opioid systems have been associated with stereotypic movements and self-injurious behavior.

Though little is known about the genetic factors affecting stereotypic movements, several genetic syndromes do predispose people to stereotypic movements and self-injurious behavior. These syndromes have unique mechanisms likely resulting in changes in the dopaminergic neurons and other changes leading to stereotypic movements.

Stereotypic movements may be understood as a form of operant behavior that is maintained and reinforced by consequences of the behavior. In addition, other factors may contribute to the timing and intensity of the behavior. For example, the behavior will be decreased in the presence of social stimulation. Stereotyped behavior is also decreased following strenuous exercise, although not following mild exercise.

Stereotypic and self-injurious behaviors may develop and persist in the absence of stimulation. Functional analysis of stereotypic behavior shows it can be maintained by positive reinforcement (e.g., sensory stimulation), negative reinforcement (e.g., removal of an unpleasant physical stimulus), or some combination of social and nonsocial reinforcement (e.g., social positive and automatic reinforcement).

Deprivation is the environmental factor most associated with stereotypic behavior. The self-stimulating effect of stereotypies has long been proposed as its function, thus explaining the increased prevalence of stereotypies in individuals living in institutions.

20.2.6 Treatments

Treatments include several classes of medication, as well as behavior plans and social interventions. In approaching treatment, the first step should be addressing the patient's deprivation with social interventions, if possible. Behavioral treatments and medications can be used secondarily as needed for management of the patient's symptoms.

No medications have been approved by the US Food and Drug Administration. However, several classes of medication have shown some efficacy in treatment of this disorder. Serotonin-reuptake inhibitors have shown some efficacy.

Antipsychotics are some of the most commonly prescribed drugs for people with mental retardation and behavioral problems. Studies and even case reports for stereotypic movements and self-injurious behaviors are sparse over the past decade, and previous studies were often seriously methodologically flawed. Despite widespread use of antipsychotics to treat stereotypies, they have limited evidence of efficacy and significant side-effects, and some scholars have suggested their use may not be appropriate. A few recent studies, however, have provided modest support for their use. In the autism literature, there are some studies that show improvement in stereotypic and self-injurious behavior with risperidone.

One study of valproic acid in the treatment of stereotypic behavior in autistic children showed a significant reduction in the stereotypic behavior in 13 patients as measured by the Children's Yale–Brown Obsessive Compulsive Scale (C-YBOCS). Opioid receptor blockers have also been used for the treatment of self-injurious behavior with some efficacy.

Behavioral therapies have been used to treat stereotypic and self-injurious behaviors. Because most stereotypic movements are automatically reinforced, interventions involving environmental enrichment, differential reinforcement, and punishment were behavioral techniques that at least temporarily decreased stereotypic movements. Much work has been done in this area and the results are often quite successful.

20.3 Reactive attachment disorder

Reactive attachment disorder is a disturbance in social relatedness that is apparent across most developmental contexts. It appears in the first 5 years of life, and it must be distinguished from pervasive developmental disorders; that is, the presence of a pervasive developmental disorder precludes the diagnosis. RAD, as defined by DSM-IV-TR, requires etiologic factors such as gross deprivation of care or successive multiple caregivers.

Two clinical patterns are apparent, an emotionally withdrawn/inhibited type and an indiscriminately social/disinhibited type. These abnormal behaviors must be due to pathogenic care that the child has received.

20.3.1 Epidemiology

Though epidemiologic data are limited, RAD is a rare disorder. Because pathogenic care is required to make the diagnosis, only children with histories of severe deprivation, such as maltreated children

Table 20-1 Signs and symptoms of reactive attachment disorder, inhibited and disinhibited types	
RAD Inhibited Type	**RAD Disinhibited Type**
Avoidance of eye contact	Excessive attention-seeking
Blunted affect, blank expression	Indiscriminate sociability
Prefers to play alone	Seeking comfort from others (strangers)
Engages in self-soothing behaviors to exclusion of seeking human comfort	Inappropriate childish behavior
Avoids physical contact	Frequent tantrums or acting-out behaviors when upset or frustrated
Hypervigilant, "guarded" or wary appearance	
Detached from environment	
Avoids receiving comfort and affection	
Inability to give and receive attention	
Failure to thrive	
Poor hygiene	
Appear bewildered, unfocused, or under-stimulated	

and those raised in institutions, are eligible. Even in high-risk groups, the diagnosis is uncommon. For example, in a study of currently and formerly institutionalized children in Bucharest, Romania, at 54 months of age, fewer than a third of the children met criteria for RAD. There are no known effects of gender or culture related to the presentation or prevalence of RAD. Age of onset is specified as within the first 5 years of life, but most likely the disorder is present from the latter part of the first year of life.

20.3.2 Etiology

Expert consensus is that the key ingredient of pathogenic care related to the development of RAD is social neglect. What remains unclear is why two distinctive subtypes of RAD arise in similar conditions of risk but are phenomenologically different and have different courses and correlates (Table 20.1).

20.3.3 Diagnostic features

In inhibited RAD, the child fails to initiate and respond to social interactions in a developmentally appropriate manner. In disinhibited RAD, the child participates in diffuse attachments, indiscriminate sociability, and excessive familiarity with strangers. Normal, developmental anxiety and concern with strangers is not present, and the infant or child superficially and uncritically accepts anyone as a caregiver (as though people were interchangeable) and acts as if the relationship had been intimate and life-long.

20.3.4 Assessment

As with most other disorders of early childhood, RAD is best assessed through a combination of interviewing and direct behavioral observation. A detailed history of the child's caregiving experiences is important in order to establish that deficiencies were sufficient to account for the child's social abnormalities. Therefore, details of the child's caregiving history, with attention to neglect, changes in primary caregiving relationships, or significant losses of primary caregivers should be determined. Standardized observational procedures that elicit the child's responses to familiar and unfamiliar caregivers in order to distinguish between the child's responses to putative attachment figures and to unfamiliar adults have been used in research and may be useful in clinical settings.

Interviews and observations should include questioning about the child having one or more adults from whom he or she seeks comfort, reassurance, nurturing, and protection, particularly in times of distress. In addition, failing to use the attachment figure for comfort, as occurs in the emotionally withdrawn/inhibited pattern, and exhibiting overly familiar behaviors with unfamiliar adults, as occurs in the indiscriminate/disinhibited pattern, should be identified.

20.3.5 Differential diagnosis

When considering a diagnosis of the emotionally withdrawn inhibited type of RAD, one must consider mental retardation and autistic spectrum disorders in the differential diagnosis. Most children with RAD will demonstrate significant concurrent developmental delays, but this may be distinguished from children who have solely delayed development.

The indiscriminately social/disinhibited type of RAD must be distinguished from nondisordered children with high levels of sociability, as well as from children with attention-deficit hyperactivity disorder.

20.3.6 Comorbidity

There are no studies to date of comorbidity in RAD. Nevertheless, reasonable speculation is possible given what is known about the etiology. Because of the conditions known to give rise to RAD, namely maltreatment and institutional deprivation, other disorders known to arise in similar conditions of risk may co-occur. Chief among these is developmental delay, particularly mental retardation and language disorders. In addition, because physical abuse may co-occur with neglect, post-traumatic stress disorder has been reported to co-occur with the emotionally withdrawn/ inhibited type of RAD.

Attention-deficit hyperactivity disorder also is known to be over-represented among children raised in institutions, and it is possible that the social impulsivity that occurs in the emotionally withdrawn inhibited type of RAD co-occurs with the more cognitive and behavioral impulsivity that occurs in attention-deficit hyperactivity disorder. This has not been examined systematically, but it remains one of the important questions about the disorder.

20.3.7 Course

Though relevant data remain scarce, findings to date suggest that the emotionally withdrawn/ inhibited and the indiscriminately social types of RAD have different courses over time. Although limited, what little data are available suggest that the emotionally withdrawn/inhibited pattern of RAD is responsive to intervention. In contrast, several studies have demonstrated that the indiscriminate social/disinhibited type of RAD is one of the most persistent social abnormalities in young children raised in institutions. Even following adoption or placement in foster care, signs of indiscriminate/disinhibited RAD may persist for years.

20.3.8 Treatments

Despite limited data, the guiding principle of treatment of RAD is that enhancing the caregiving environment of the child leads to elimination of signs of disordered attachment behavior. The primary goal of treatment for the emotionally withdrawn/inhibited type of RAD is creating the possibility for the child to develop a focused attachment relationship to a primary caregiver. Ordinarily, this happens quickly once a child is in a reasonably typical caregiving environment. Attachment behaviors in young children placed into foster care, for example, begin to develop within days of initial placement. The goal for treatment of the indiscriminate disinhibited type of RAD is to increase the child's reliance on attachment figures and decrease engagement with unfamiliar adults. Clinicians often advise that adoptive families limit the contacts of children adopted out of institutions for a period of several months, in order to give the child an opportunity to form selective attachments to them and to reduce the confusion of transitioning from an institutional setting to a family. There are, however, no studies that have addressed this advice. Indeed, from studies of children adopted out of institutions, long-term stability of indiscriminate/disinhibited behavior is clear.

Over the past decade, so-called attachment therapy (AT) has been promoted by clinicians in the absence of any legitimate theoretical underpinnings or research. AT practices routinely use restraint and physical and psychological abuse to seek their desired results. Sessions of attachment holding therapy, and rage reduction, have been noted to last as long as 12 hours per session. In 2000, a "re-birthing" therapy, a bizarre plan to re-enact the birth process so that the child could be "reborn" to her adoptive mother, resulted in the death of a 10-year-old child at a "treatment center" in Colorado. Parents who are desperate to find help for their children are taken in by the advertisements of these AT centers and their "therapists," some of whom claim a 75% success rate on the internet. Clinicians should be aware of the dangers of these purveyors of quackery and educate parents appropriately.

No medications are indicated for RAD. Somatic treatments are used only to treat comorbid disorders.

The American Academy of Child and Adolescent Psychiatry has an extensively developed practice parameter on RAD. However, there are no solid empirical data about successful treatment of RAD, and managing the disorder is a long-term challenge that can be demanding for parents and caregivers.

Clinical Vignette

Lindsey, a 41-month-old girl, was removed from her mother at age 32 months and placed in foster care. Before that, she had a history of neglect and witnessing extensive partner violence between her mother and mother's boyfriend. She was dismissed from her childcare center for spitting, hitting, biting, and having a "demonic look" earlier in the year. At the time she came into care, Lindsey did not check back with her foster mother in unfamiliar settings, showed affection towards total strangers, and her foster mother reported having to hold her hand in public settings (such as the mall) to prevent her from "wandering off" with strangers. This caused the foster mother considerable worry and restricted the number of times she was willing to take Lindsey out in public.

When seen for evaluation, Lindsey was active, running, climbing, and doing summersaults, repeatedly calling attention to herself. Despite her foster mother's admonitions, she ran into the offices of other clinicians several times, and she approached and tried to kiss several adults in the waiting area. She walked into the receptionist's area and linked her arm around the receptionist's arm. In the office, she made a show of falling down and stating she was hurt, expressing the desire to be rescued.

A behavioral plan was implemented to assist her foster mother in managing Lindsey's behavior. Her foster mother was advised to restrict Lindsey's contact with unfamiliar adults and to talk with her about appropriate behavior with strangers. In a follow-up 3 months later, the foster mother reported that in a new daycare setting that was warmer but more structured than the initial setting, Lindsey's behavior settled down considerably. Her eagerness to hug and kiss strangers was reported to be declining, but she continued to approach unfamiliar adults.

KEY POINTS

- Stereotypic movement disorder involves repetitive habitual behaviors that cause impairment to the individual.

- Certain genetic syndromes are associated with repetitive behaviors (e.g., skin picking in Prader–Willi syndrome, hand-flapping and wringing in Rett syndrome, hand-flapping in fragile X syndrome).

- The differential diagnosis of stereotypic movement disorder requires the clinician to rule out a number of other psychiatric conditions in which repetitive behaviors are core features.

- Stereotypies are most often observed in individuals who are institutionalized and have profound mental retardation, and to some degree in people who live in the community and have moderate mental retardation, as well as autism.

- Repetitive or habitual behaviors may be associated with an underlying condition, such as a sensory impairment or developmental disorder, unrecognized medical or neurologic condition, the side-effect of a medication, or a psychiatric disorder.

- Behavior therapy is the mainstay in the treatment for children with habit behaviors.

- Attachment disorders are the psychological result of negative experiences with caregivers, usually since infancy, that disrupt the exclusive and unique relationship between children and their primary caregiver(s).

- Reactive attachment disorder requires etiologic factors, such as gross deprivation of care or successive multiple caregivers, for diagnosis.

- In inhibited RAD, the child does not initiate and respond to social interactions in a developmentally appropriate manner. In disinhibited RAD, the child participates in diffuse attachments, indiscriminate sociability, and excessive familiarity with strangers.

- There are no solid empirical data about successful treatment of RAD, and managing the disorder is a long-term challenge that can be demanding for parents and caregivers.

Further Reading

American Academy of Child and Adolescent Psychiatry (2005) Practice parameter for the assessment and treatment of children with reactive attachment disorder of infancy and early childhood. *Journal of American Academy of Child and Adolescent Psychiatry*, **44**, 1206–1219.

Rapp, J.T. and Vollmer, T.R. (2005a) Stereotypy I: a review of behavioral assessment and treatment. *Research in Developmental Disabilities*, **26** (6), 527–547.

Rapp, J.T. and Vollmer, T.R. (2005b) Stereotypy II: a review of neurobiological interpretations and suggestions for an integration with behavioral methods. *Research in Developmental Disabilities*, **26** (6), 548–564.

Adjustment Disorder

21.1 Introduction

Adjustment disorder (AD) is considered one of the subthreshold disorders, which are less well defined and share characteristics of other diagnostic groups. Subthreshold disorders fall between defined disorders and problem level (V Code) diagnosis. Because of insufficient behavioral criteria for patients with AD, diagnostic reliability and validity of this disorder remain problematic. This chapter discusses AD in its various manifestations, in addition to its epidemiology and treatment.

21.2 Diagnostic criteria

DSM-IV-TR states that the essential feature of adjustment disorder is the development of clinically significant emotional or behavioral symptoms in response to an identifiable psychosocial stressor. The symptoms must develop within 3 months after the onset of the stressor. The clinical significance of the reaction is indicated either by marked distress that is in excess of what would be expected given the nature of the stressor or by significant impairment in social or occupational (academic) functioning. This category should not be used if the emotional and cognitive disturbances meet the criteria for *another* specific Axis I disorder (e.g., a specific anxiety or mood disorder) or are merely an exacerbation of a pre-existing Axis I or Axis II disorder. Adjustmnet disorder may be diagnosed if other Axis I or II disorders are present, but do not account for the pattern of symptoms that have occurred in response to the stressor. The diagnosis of AD does not apply when the symptoms represent bereavement (criterion D). By definition, AD must resolve within 6 months of termination of the stressor or its consequences. However, the symptoms may persist for a prolonged period (i.e., longer than 6 months) if they occur in response to a chronic stressor (e.g., a chronic, disabling general medical condition) or to a stressor that has enduring consequences (e.g., the financial and emotional difficulties resulting from a divorce).

Each of the diagnostic constructs required for the diagnosis of AD is difficult to assess and measure: (1) the stressor, (2) the maladaptive reaction to the stressor, and (3) the time and relationship between the stressor and the psychological response. None of these three components has been operationalized.

Adjustment disorder is described as being a maladaptive response to a psychosocial stressor, but there are no specific symptoms of AD. The nature of the symptomatology is described by a variety of possible "subtypes" (Table 21.1).

Disorders that do not fulfill the criteria for a specific mental disorder may be accorded a lesser interest by mental-health care workers, research institutes, and third-party payers, even though they present with serious (or incipient) symptoms that require intervention or treatment. However, attention to less severe mental symptoms (and psychiatric morbidity) may forestall the evolution to

Fundamentals of Psychiatry, First Edition. Allan Tasman and Wanda K. Mohr.
© 2011 John Wiley & Sons, Ltd. Published 2011 by John Wiley & Sons, Ltd.
This chapter is based on Chapter 81 (James J. Strain, Kim Klipstein, Jeffrey H. Newcorn) of *Psychiatry, Third Edition*

Table 21-1   Subtypes of adjustment disorder (AD)

Subtype	Symptomatology
With depressed mood	Symptoms are that of a minor depression
With anxious mood	Symptoms of anxiety dominate the clinical picture
With mixed anxiety and depressed mood	Symptoms are a combination of depression and anxiety
With disturbance of conduct	Symptoms are demonstrated in behaviors that break societal norms or violate the rights of others
With mixed disturbance of emotions and conduct	Symptoms include combined affective and behavioral characteristics of AD with mixed emotional features and AD with disturbance of conduct
AD not otherwise specified	This residual diagnosis is used when a maladaptive reaction that is not classified under other ADs occurs in response to stress

more serious disorders and allow remediation before relationships, work, and functioning are so impaired that they are disrupted or permanently impaired.

With respect to course, most studies point to a benign prognosis for the AD. But it is important to realize that the risk of serious morbidity and mortality still exists. Several recent studies investigating the association between suicide and AD have underscored the importance of monitoring patients closely for suicidality, especially in younger populations.

21.3 Epidemiology

Adjustment disorder has principally been studied in clinical samples. Epidemiologic data in adults are not available. The AD diagnosis was not included in the Epidemiologic Catchment Area Study conducted in five disparate sites throughout the United States, and there are only a few studies in children and adolescents. The prevalence of AD in children and adolescents may be somewhat higher than it is in adults, but varies considerably according to the population studied.

Adjustment disorder is thought to be common, although few studies support this assertion. Some studies suggest rates as high as 22.6% in clinical patient populations, with depressed mood being the most common subtype.

21.4 Etiology

By definition, adjustment disorders are stress-related phenomena in which a psychosocial stressor results in the development of maladaptive states and psychiatric symptoms. The condition is presumed to be a transitory reaction; symptoms recede when the stressor is removed or a new state of adaptation is defined. There are also other stress-related disorders in DSM-IV-TR, such as posttraumatic and acute stress disorders whose stress reactions follow a disaster or cataclysmic personal event (see Chapter 15). These stress disorders are among the few conditions in DSM-IV-TR, along with substance-induced disorders and mental disorders due to a general medical condition, with a *known cause* and for which the etiological agent is *essential* to establishing the diagnosis. The relationship between stress and the occurrence of a psychiatric disorder is both complex and uncertain, which has caused many to question the theoretical basis of AD.

There may be multiple stressors, insidious or chronic, as opposed to discrete events. Furthermore, relatively minor precipitating events may generate a disturbance in an individual who has previously been sensitized to stress. Proper use of the AD diagnosis also requires a careful understanding of the timing of the stressor and the subsequent emotional or behavioral symptoms.

21.5 Treatments

There are few reported randomized controlled trials with regard to the psychologic, social, or pharmacologic treatment of AD, so the choice of intervention remains a clinical decision. With no evidence from randomized controlled trials, the treatment recommendations for the AD remain based on *consensus* rather than evidence. However, there has not been an official consensus conference on the optimal way to treat this disorder.

There are two clinical empirical approaches to treatment. One is based on the understanding that this disorder emanates from a psychological reaction to a stressor. The stressor needs to be identified, described, and shared with the patient; plans must be made to mitigate it, if possible. The abnormal response may be attenuated if the stressor can be eliminated or reduced. For example, in the medically ill, the most common stressor is the medical illness itself; and the AD may remit when the medical illness improves or a new level of adaptation is reached. The other approach to treatment is to provide intervention for the symptomatic presentation, despite the fact that it does not reach threshold level for a specific disorder, on the premise that it is associated with impairment and that treatments that are effective for more pronounced presentations of similar pathology are likely to be effective. This may include psychotherapy, pharmacotherapy, or a combination of the two.

Clinical Vignette

Mrs K, a 35-year-old married woman and mother of three children, was desperate when she learned she had cancer and would need a mastectomy followed by chemotherapy and radiation. She was convinced that she would not recover, that her body would be forever distorted and ugly, that her husband would no longer find her attractive, and that her children would be ashamed of her baldness and the fact that she had cancer. She wondered whether anyone would ever want to touch her again. Because her mother and sister had also experienced breast cancer, Mrs K felt she was fated to an empty future.

Despite several sessions dealing with her feelings, the patient's dysphoria remained profound. It was decided to add antidepressant medication (fluoxetine 20 mg/day) to her psychotherapy to decrease the continuing unpleasant symptoms. Two weeks later, Mrs K reported that she was feeling less despondent and less concerned about the future and that she had a desire to start resuming her former activities with her family. As she came to terms with the overwhelming stressor and, assisted with antidepressant agents, her depressed mood improved, more adequate coping strategies to handle her serious medical illness were mobilized.

Although it is uncommon to use psychotropic medication for the majority of the adjustment disorderss, this clinical vignette illustrates the effective use of antidepressant therapy in a patient who was not responding to counseling and psychotherapy; she never had symptoms that met the DSM-IV-TR criteria for a major depressive disorder. It has been found that the addition of a psychotropic medication in AD, on the basis of the mood disturbance, may assist those patients who continue to experience disordered mood and adjustment to the stressor despite treatment with verbal therapies. The antidepressant medications have also been found helpful in the terminally ill who exhibit AD with depressed mood and who have not responded to counseling alone.

KEY POINTS

- Adjustment disorder is considered one of the subthreshold disorders, which are less well defined and share characteristics of other diagnostic groups.

- The essential feature of AD is the development of clinically significant emotional or behavioral symptoms in response to an identifiable psychosocial stressor, but there are no *specific* symptoms of AD.

- The symptomatology of AD is described by a variety of possible subtypes that include: AD with depressed mood; AD with anxious mood; AD with mixed anxiety and depressed mood; AD with disturbances of conduct; AD with mixed disturbance of emotions and conduct; and AD not otherwise specified.

- Treatment of AD includes identification and mitigation of the stressor and providing intervention for the symptomatic presentation which may include psychotherapy, pharmacotherapy, or a combination of the two.

Further Reading

Araoz, D.L. and Carrese, M.A. (1996) *Solution Oriented Brief Therapy for Adjustment Disorders: A Guide for Providers Under Managed Care*, Taylor & Francis, New York.

22 Impulse Control Disorders

22.1 Introduction

The disorders in this chapter share the feature of impulse dyscontrol despite their being dissimilar in behavioral expressions. Individuals who experience such dyscontrol are overwhelmed by the urge to commit certain acts that are often apparently illogical or harmful. These conditions include intermittent explosive disorder (failure to resist aggressive impulses), kleptomania (failure to resist urges to steal items), pyromania (failure to resist urges to set fires), pathological gambling (failure to resist urges to gamble), and trichotillomania (failure to resist urges to pull one's hair).

Behaviors characteristic of these disorders may be prominent in individuals as symptoms of another mental disorder. If these symptoms progress to such a point that they occur in distinct, frequent episodes and begin to interfere with the person's normal functioning, they may then be classified as a distinct impulse control disorder (ICD).

In DSM-IV-TR there are also a number of other disorders that are not included as a distinct category but are categorized as ICDs "not otherwise specified." These include sexual compulsions (impulsive–compulsive sexual behavior), compulsive shopping (impulsive–compulsive buying disorder), skin-picking (impulsive–compulsive psychogenic excoriation), and internet addiction (impulsive–compulsive computer usage disorder). These disorders, some of which may not be included in the next version of the DSM, are unique in that they share features of both impulsivity and compulsivity and might be labeled as ICDs. Patients with these disorders engage in the behavior to increase arousal. However, there is a compulsive component in which the patient continues to engage in the behavior to decrease dysphoria.

Because of the limited body of systematically collected data, the following sections largely reflect accumulated clinical experience. Therefore, the clinician should be particularly careful to consider the exigencies of individual patients in applying treatment recommendations.

22.2 Impulsivity

The trait of impulsivity has been the subject of ongoing interest in psychiatry and the very concept is still in flux. Impulsivity is a defining characteristic of many psychiatric illnesses, even those not classified as ICDs. Examples of these are borderline personality disorder, conduct disorder, binge-eating disorder, among many others.

Impulsivity is the failure to resist an impulse, drive, or temptation that is potentially harmful to oneself or others and is a common clinical problem and a core feature of human behavior. An

Fundamentals of Psychiatry, First Edition. Allan Tasman and Wanda K. Mohr.
© 2011 John Wiley & Sons, Ltd. Published 2011 by John Wiley & Sons, Ltd.
This chapter is based on Chapter 80 (Daphne Simeon, Heather Berlin) of *Psychiatry, Third Edition*

impulse is rash and lacks deliberation. It may be sudden and ephemeral, or a steady rise in tension that may reach a climax in an explosive expression of the impulse, which may result in careless actions without regard to the consequences to self or others. Impulsivity is evidenced behaviorally as an underestimated sense of harm, carelessness, extroversion, impatience, including the inability to delay gratification, and a tendency toward risk-taking and sensation-seeking. What makes an impulse pathological is the person's inability to resist it and its expression.

22.3 Intermittent explosive disorder

22.3.1 Diagnostic features

Intermittent explosive disorder (IED) is a DSM diagnosis used to describe people with pathologic impulsive aggression. Impulsive aggression, however, is not specific to IED. It is a key feature of several psychiatric disorders and and may emerge during the course of yet other psychiatric disorders. Therefore, IED as formulated in DSM-IV-TR is essentially a diagnosis of exclusion.

The individual may describe the aggressive episodes as "spells" or "attacks." The symptoms appear within minutes to hours and, regardless of the duration of the episode, may remit almost as quickly. As in other ICDs, the explosive behavior may be preceded by a sense of tension or arousal and is followed immediately by a sense of relief or release of tension.

Although not explicitly stated in the DSM-IV-TR definition of IED, impulsive aggressive behavior may have many motivations that are not meant to be included within this diagnosis. IED should not be diagnosed when the purpose of the aggression is monetary gain, vengeance, self-defense, social dominance, or expressing a political statement or when it occurs as a part of gang behavior. Typically, the aggressive behavior is ego-dystonic to individuals with IED, who feel genuinely upset, remorseful, regretful, bewildered, or embarrassed about their impulsive aggressive acts.

In one very small study, most of the subjects diagnosed with IED identified their spouse, lover, or girl/boy friend as a provocateur of their violent episodes. Only one was provoked by a stranger. For most, the reactions occurred immediately and without a noticeable prodromal period. All subjects with IED denied that they intended the outburst to occur in advance. Most subjects remained well-oriented during the outbursts, although two claimed to lose track of where they were. None lost control of urine or bowel function during the episode. Subjects reported various degrees of subjective feelings of behavioral dyscontrol. Only four felt that they completely lost control. Six had good recollection of the event afterward, eight had partial recollection, and one lost memory of the event afterward. Most IED subjects tried to help or comfort the victim afterward.

22.3.2 Epidemiology

Little is known about the epidemiology of intermittent explosive disorder. Historically it has been thought uncommon, but the National Comorbidity Survey Replication (NCS-R) study found that IED is much more common than previously thought. Lifetime and 12-month prevalence estimates of DSM-IV-defined IED were 7.3% and 3.9%, with a mean 43 lifetime attacks. IED-related injuries occurred 180 times per 100 lifetime cases. Mean age at onset was 14 years.

22.3.3 Assessment and differential diagnoses

The differential diagnosis of IED covers the differential diagnosis of impulsivity and aggressive behavior in general. The DSM-IV-TR diagnosis of IED is essentially a diagnosis of exclusion, and the clinician should evaluate and carefully rule out more common diagnoses that are associated with impulsive violence. For example, a careful history and attention to detail may help to distinguish IED from conditions such as antisocial personality disorder (ASPD) or borderline personality disorder (BPD). Patients with IED are usually genuinely distressed by their impulsive aggressive outbursts and may voluntarily seek psychiatric help to control them. In contrast, patients with ASPD do not feel true remorse for their actions and view them as a problem only insofar as they suffer their consequences, such as incarceration and fines. Although patients with BPD, like those with IED, are often distressed by their impulsive actions, the rapid development of intense and unstable transference toward the clinician during the evaluation period of patients with BPD may be helpful in distinguishing it from IED.

Other causes of episodic impulsive aggression are substance-use disorders, in particular alcohol abuse and intoxication. When the episodic impulsive aggression is associated only with intoxication, IED is ruled out. However, IED and alcohol abuse may be related, and the diagnosis of one should lead the clinician to search for the other.

Neurologic conditions such as dementias, focal frontal lesions, partial complex seizures, and post-concussion syndrome after recent head trauma may all present as episodic impulsive aggression and need to be differentiated from IED. Other neurologic causes of impulsive aggression include encephalitis, brain abscess, normal-pressure hydrocephalus, subarachnoid hemorrhage, and stroke. In these instances, the diagnosis would be personality change due to a general medical condition, aggressive type, and it may be made with a careful history and the characteristic physical and laboratory findings.

22.3.4 Comorbidity

Subjects with IED most frequently have other Axis I and II disorders. The most frequent Axis I diagnoses comorbid with IED include mood, anxiety, substance, eating, and other ICDs ranging in frequency from 7% to 89%. Such Axis I comorbidity rates raise the question of whether IED constitutes a separate disorder. However, recent data finding earlier onset of IED compared with all disorders, except for phobic-type anxiety disorders, suggest that IED is not secondary to these other disorders. Individuals with IED may have comorbid mood disorders. Although the diagnosis of a manic episode excludes IED, the evidence for serotonergic abnormalities in both major depressive disorder and ICDs supports the clinical observation that impulsive aggression may be increased in depressed patients, leading ultimately to completed suicide.

22.3.5 Course

Limited research is available concerning the age at onset and natural course of IED. But, according to DSM IV-TR and anecdotal case reports, the onset appears to be from childhood to the early twenties, and may be abrupt and without a prodromal period. The age of onset and course of IED distinguish it as separate from its comorbid diagnoses. The course of IED is variable, with an episodic course in some and a more chronic course in others. IED may persist well into middle life unless treated successfully. In some cases, it may decrease in severity or remit completely with old age.

Episodes typically last less than 30 minutes and involve one or a combination of physical assault, verbal assault, or destruction of property. If there is provocation it is usually from a known person and is seemingly minor in nature. Many individuals frequently have minor aggressive episodes in the interim between severely aggressive/destructive episodes. Considerable distress, social, financial, occupational, or legal or impairments typically result from these episodes.

22.3.6 Treatments

22.3.6.1 Psychological treatments

Few systematic data are available on response to treatment. Some of the recommended treatment approaches to IED are based on treatment studies of impulsivity and aggression in the setting of other mental disorders and general medical conditions. Thus, no standard regimen for the treatment of IED can currently be recommended. Both psychological and somatic therapies have been employed. A prerequisite for both modalities is the willingness of the individual to acknowledge some responsibility for the behavior and participate in attempts to control it.

The major psychotherapeutic task of treating this population involves teaching them how to recognize their own feeling states and especially the affective state of rage. Lack of awareness of their own mounting anger is presumed to lead to the buildup of intolerable rage that is then discharged suddenly and inappropriately in a temper outburst. Patients are therefore taught how to first recognize and then verbalize their anger appropriately. In addition, during the course of insight-oriented psychotherapy, they are encouraged to identify and express the fantasies surrounding their rage. Group psychotherapy for temper-prone patients has also been described. The cognitive–behavioral model of psychological treatment, or versions of CBT such as dialectic behavior therapy, may be usefully applied to problems with anger and rage management.

22.3.6.2 Somatic treatments

Several classes of medications have been used to treat IED and impulsive aggression in the context of other disorders. These included beta-blockers (propranolol and metoprolol), anticonvulsants (carbamazepine and valproic acid), lithium, antidepressants (tricyclic antidepressants and serotonin-reuptake inhibitors), and antianxiety agents (lorazepam, alprazolam, and buspirone).

A substantial body of evidence supports the use of propranolol, often in high doses for impulsive aggression in patients with chronic psychotic disorders and mental retardation. Lithium has been shown to have antiaggressive properties and may be used to control temper outbursts. In patients with comorbid major depressive disorder, OCD, or Cluster B and C personality disorders (see Chapter 19), SSRIs may be useful. Overall, in the absence of more controlled clinical trials, the best approach may be to tailor the psychopharmacologic agent to coexisting psychiatric comorbidity. In the absence of comorbid disorders, carbamazepine, titrated to antiepileptic blood levels, may be used.

22.4 Kleptomania

22.4.1 Diagnosis and diagnostic features

Kleptomania shares with all other ICDs the recurrent failure to resist impulses. Unfortunately, in the absence of epidemiologic studies, little is known about kleptomania. Clinical case series and case reports are limited. Family, neurobiologic, and genetic investigations are not available. There are no established treatments of choice. The reader of this secton must keep that in mind.

Kleptomania was designated a psychiatric disorder in 1980. It is currently classified in DSM-IV-TR as an ICD but is still poorly understood. The diagnostic criterion, which focuses on the senselessness of the items stolen, has often been considered the criterion that distinguishes kleptomania patients from ordinary shoplifters, but interpretation of this criterion is controversial. Patients with kleptomania may in fact desire the items they steal and be able to use them, but do not need them. This may be particularly the case with kleptomania patients who hoard items, for which multiple versions of the same item are usually not needed, but the item itself may be desired and may be of practical use to the patient. People with kleptomania often report amnesia surrounding the shoplifting act, and deny feelings of tension or arousal prior to shoplifting and feelings of pleasure or relief after the thefts. They often recall entering and leaving a store but have no memory of events in the store, including the theft. Others, who are not amnestic for the thefts, describe shoplifting as"automatic" or "a habit," and may also deny feelings of tension prior to a theft or pleasure after the act, although they report an inability to control their shoplifting. Some report that they felt tension and pleasure when they started stealing, but it became a "habit" over time. Some speculate that patients who are amnestic for shoplifting or who do so "out of habit" represent two subtypes of kleptomania.

At presentation, the typical patient suffering from kleptomania is a 35-year-old woman who has been stealing for about 15 years and may not mention kleptomania as the presenting complaint or in the initial history. The patient may complain instead of anxiety, depression, lability, dysphoria, or manifestations of character pathology. There is often a history of a tumultuous childhood and poor parenting, and in addition acute stressors may be present, such as marital or sexual conflicts. The patient experiences the urge to steal as irresistible, and the thefts are commonly associated with a thrill, a "high," a sense of relief, or gratification. Generally, the behavior has been hard to control and has often gone undetected by others. The kleptomania may be restricted to specific settings or types of object, and the patient may or may not be able to describe rationales for these preferences. Quite often, the objects taken are of inherently little financial value, or have meaningless financial value relative to the income of the person who has taken the object. Moreover, the object may never actually be used. These factors often help distinguish criminal theft from kleptomania. The theft is followed by feelings of guilt or shame and, sometimes, attempts at atonement.

The frequency of stealing episodes may greatly fluctuate in concordance with the degree of depression, anxiety, or stress. There may be periods of complete abstinence. The patient may have a past history of psychiatric treatments including hospitalizations or of arrests and convictions.

22.4.2 Epidemiology

Kleptomania prevalence can be estimated only grossly and indirectly. In a study of shoplifters, the estimate ranged from 0% to 24%. Kleptomania occurs transculturally and has been described in various Western and Eastern cultures.

The frequency of kleptomania may be indirectly extrapolated from incidence rates of kleptomania in comorbid disorders with known prevalence, like bulimia nervosa. Such speculations suggest at least a 0.6% prevalence of kleptomania in the general population. However, given that people who shoplift are often not caught, this is almost certainly an underestimate. Also, the shame and embarrassment associated with stealing prevents most people from voluntarily reporting klepto-mania symptoms.

22.4.3 Course

Kleptomania may begin in childhood, adolescence, or adulthood, and sometimes in late adulthood. However, most patients have an onset of symptoms before the age of 21 years, that is, by late adolescence. The disorder appears to be chronic, but with varying intensity. The majority of patients may eventually be apprehended for stealing once or more, and a minority may even be imprisoned; usually these repercussions do not result in more than a temporary remission of the behavior. People with kleptomania may also have extensive histories of psychiatric treatments, including hospitalization for other conditions, most commonly depression or eating disorders. Because of the unavailability of longitudinal studies, the prognosis is unknown. However, it appears that without treatment the behavior may be likely to persist for decades, sometimes with significant associated morbidity, despite multiple convictions for shoplifting (arrest or imprisonment), with transient periods of remission.

Three typical courses have been described: sporadic with brief episodes and long periods of remission; episodic with protracted periods of stealing and periods of remission; and chronic with varying intensity.

22.4.4 Etiology and pathophysiology

The etiology of kleptomania is essentially unknown, although various models have been proposed in an effort to conceptualize the disorder. At present, the available empirical data are insufficient to substantiate any of these models.

22.4.5 Assessment

Making a diagnosis of kleptomania is not a complicated matter. However, kleptomania may frequently go undetected because the patient may not mention it spontaneously and the clinician may fail to inquire about it as part of the routine history. The index of suspicion should rise in the presence of commonly associated symptoms such as chronic depression, other impulsive or compulsive behaviors, tumultuous relationships, or unexplained legal troubles. A cursory review of compulsivity and impulsivity, citing multiple examples for patients, should be a part of any thorough and complete psychiatric evaluation.

22.4.6 Differential diagnosis

It is important to do a careful differential diagnosis and pay attention to the various exclusion criteria before diagnosing theft as kleptomania. Possible diagnoses of sociopathy, mania, or psychosis should be carefully considered. The clinician should inquire about the affective state of the patient during the episodes, the presence of delusions or hallucinations associated with the occurrence of the behavior, and the motivation behind the behavior. Atypical presentations should raise a greater suspicion of an organic etiology for which a medical evaluation would then be indicated. Medical conditions that have been associated with kleptomania include cortical atrophy, dementia, intra-cranial mass lesions, encephalitis, normal-pressure hydrocephalus, benzodiazepine withdrawal, and temporal-lobe epilepsy. A complete evaluation when such suspicions are present includes a physical and neurologic examination, general serum chemistry and hematologic panels, and an EEG with temporal leads or computed tomography of the brain.

22.4.7 Comorbidity

High rates of other psychiatric disorders found in patients with kleptomania have sparked debate over the proper characterization of this disorder. Among those with kleptomania who present for treatment, there is a high incidence of comorbid mood, anxiety, and eating disorders, when compared with rates in the general population.

22.4.8 Treatments

The acute treatment of kleptomania has not been, to date, systematically investigated. Recommendations are based on retrospective reviews, case reports, and small case series. Maintenance treatment for kleptomania has not been investigated either, and only anecdotal data exist for patients who have been followed for significant periods after initial remission. No treatments have been systematically shown to be effective. In general, it appears that thymoleptic medications and behavioral therapy may be the most efficacious treatments for the short term, while long-term psychodynamic psychotherapy may be indicated and have good results for selected patients.

22.4.8.1 Somatic treatments

No medication is currently approved by the US Food and Drug Administration for treating kleptomania. So, it is important to inform patients of "off-label" uses of medications for this disorder. The findings from case reports have not been consistent. Seven cases of fluoxetine, three of imipramine, two of lithium as monotherapy, two of lithium augmentation, four of tranylcypromine, and one of carbamazepine combined with clomipramine all failed to reduce kleptomania symptoms. Some evidence suggests that selective serotonin-reuptake inhibitors may even induce kleptomania symptoms. One case series found that kleptomania symptoms respond to topiramate.

Opioid antagonists such as naltrexone may be effective in reducing both the urges to shoplift and shoplifting behavior, by reducing the "thrill" associated with shoplifting and thus preventing the positive reinforcement of the behavior.

22.4.8.2 Psychosocial treatments

Formal studies of psychosocial interventions for kleptomania have not been performed. However, a number of clinical reports have supported behavioral therapy. Different behavioral techniques have been employed with some success, including aversive conditioning, systematic desensitization, covert sensitization, and behavior modification.

22.5 Pyromania and fire-setting behavior

22.5.1 Diagnostic features

The primary characteristics of pyromania are recurrent, deliberate fire-setting, the experience of tension or affective arousal before the fire-setting, an attraction or fascination with fire and its contexts, and a feeling of gratification or relief associated with the fire-setting or its aftermath. True pyromania is present in only a small subset of fire-setters. The diagnosis of pyromania emphasizes the affective arousal, thrill, or tension preceding the act, as well as the feeling of tension relief or pleasure in witnessing the outcome. This is useful in distinguishing between pyromania and fire-setting elicited by other motives (financial gain, concealment of other crimes, political, arson related to other mental illness, revenge, attention-seeking, erotic pleasure, or a component of conduct disorder).

22.5.2 Epidemiology

Most epidemiologic studies have not directly focused on pyromania but instead on various populations of arsonists or fire-setters. Most studies suggest that true pyromania is rare and reveal a preponderance of males with a history of fire fascination. Men greatly outnumber women with the disorder.

22.5.3 Course

Pyromania onset has been reported to occur as early as age 3 years, but it may initially present in adulthood. Because of the legal implications of fire-setting, individuals may not admit previous events, which may result in biased perceptions of the common age at onset.

22.5.4 Comorbidity

Limited data are available regarding individuals with pyromania. Reported data of comorbid diagnoses are generally derived from forensic samples and do not distinguish between criminally motivated and compulsive fire-setters. Fire-setting behavior may be associated with other mental conditions such as mental retardation, conduct disorder, alcohol and other substance use disorders, personality disorders, and schizophrenia. In most cases, fire-setting behavior is not directly related to pyromania.

22.5.5 Course

According to DSM-IV-TR, there are insufficient data to establish a typical age at onset of pyromania and to predict the longitudinal course. However, the impulsive nature of the disorder suggests a repetitive pattern. Again, because legal consequences may occur, the individual may be motivated to represent the index episode as a unique event. Fire-setting for non-psychiatric reasons may be more likely to be a single event. In individuals with pyromania, fire-setting incidents are episodic and may wax and wane in frequency. Studies indicate that the recidivism rate for fire-setters is up to 28%.

22.5.6 Differential diagnosis

Other causes of fire-setting must be ruled out. Fire-setting behavior may be motivated by circumstances unrelated to mental disorders. Such motivations include profit, crime concealment, revenge, vandalism, and political statement or action. Furthermore, fire-setting may be a part of ritual, cultural, or religious practices in some cultures. Fire-setting may occur in the presence of other mental disorders. A diagnosis of fire-setting is not made when the behavior occurs as part of conduct disorder, antisocial personality disorder, or a manic episode or if it occurs in response to a delusion or hallucination. The diagnosis is also not given if the individual suffers from impaired judgment associated with mental retardation, dementia, or substance intoxication.

22.5.7 Etiology and pathophysiology

Because pyromania is rare, there is little reliable scientific literature available on individuals who fit diagnostic criteria. Impulse fire-setters who are violent offenders are often dependent on alcohol and have an alcohol-dependent father. Children at risk of pyromania were more often involved than control subjects in fire-setting, threatening to set a fire, sounding a false fire alarm, or calling the fire department with a false report of fire. Thus, there may be a continuum between excessive interest in fire and "pure" pyromania.

22.5.8 Treatments

Because of the danger inherent in fire-setting, the primary goal is elimination of the behavior. The treatment literature does not distinguish between pyromania and fire-setting behavior of other causes. Much of the literature is focused on controlling fire-setting behavior in children and adolescents.

22.5.8.1 Somatic treatments

There are no reports of pharmacologic treatment of pyromania. Because fire-setting may be frequently embedded in other psychiatric illness, therapeutic attention may be directed primarily to the underlying disorder. However, the dangerous nature of fire-setting requires that the behavior be controlled. Much in the same fashion that one would seek to educate impaired patients about the functional risks associated with their symptoms – and to establish boundaries of acceptable behavior – the fire-setting behavior must be directly addressed, even if it is not a core symptom of the associated disorder.

22.5.8.2 Psychosocial treatments

Treatment for fire-setters is problematic because they frequently refuse to take responsibility for their acts, are in denial, have alcoholism, and lack insight. It has been estimated that up to 60% of childhood fire-setting is motivated by curiosity. Such behavior often responds to direct educational efforts. In children and adolescents, focus on interpersonal problems in the family and clarification of events preceding the behavior may help to control the behavior. Principles of cognitive–behavioral therapy have been also applied to childhood fire-setting. Treatments are largely behavioral or focused on intervening in family or intrapersonal stresses that may precipitate episodes of fire-setting. Behavioral treatments such as aversive therapy have helped. Other treatment methods rely on positive reinforcement with threats of punishment and stimulus satiation.

22.6 Pathological gambling

22.6.1 Diagnostic features

Pathological gambling disorder is characterized by uncontrollable gambling well beyond the point of a social or recreational activity, such that the gambling has a major disruptive effect on the gambler's life. People who are pathological gamblers may lose their life savings, and may commit crimes (stealing, embezzling, or forging checks) to get money for their "habit." Relationships and jobs may also be lost as a result. The person is often unable to control the gambling behavior, continuing to place bets or go to casinos in spite of attempts to cut back or stop. A common behavior is "chasing," which refers to betting larger sums of money or taking greater risks in order to undo or make up for previous losses. The person may also lie about gambling or engage in such antisocial behaviors as stealing, credit card fraud, check forgery, embezzling from an employer, or similar dishonest behaviors.

22.6.2 Assessment

It is not difficult to diagnose pathological gambling once one has the facts. It is much more of a challenge to elicit the facts, because the vast majority of patients with pathological gambling view their impulses as ego-syntonic and may often lie about the extent of their gambling.

People with pathological gambling may first seek help because of comorbid disorders. Given the high prevalence of addictive disorders in pathological gambling and the increased prevalence of pathological gambling in those with alcoholism and other substance abuse, an investigation of gambling patterns and their consequences is warranted for any patient who presents with a substance abuse problem. Likewise, the high rates of comorbidity with mood disorders suggest the utility of investigating gambling patterns of patients presenting with an affective episode. The spouses and significant others of patients with pathological gambling deserve special attention. Individuals with pathological gambling usually feel entitled to their behavior and often rely on their families to bail them out. As a consequence, it is often the partner of the patient with pathological gambling who first realizes the need for treatment and who bears the consequences of the disorder.

22.6.3 Epidemiology

Pathological gambling is considered to be the most common of the ICDs not elsewhere classified. The number of people whose gambling behavior meets criteria for pathological gambling in the US is estimated to be up to 6 million.

22.6.4 Etiology

There are no known biological causes of pathological gambling disorder. The incidence of pathological gambling among first-degree family members of pathological gamblers appears to be approximately 20%. Some studies have found interesting differences between compulsive gamblers and the general population on the biologic level, for example in the dopaminergic reward pathways, but none that is thought to be an actual cause of pathological gambling. Learning theories of pathological gambling have focused on the learned and conditioned aspects of gambling.

22.6.5 Comorbidity

Overall, patients with pathological gambling have high rates of comorbidity with several other psychiatric disorders and conditions. Individuals presenting for clinical treatment of pathological gambling apparently have impressive rates of comorbidity. A recent study reported 62.3% of one group of problem gamblers seeking treatment had a comorbid psychiatric disorder. The most frequent were personality disorders (42%), alcohol abuse or dependence (33.3%), adjustment disorders (17.4%), and mood disorders (8.7%). Lifetime comorbid diagnoses included alcohol abuse or dependence (34.8%), mood disorders (15.9%), and anxiety disorders (7.2%).

22.6.6 Course

The onset of pathologic gambling is usually insidious, although some may be "hooked" by their first bet. There may be years of social gambling with minimal or no impairment followed by an abrupt onset of pathologic gambling that may be precipitated by greater exposure to gambling or by a psychosocial stressor. The gambling pattern may be regular or episodic, and the course tends to be chronic. Over time, there is usually a progression in the frequency of gambling, the amounts wagered, and the preoccupation with gambling and with obtaining money with which to gamble. The urge to gamble and gambling activity generally increase during periods of stress or depression, as an attempted escape or relief.

Pathologic gambling usually begins in adolescence in men with gradual development of dependence, and may remain undiagnosed for years; they often present with a 20- to 30-year gambling history. In contrast, onset in females is usually later in life. Prior to seeking treatment, the duration of pathologicl gambling is about 3 years. Thus, as a result of the differences in onset and duration, female pathologic gamblers generally have a better prognosis than males. Females also tend to be depressed and may use gambling as an anesthetic.

Psychiatric disorders such as major depression and alcohol or substance abuse and dependence may develop from, or be exacerbated by, pathologic gambling. There is also a mortality risk associated with the disorder: estimates of suicide attempts range from 17% to 24%.

22.6.7 Differential diagnosis

The differential diagnosis of pathological gambling is relatively straightforward. It should be differentiated from professional gambling, social gambling, and a manic episode.

22.6.8 Treatments

The goals of treatment are the achievement of abstinence from gambling, rehabilitation of the damaged family and work roles and relationships, treatment of comorbid disorders, and relapse prevention. This approach echoes the goals of treatment of an individual with substance dependence. No standard treatment has emerged. Despite many reports of behavioral and cognitive interventions, there are minimal data available from well-designed or clearly detailed treatment studies.

22.6.8.1 Psychosocial treatments
The most popular intervention for problem gambling is GA, a 12-step group built on the same principles as AA, which employs empathic confrontation by peers who struggle with the same impulses. Inpatient and outpatient programs have included various combinations of individual and group psychotherapy and substance-use treatment. Behavioral, cognitive, and combined cogniti-ve–behavioral methods have been used. Aversion therapy has been employed to reach the goal of total abstinence of gambling, as have behavior monitoring, contingency management, contingency contracting, covert sensitization, systematic desensitization, image desensitization, *in vivo* expo-sure, image relaxation, psychoeducation, cognitive restructuring, and teaching problem-solving skills.

22.6.8.2 Somatic treatments
Although research reports of the pharmacologic treatment of pathologic gambling have reported some efficacy, there are still insufficient data to come to any conclusions about the utility of medication. Treatment studies have demonstrated some promising results with the use of selective serotonin-reuptake inhibitors.

22.7 Trichotillomania

22.7.1 Diagnostic features

The essential feature of trichotillomania is the recurrent failure to resist impulses to pull out one's own hair. Resulting hair loss may range in severity from negligible to severe (complete baldness and involving multiple sites on the scalp or body). Individuals with this condition do not want to engage in the behavior, but attempts to resist the urge result in great tension. Thus, hair-pulling is motivated by a desire to reduce this dysphoric state. In some cases, the hair-pulling results in a pleasurable sensation, in addition to the relief of tension. Tension may precede the act or may occur when attempting to stop. Distress over the symptom and the resultant hair loss may be severe.

Typically, the person complaining of unwanted hair-pulling is a young adult or parent of a child who has been seen pulling out hair. Hair-pulling tends to occur in small bursts that may last minutes to hours. Episodes may occur once or many times each day. Hairs are pulled out individually and may be pulled out rapidly and indiscriminately. Often, however, the hand of the individual may roam the afflicted area of scalp or body, searching for a shaft of hair that may feel particularly coarse or thick. Satisfaction with having pulled out a complete hair (shaft and root) is often expressed. Occasionally the experience of hair-pulling is described as pleasurable. Some experience an itch-like sensation in the scalp that is eased by the act of pulling. The person may then toss away the hair shaft or inspect it. A substantial number of people then chew or consume the hair (trichophagia).

Hair-pulling is most commonly limited to the eyebrows and eyelashes. The scalp is the next most frequently afflicted site. However, hairs in any location of the body may be the focus of hair-pulling urges.

Anxiety is almost always associated with the act. Such anxiety may occur in advance of the hair-pulling behavior. A state of tension may occur spontaneously, driving the person to pull out hair in an attempt to reduce dysphoric feelings. Circumstances that seem to predispose to episodes include both states of stress and, paradoxically, moments of relaxation. The distress that usually accompanies trichotillomania varies in severity.

Concerns tend to focus on the social and vocational consequences of the behavior. Themes of worry include fear of exposure, feeling that "something is wrong with me," anxiety about intimate relationships, and sometimes inability to pursue a vocation.

22.7.2 Course

The age at onset typically ranges from early childhood to young adulthood. Peak ages at presentation may be bimodal, with an earlier peak about age 5 to 8 years among children in whom it has a self-limited course, whereas among patients who present to clinicians in adulthood the mean age at onset is approximately 13 years. Initial onset after young adulthood seems to be uncommon. There have been reports of onset as early as 14 months of age and as late as 61 years. Tricotillomania in adolescents and adults typically follows a chronic course, involves multiple hair sites, and frequent associated comorbidities.

22.7.3 Assessment

In general, the diagnosis of trichotillomania is not complicated. The essential symptom – recurrently pulling out hair in response to unwanted urges – is easily described by patients. When patients acknowledge the behavior and areas of patchy hair loss are evident, the diagnosis is not usually in doubt. Problems in diagnosis may arise when the diagnosis is suspected but the patient denies it. Such denial may occur in younger individuals and some adults. When the problem is suspected but denied by the patient, a skin biopsy from the affected area may aid in making the diagnosis.

22.7.4 Differential diagnosis

Among individuals presenting with alopecia who complain of hair-pulling urges, the diagnosis is not usually in doubt. When patients deny hair-pulling, dermatologic causes of alopecia should be considered. These include alopecia areata, male-pattern hair loss, chronic discoid lupus erythematosus, lichen planopilaris, folliculitis decalvans, pseudopelade, and alopecia mucinosa. Trichotillomania is not diagnosed when hair-pulling occurs in response to a delusion or hallucination.

22.7.5 Etiology

The etiology of trichotillomania is unknown, but the phenomenologic similarities between trichotillomania and OCD have prompted speculations that the pathophysiology of the two conditions may be related.

22.7.6 Comorbidities

Individuals with trichotillomania have increased risk for mood disorders (major depressive disorder, dysthymic disorder) and anxiety symptoms. The frequency of specific anxiety disorders (e.g., generalized anxiety and panic disorders, and OCD) may be increased as well.

22.7.7 Treatments

Treatments typically occur in an outpatient setting. Eradication of hair-pulling behavior is the general focus. Distress, avoidant behaviors, and cosmetic impairment are secondary to the hair-pulling and would be likely to remit if it is controlled.

22.7.7.1 Psychosocial treatments

Various behavioral techniques have been tried. The most successful, habit reversal, is based on designing competitive behaviors that should inhibit the hair-pulling behavior. For example, if hair-pulling requires raising the arm to the scalp and contracting the muscles of the hand to grasp a hair, the behaviorist may design a behavioral program in which the patient is taught to lower the arm and extend the muscles of the hand. As with most behavioral techniques, these interventions are most successful when the patient is strongly motivated and adherent to treatment. Also, the treating clinician should be experienced in the use of such techniques. If necessary, a referral should be made to an experienced individual.

22.7.7.2 Somatic treatments

The literature on somatic treatments is generally made up of case studies. In general, knowledge about trichotillomania treatments is limited by small sample sizes, lack of specificity regarding sample characteristics, nonrandom assignment to treatment, dearth of long-term follow-up data, exclusive reliance on patient self-report measures, and lack of information regarding rates of treatment refusal and dropout. A variety of medications have been used. Initial reports demonstrated the apparent benefits of fluoxetine and clomipramine. Clomipramine was found to be superior to desipramine. Fluoxetine was reported beneficial in open treatment. Although reports for more than 60 patients have subsequently added support for the use of these medications, the two double-blind studies in which fluoxetine has been compared with placebo did not demonstrate any improvement compared to placebo.

Clinical Vignette

Mr A, a 42-year-old separated man, worked as a bank clerk. He sought outpatient psychiatric treatment after an angry outburst that led to the breakdown of his second marriage: his wife issued an order of protection against him after a rage attack in which he slapped her across the face and destroyed most of the kitchen and living room furniture. His rage was triggered by his wife's decision to buy a new microwave oven without consulting him. Mr A, who remembered the episode clearly and with remorse, said that he realized how angry he was only after he actually struck at his wife.

During the course of his evaluation, Mr A became tearful and admitted to several similar episodes during the course of his current and previous marriages. These episodes were rare, occurring once or twice a year. They were brief and apparently unpredictable and resulted in his separation from his first wife. Except during those episodes, he was a pleasant, rather timid man who deferred to his wife in most important decisions. There was no history suggestive of antisocial or borderline personality disorder.

Mr A, who described himself as a shy, withdrawn child, gave a history of head trauma at the age of 12 years, while he was ice-skating, with loss of consciousness for 10 minutes. Other than this, his medical history was normal. There were no neurologic or behavioral sequelae. Mr A also described prolonged physical abuse by his alcoholic father. Mr A himself denied a history of substance abuse, involvement with the criminal justice system, or prior psychiatric treatment. He denied a history of manic and depressive episodes. He had few friends and was not popular at his job. Although he had never lost his temper there, he believed that his boss and coworkers could sense his "stress" while dealing with clients.

Mr A's physical and neurological examination was notable only for mild bilateral difficulty with rapid alternating hand movements. Except for his tearfulness while describing the episode, his Mental Status Examination was unremarkable. Results of routine laboratory blood work and computed tomography of the head were within normal limits. An EEG was notable for diffuse slowing without an epileptic focus.

Mr A's treatment was started with carbamazepine at standard dosage. He also received a short course of psychotherapy that focused on recognizing his anger and venting it appropriately, on his memories of childhood physical abuse, and on his current sense of himself as a helpless person who was being controlled by his wife and boss. In addition, it was recommended that he transfer to a position that would not involve contact with clients.

During a 2-year follow-up, Mr A had no further rage episodes. He continued to have few friends but was able to maintain a long-term relationship with a woman he was planning to marry.

KEY POINTS

- Impulse control disorders include intermittent explosive disorder, kleptomania, pathological gambling, pyromania, and trichotillomania.

- The onset of these disorders usually occurs between the ages of 7 and 15 years and they are understudied.

- Impulsivity is the key feature of these disorders.

- Impulse control disorders may be part of the obsessive–compulsive disorder spectrum.

- Little empirical literature exists regarding their treatment and information regarding their treatment is often derived from case reports.

Further Reading

Franklin, M.E. and Tolin, D.F. (2007) *Treating Trichotillomania*, Springer-Verlag, New York.
Hollander, H. and Stein, D.J. (2005) *Clinical Manual of Impulse Control Disorders*, American Psychiatric Publishing, Washington, DC.
Libal, A., Johnson, M.A., and Esherick, D. (2003) *Drug Therapy and Impulse-Control Disorders*, Mason Crest Publishers, Broomall, PA.

23   Mental Disorders due to a Medical Condition

23.1 Introduction

In evaluating patients with mental symptoms of any sort, one of the first questions to ask is whether those symptoms are occurring as part of a primary psychiatric disorder or are caused by a general medical condition. This chapter discusses disorders characterized by mental symptoms that occur due to the direct physiologic effect of a general medical condition.

23.2 Clinical considerations

The first step in a complete assessment is to review the history, physical examination, and laboratory tests. The thorough clinician not only looks for a temporal correlation (e.g., the onset of a psychosis shortly after starting or increasing the dose of a medication), but also keeps in mind well-documented associations between certain mental symptoms (e.g., depression) and certain general medical conditions (e.g., Cushing's syndrome). If it appears, at this point, that the mental symptoms could indeed be occurring secondary to a medical condition, the next step involves determining whether or not these symptoms could be better accounted for by a primary psychiatric disorder.

In cases where the mental symptoms do not present an emergency, one looks to whether the underlying medical condition is treatable. If the underlying condition is not treatable, one generally proceeds directly to symptomatic treatment. In cases where the underlying condition is treatable, one must make a judgment as to whether, with treatment of the medical condition, the mental symptoms will resolve at a clinically acceptable rate. For example, in the case of a patient with anxiety due to hyperthyroidism who has just begun treatment with an antithyroid drug, the decision as to whether to offer a benzodiazepine as symptomatic treatment for the anxiety depends not only on the severity and tolerability of the anxiety, but also on the expected time required for the antithyroid drug to resolve the hyperthyroidism; here, clearly, considerable clinical judgment is required.

23.3 Psychotic disorders

23.3.1 Clinical patterns

A psychotic disorder due to a general medical condition is characterized clinically by hallucinations or delusions occurring in a clear sensorium, without any associated decrement in intellectual abilities. Furthermore, one must be able to demonstrate, by history, physical examination, or laboratory findings, that the psychosis is occurring on the basis of a general medical disorder.

Fundamentals of Psychiatry, First Edition. Allan Tasman and Wanda K. Mohr.
© 2011 John Wiley & Sons, Ltd. Published 2011 by John Wiley & Sons, Ltd.
This chapter is based on Chapter 52 (David P. Moore) of *Psychiatry, Third Edition*

Box 23.1 lists the various secondary causes of psychosis, dividing them into those occurring *secondary to precipitants* (e.g., medications), those occurring *secondary to diseases with distinctive features* (e.g., the chorea of Huntington's disease), and finally a group occurring *secondary to miscellaneous causes* (e.g., cerebral tumors).

Box 23.1 Causes of Psychosis Due to a General Medical Condition.

Secondary to precipitants
Medications:
    Neuroleptics (supersensitivity psychosis)
    Dopaminergic drugs
    Disulfiram
    Sympathomimetics
    Bupropion
    Fluoxetine
    Baclofen (on discontinuation)
    Levetiracetam
    Topiramate
Other precipitants
    Postencephalitic psychosis
    Post-traumatic brain injury

Secondary to diseases with specific features
Associated with epilepsy:
    Ictal psychosis
    Postictal psychosis
    Psychosis of forced normalization
    Chronic interictal psychosis
Encephalitic onset:
    Herpes simplex encephalitis
    Encephalitis lethargica
    Infectious mononucleosis
With other specific features:
    Huntington's disease (chorea)
    Sydenham's chorea
    Chorea gravidarum
    Manganism (parkinsonism)
    Creutzfeldt–Jakob disease (myoclonus)
    Hashimoto's encephalopathy (myoclonus)
    Wilson's disease (various abnormal involuntary movements)
    AIDS
    Systemic lupus erythematosus
    Hyperthyroidism
    Hypothyroidism (cold intolerance, voice change, constipation, hair loss, myxedema)
    Cushing's syndrome
    Adrenocortical insufficiency
    Hepatic porphyria
    Spinocerebellar ataxia
    Dentatorubro-pallidoluysian atrophy
    Prader–Willi syndrome

Secondary to miscellaneous causes
Cerebral tumors
Cerebral infarction
Multiple sclerosis
Neurosyphilis
Vitamin B_{12} deficiency
Metachromatic leukodystrophy
Subacute sclerosing panencephalitis
Fahr's syndrome
Thalamic degeneration
Velo–cardio–facial syndrome

Psychosis occurring *secondary to precipitants* is perhaps the most common form of secondary psychosis. Among the various possible precipitants, substances (drugs of abuse) are perhaps the most common. These are considered in the chapters on stimulants, hallucinogens, phencyclidine, cannabis, and alcohol. After drugs of abuse, various medications are the next most common precipitants, and the most problematic are the neuroleptics themselves. It appears that, in a very small minority of patients treated chronically with neuroleptics, a "supersensitivity psychosis" (or, as it has also been called, on analogy with tardive dyskinesia, "tardive psychosis") may occur. Making such a diagnosis in the case of patients with schizophrenia may be difficult, as one may well say that any increase in psychotic symptoms, rather than evidence for a supersensitivity psychosis, may merely represent an exacerbation of the schizophrenia. In the case of patients treated with antipsychotics for other conditions (e.g., Tourette's syndrome), however, the appearance of a psychosis is far more suggestive, as it could not be accounted for on the basis of the disease for which the neuroleptic was prescribed. Of the dopaminergic drugs capable of causing a psychosis, levodopa is the most common, and although direct-acting dopamine agonists such as bromocriptine and lergotrile and pramipexole may also be at fault, they are much less likely causes than is levodopa itself. The other medications noted in Box 23.1 only very rarely cause a psychosis.

Of the encephalitides that may have a psychosis as a sequela, the most classic is encephalitis lethargica (von Economo's disease), a disease that, though no longer occurring in epidemic form, may still be seen sporadically. Other encephalitides, such as herpes simplex encephalitis, may also (albeit rarely) have a psychosis as one of their sequelae.

Of the psychoses *secondary to diseases with distinctive features*, the psychoses of epilepsy are by far the most important, and these may be ictal, postictal, or interictal. Ictal psychoses represent complex partial seizures and are immediately suggested by their exquisitely paroxysmal onset.

Postictal psychoses are typically preceded by a "flurry" of grand mal or complex partial seizures and, importantly, are separated from the last of this "flurry" of seizures by a "lucid" interval lasting from hours to days. Interictal psychoses appear in one of two forms, namely, the psychosis of forced normalization and the chronic interictal psychosis. The psychosis of forced normalization appears when anticonvulsants have not only stopped seizures but have essentially "normalized" the EEG: a disappearance of the psychosis with the resumption of seizure activity secures the diagnosis. The chronic interictal psychosis, often characterized by delusions of persecution and reference and auditory hallucinations, appears subacutely, over weeks or months, in patients with longstanding, uncontrolled grand mal or complex partial seizures.

Encephalitic psychoses are suggested by such typical "encephalitic" features as headache, lethargy, and fever. Prompt diagnosis is critical, especially in the case of herpes simplex encephalitis, given its treatability. The other specific features listed in Box 23.1 are fairly straightforward.

Of the *miscellaneous causes* capable of causing psychosis, cerebral tumors are perhaps the most important, with psychosis being noted with tumors of the frontal lobe, corpus callosum, and temporal lobe. Suggestive clinical evidence for such a cause includes prominent headache, seizures, or certain focal signs, such as aphasia. Cerebral infarction is likewise an important cause, and is suggested not only by accompanying focal signs, but also by its acute onset: infarction of the frontal lobe, temporoparietal area, and thalamus have all been implicated. Neurosyphilis should never be forgotten as a differential possibility in cases of psychosis of obscure origin. Vitamin B_{12} deficiency should be borne in mind, especially as this may present with psychosis without any evidence of spinal cord or hematologic involvement. The remaining disorders listed in Box 23.1 are extremely rare causes of psychosis.

23.3.2 Assessment

In most cases, a thorough history and physical examination will disclose evidence of the underlying cause of the psychosis. When the patient's symptomatology is atypical for one of the primary causes of psychosis (e.g., schizophrenia), yet the history and physical examination fail to disclose clear evidence for another cause, a "laboratory screen" as listed in Box 23.2 may be appropriate. Clearly, one does not order all these tests at once, but begins with those most likely to be informative, given the overall clinical picture.

Box 23.2 A "Laboratory Screen" for Secondary Psychosis.

Serum or urine drug screen
Testosterone level (reduced in anabolic steroid abusers)
Red-blood-cell mean corpuscular volume (elevated in alcoholism and many cases of B_{12} deficiency)
Liver transaminases (elevated in alcoholism)
HIV testing
FTA (fluorescent *Treponema pallidum* antibody)
B_{12} levels (or, for increased sensitivity, a methylmalonic acid level)
ANA (antinuclear antibody)
Antithyroid antibodies (antithyroid peroxidase and antithyroglobulin) – present in Hashimoto's
   encephalopathy
Free T4, TSH
Cortisol and ACTH levels and 24-hour urine for free cortisol
Copper and ceruloplasmin levels
MRI
EEG
Lumbar puncture

23.3.3 Treatments

Treatment, if possible, is directed at the underlying cause. When such treatment is unavailable or ineffective, or where control of the psychosis is urgently required, neuroleptics are indicated. Although conventional neuroleptics, such as haloperidol, have long been used successfully, a second-generation antipsychotic (SGA), such as olanzapine or risperidone, may be better tolerated. In general, it is best to start with a low dose (e.g., 2.5 mg of haloperidol, 5 mg olanzapine, or 1 mg of risperidone) with incremental increases, if necessary, introduced slowly.

23.4 Mood disorder with depressive features

23.4.1 Clinical patterns

A mood disorder with depressive features is characterized by a prominent and persistent depressed mood or loss of interest, and by the presence of evidence – from the history, physical examination, and/or laboratory tests – of a general medical condition capable of causing such a disturbance. Although other depressive symptoms (e.g., lack of energy, sleep disturbance, appetite change, psychomotor change) may be present, they are not necessary for the diagnosis. The various secondary causes of depression are listed in Box 23.3.

In using Box 23.3, the first question to ask is whether the depression could be *secondary to precipitants*. Of the various possible precipitants, substances of abuse (e.g., as seen in alcoholism or during stimulant withdrawal) are very common causes, and these are covered in their respective chapters. Medications are particularly important; however, it must be borne in mind that most patients are able to take the medications listed in Box 23.3 without untoward effect: consequently,

Box 23.3 Causes of Depression Due to a General Medical Condition.

Secondary to precipitants
Medications:
  Propranolol
  Interferon
  ACTH
  Prednisone
  Reserpine
  Alpha-methyldopa
  Levetiracetam
  Nifedipine
  Ranitidine
  Metoclopramide
  Bismuth subsalicylate
  Pimozide
  Subdermal estrogen/progestin
  Anticholinergic withdrawal ("cholinergic rebound")
Poststroke depression
Traumatic brain injury
Whiplash

Secondary to diseases with specific features
Hypothyroidism
Hyperthyroidism
Cushing's syndrome
Chronic adrenocortical insufficiency
Obstructive sleep apnea (severe snoring)
Multiple sclerosis (various focal findings)
Down's syndrome
Epilepsy:
  Ictal depression
  Chronic interictal depression

Occuring as part of certain neurodegenerative or dementing disorders
Alzheimer's disease
Multi-infarct dementia
Diffuse Lewy-body disease
Parkinson's disease
Fahr's syndrome
Tertiary neurosyphilis
Limbic encephalitis

Secondary to miscellaneous or rare causes
Cerebral tumors
Hydrocephalus
Pancreatic cancer
New-variant Creutzfeldt–Jakob disease
Hyperparathyroidism
Systemic lupus erythematosus
Pernicious anemia
Pellagra
Lead encephalopathy
Hyperaldosteronism

before ascribing a depression to any medication it is critical to demonstrate that the depression did not begin before the medication was begun, and ideally, to demonstrate that the depression resolved after the medication was discontinued.

Anticholinergic withdrawal may occur within days after abrupt discontinuation of highly anticholinergic medications, such as benztropine or certain tricyclic antidepressants, and is characterized by depressed mood, malaise, insomnia, and gastrointestinal symptoms such as nausea, vomiting, abdominal cramping, and diarrhea. Poststroke depression is not uncommon, and may be more likely when the anterior portion of the left frontal lobe is involved; although spontaneous remission within a year is the rule, depressive symptoms, in the meantime, may be quite severe. Both head trauma and whiplash injuries may be followed by depressive symptoms in nearly half of all cases. Depression may occur secondary to diseases with distinctive features, and keeping such features in mind when evaluating depressed patients will lead to a gratifying number of diagnostic "pickups." These features are noted in Box 23.3 and are for the most part self-explanatory; depression associated with epilepsy, however, merits some further discussion.

Ictal depressions are, in fact, simple partial seizures whose symptomatology is for the most part restricted to affective changes. The diagnosis of ictal depression is suggested by the paroxysmal onset of depression (literally over seconds); although such simple partial seizures may last only minutes, longer durations, up to months, have also been reported. Interictal depressions, rather than occurring secondary to paroxysmal electrical activity within the brain, occur as a result of longlasting changes in neuronal activity, perhaps related to "kindling" within the limbic system, in patients with chronically recurrent seizures, either grand mal or, more especially, complex partial. Such interictal depressions are of gradual onset and are chronic. Depression *occurring as part of certain neurodegenerative or dementing disorders* is immediately suggested by the presence of other symptoms of these disorders, such as dementia or distinctive physical findings (e.g., parkinsonism). The *miscellaneous or rare causes* represent, for the most part, uncommon etiologies in the differential for depression, and should be considered when, despite a thorough investigation, the diagnosis of a particular case of depression remains unclear.

23.4.2 Assessment and differential diagnosis

Although the foregoing list of possible causes of depression due to a general medical condition is long, using it in the clinical evaluation of depressed patients need not be burdensome. Evidence for most of the *precipitants, diseases with distinctive features,* and *neurodegenerative or dementing disorders* will be uncovered in the course of a standard interview and examination and, after using the list a few times, clinicians will recognize their diagnostic relevance.

The *miscellaneous or rare* causes, as in any other branch of medicine, are only considered when one is at the end of one's diagnostic rope, a situation often reached when patients fail to respond to treatment that, if the diagnosis were correct, should have led to relief but did not.

23.4.3 Treatments

Treatment efforts should be directed at relieving, if possible, the underlying cause. When this is not possible, antidepressants should be considered. Controlled studies have demonstrated the effectiveness of both nortriptyline and citalopram for poststroke depression, and nortriptyline for depression seen in Parkinson's disease. For other secondary depressions, citalopram is probably a good choice, given its benign side-effect profile and notable lack of drug interactions. Nortriptyline should be used with caution in patients with cardiac conduction defects (as it may prolong conduction time) and in those at risk for seizures as in head trauma, as this agent may also lower the seizure threshold.

23.5 Manias

23.5.1 Clinical patterns

A mood disorder is characterized by a prominent and persistently elevated, expansive, or irritable mood, which – on the basis of the history, physical or laboratory examinations – can be attributed to an underlying general medical condition. Other manic symptoms, such as increased energy, decreased need for sleep, hyperactivity, distractibility, pressured speech and flight of ideas, may or may not be present. Cases of elevated or irritable mood secondary to other causes (e.g., secondary to treatment with corticosteroids) are much less common.

Box 23.4 lists secondary causes of elevated or irritable mood, with these causes divided into categories designed to facilitate the task of differential diagnosis.

Box 23.4 Causes of Mania Due to a General Medical Condition.

Secondary to precipitants
Medications:
   Corticosteroids or adrenocorticotrophic hormone
   Anabolic steroids
   Levodopa
   Pramipexole
   Ropinirole
   Zidovudine
   Interferon alpha
   Oral contraceptives
   Isoniazid
   Clarithromycin
   Buspirone
   Procyclidine
   Procarbazine
   Propafenone
   Baclofen (on discontinuation after long-term use)
   Reserpine (on discontinuation after long-term use)
   Methyldopa (on discontinuation after long-term use)
Other precipitants
Closed head injury
Hemodialysis
Encephalitis
Aspartame
Metrizamide

Secondary to diseases with specific features
Hyperthyroidism
Cushing's syndrome
Multiple sclerosis
Cerebral infarction
Sydenham's chorea
Chorea gravidarum
Hepatic encephalopathy
Uremia (asterixis, delirium)
Epilepsy:
   Ictal mania
   Postictal mania

Occuring as part of a neurodegenerative or dementing disease
Alzheimer's disease
Neurosyphilis
Huntington's disease
Creutzfeldt–Jakob disease

Secondary to miscellaneous causes
Cerebral tumors
Systemic lupus erythematosus
Vitamin B_{12} deficiency
Metachromatic leukodystrophy
Adrenoleukodystrophy
Tuberous sclerosis

It is very rare for mania to constitute the initial presentation of any of the diseases or disorders listed in Box 23.4. In most cases of mania *secondary to precipitants*, the cause (e.g., treatment with high-dose prednisone) is fairly straightforward. In cases *secondary to diseases with distinctive features or occurring as part of certain neurodegenerative or dementing diseases*, the cause is generally readily discernible if the clinician is alert to the tell-tale distinctive features (e.g., a Cushingoid habitus) and to the presence of dementia indicating one of the dementing disorders listed in Box 23.4. *The miscellaneous or rare causes* are generally only resorted to when other investigations prove unrewarding.

In using Box 23.4, the first step is to determine whether the mania could be *secondary to precipitants*. Substance-induced mood disorder related to drugs of abuse is covered in the relevant substance-related disorders chapters in this book. Of the precipitating factors listed in Box 23.4, medications are the most common offenders. Before, however, attributing the mania to one of these medications, it is critical to demonstrate that the mania occurred only after initiation of that medication; ideally, one would also want to show that the mania spontaneously resolved subsequent to the medication's discontinuation. Of the medications listed, corticosteroids such as prednisone are likely to cause mania, with the likelihood increasing in direct proportion to dose. Levodopa is the next most likely cause, and in the case of levodopa the induced mania may be so pleasurable that some patients have ended up abusing the drug. Anabolic steroid abuse may cause an irritable mania, and such a syndrome occurring in a "bulked up" patients should prompt a search for other clinical evidence of abuse, such as gynecomastia and testicular atrophy. Closed head injury may be followed by mania either directly upon emergence from post-coma delirium, or after an interval of months. Hemodialysis may cause mania, and has been reported to have occurred as the presenting sign of an eventual dialysis dementia. Encephalitis may cause mania, as for example in postinfectious encephalomyelitis, with the correct diagnosis eventually being suggested by more typical signs such as delirium or seizures. Encephalitis lethargica (von Economo's disease) may also be at fault, with the diagnosis suggested by classic signs such as sleep reversal or oculomotor paralyses. Aspartame taken in very high dose caused mania and a seizure in one report, and metrizamide myelography prompted mania in another.

Mania occurring *secondary to disease with distinctive features* is immediately suggested by these features, as listed in Box 23.4. Ictal mania is characterized by its paroxysmal onset, over seconds, and the diagnosis of postictal mania is suggested when mania occurs shortly after a "flurry" of grand mal or complex partial seizures.

Mania *occurring as part of certain neurodegenerative or dementing diseases* is suggested, in general, by a concurrent dementia, and in most cases the mania plays only a minor role in the overall clinical picture. Neurosyphilis, however, is an exception to this rule, for in patients with general paresis of the insane (dementia paralytica) mania may dominate the picture. Of the *miscellaneous or rare causes* of mania, cerebral tumors are the most important to keep in mind, with mania being noted with tumors of the midbrain, tumors compressing the hypothalamus (e.g., a craniopharyngioma) or a pituitary adenoma, and tumors of the right thalamus, right cingulate gyrus, or one or both frontal lobes.

23.5.2 Treatments

Treatment, if possible, is directed at the underlying cause. In cases where such etiologic treatment is not possible, or not rapidly effective enough, pharmacologic measures should be considered. Mood stabilizers, such as lithium or divalproex used in the same manner as when treating primary mania in bipolar disorder, is the pharmacotherapy of choice. In choosing between lithium and divalproex, in cases where there is a risk for seizures (e.g., head injury, encephalitis, stroke, or tumors), divalproex clearly is preferable. In cases where emergent treatment is required, before lithium or divalproex could have a chance to become effective, oral or intramuscular haloperidol or olanzapine, or oral risperidone, may be employed, again much as in the treatment of mania in bipolar disorder.

23.6 Anxiety disorder with panic attacks or with generalized anxiety

23.6.1 Clinical patterns

Although epidemiologic studies are lacking, the clinical impression is that anxiety secondary to a general medical condition is common. Pathologic anxiety secondary to a general medical condition may occur in the form of well-circumscribed and transient panic attacks or in a generalized, more chronic form. As the differential diagnoses for these two forms of anxiety are quite different, it is critical to clearly distinguish them.

Panic attacks have an acute or paroxysmal onset, and are characterized by typically intense anxiety or fear, which is accompanied by various "autonomic" signs and symptoms, such as tremor, diaphoresis, and palpitations. Symptoms rapidly crescendo over seconds or minutes and in most cases the attack will clear within anywhere from minutes up to a half-hour. Although attacks tend to be similar to one another in the same patient, there is substantial inter-patient variability.

Generalized anxiety tends to be of subacute or gradual onset, and may last for long periods – from days to months – depending on the underlying cause. Here, some patients, rather than complaining of feeling anxious *per se*, may complain of being worried, tense, or ill at ease. Autonomic symptoms tend not to be as severe or prominent as those seen in panic attacks: shakiness, palpitations (or tachycardia), and diaphoresis are perhaps most common.

Panic attacks are most commonly seen in one of the primary anxiety disorders, namely, panic disorder, agoraphobia, specific phobia, social phobia, obsessive–compulsive disorder, or post-traumatic stress disorder, all of which are covered elsewhere in this book. The causes of secondary panic attacks are listed in Box 23.5. Substance-induced anxiety disorder related to drugs of abuse can also occur as a result of cocaine, cannabis, or LSD use. Clozapine has also been associated with panic attacks. Partial seizures and paroxysmal atrial tachycardia are both characterized by their exquisitely paroxysmal onset, over a second or two; in addition, paroxysmal atrial tachycardia is distinguished by the prominence of the tachycardia and by an ability, in many cases, to terminate the attack with a Valsalva maneuver. Hypoglycemia is often suspected as a cause of anxiety, but before the diagnosis is accepted one must demonstrate the presence of "Whipple's triad": hypoglycemia (blood glucose ≤ 45 mg/dL), typical symptoms, and the relief of those symptoms with glucose. Angina or acute myocardial infarction can present with a panic attack, with the diagnosis being suggested by the clinical setting, for example, multiple cardiac risk factors. A pulmonary embolus, at the moment of its lodgment in a pulmonary artery, may also present with a panic attack, and again the correct diagnosis is suggested by the clinical setting (e.g., situations, such as prolonged immobilization,

---

Box 23.5 Causes of Panic Attacks Due to a General Medical Condition.

Partial seizures
Paroxysmal atrial tachycardia
Hypoglycemia
Angina or acute myocardial infarction
Pulmonary embolus
Acute asthmatic attack
Pheochromocytoma
Parkinson's disease
Certain medications or substances of abuse

which favor deep venous thrombosis). Acute asthmatic attacks are suggested by wheezing, and pheochromocytoma by associated hypertension. Parkinson's disease patients treated with levodopa may experience panic attacks during "off" periods.

Generalized anxiety is most commonly seen in the primary psychiatric disorder, generalized anxiety disorder, and is discussed elsewhere in this book. It may also be an integral part of withdrawal from alcohol and sedative/hypnotics, also discussed elsewhere in this text. The secondary causes of generalized anxiety are listed in Box 23.6.

Box 23.6 Causes of Generalized Anxiety Due to a General Medical Condition.

Sympathomimetics
Theophylline
Caffeine
Various antidepressants (e.g., tricyclics, SSRIs)
Hyperthyroidism
Cushing's syndrome
Hypocalcemia
Chronic obstructive pulmonary disease
Congestive heart failure
Poststroke
Posthead traumatic brain injury

Sympathomimetics and theophylline, as used in asthma and COPD, are frequent causes, as is caffeine and many of the antidepressants. Hyperthyroidism is suggested by heat intolerance and proptosis, and Cushing's syndrome by the typical Cushingoid habitus (i.e., moon facies, hirsutism, acne, "buffalo hump," and abdominal striae). Hypocalcemia may be suggested by a history of seizures or tetany. Both chronic obstructive pulmonary disease and congestive heart failure are suggested by marked dyspnea. Stroke and traumatic brain injury may be followed by chronic anxiety, but this is seen in only a minority of these patients.

23.6.2 Treatments

Treatment is directed at the underlying cause, and this is sufficient for all cases of secondary panic attacks and most cases of secondary generalized anxiety; exceptions include poststroke and posttraumatic brain injury anxiety, and in these cases benzodiazepines have been used with success.

23.7 Obsessive–compulsive disorder

23.7.1 Clinical patterns

Obsessions and compulsions are features of obsessive–compulsive disorder. Obsessions consist of unwanted, and generally anxiety-provoking, thoughts, images, or ideas that repeatedly come to mind despite the person's attempts to stop them. Allied with these are compulsions, which consist of anxious urges to do or undo things, urges that, if resisted, are followed by rapidly increasing anxiety, which can often only be relieved by giving into the compulsion to act.

Those rare instances where obsessions and compulsions are secondary to a general medical condition or medication are listed in Box 23.7.

In most cases, the causes of secondary obsessions or compulsions are readily discerned as, for example, a history of encephalitis, anoxia, traumatic brain injury, or treatment with certain second-generation antipsychotics such as clozapine, olanzapine, or risperidone. Sydenham's chorea is immediately suggested by the appearance of chorea; however, it must be borne in mind that obsessions and compulsions may constitute the presentation of Sydenham's chorea, with the

Box 23.7 Causes of Obsessions and Compulsions Due to a General Medical Condition.

Postencephalitic
Postanoxic
Post-traumatic brain injury
Clozapine
Olanzapine
Risperidone
Sydenham's chorea
Huntington's disease
Simple partial seizures
Infarction of the basal ganglia or right parietal lobe
Fahr's syndrome

appearance of chorea being delayed for days. Ictal obsessions or compulsions, constituting the sole clinical manifestation of a simple partial seizure, may, in themselves, be indistinguishable from the obsessions and compulsions seen in obsessive–compulsive disorder, but are suggested by a history of other seizure types, such as complex partial or grand mal seizures.

Infarction of the basal ganglia or parietal lobe is suggested by the subacute onset of obsessions or compulsions accompanied by "neighborhood" symptoms such as abnormal movements or unilateral sensory changes. Fahr's syndrome, unlike the foregoing, may be an elusive diagnosis, only suggested perhaps when CT imaging incidentally reveals calcification of the basal ganglia.

23.7.2 Treatments

Most causes of secondary obsessions and compulsions are picked up on the routine history and physical examination, with the possible exception of ictal cases, and here it is critical to make a close inquiry as to a history of other seizure types: ictal EEGs are not reliable because they are often normal in the case of simple partial seizures. In doubtful cases a "diagnosis by treatment response" to a trial of an anticonvulsant may be appropriate. When treatment of the underlying cause is not possible, a trial of a selective serotonin-reuptake inhibitor, as used for obsessive–compulsive disorder, might be appropriate.

23.8 Catatonic disorders

23.8.1 Clinical patterns

Stuporous catatonia, in the majority of cases, occurs as part of such primary psychiatric disorders as schizophrenia, a depressive episode of either major depression or bipolar disorder, or a manic episode of bipolar disorder, and these are discussed elsewhere in other chapters. The causes of catatonia due to a general medical condition or medications are listed in Box 23.8.

Focal lesions capable of causing catatonia are typically found in the medial or inferior portions of the frontal lobes. The miscellaneous conditions listed are all quite rare causes of catatonia.

Stuporous catatonia occurring in association with epilepsy is often suggested by a history of grand mal or complex partial seizures. Ictal catatonia is further suggested by its exquisitely paroxysmal onset, and postictal catatonia by an immediately preceding "flurry" of grand mal or complex partial seizures. Psychosis of forced normalization is an interictal condition distinguished by the appearance of symptoms subsequent to effective control of seizures. The chronic interictal psychosis is also, as suggested by the name, an interictal condition, which, however, appears not after seizures are controlled but rather in the setting of ongoing, chronic uncontrolled

Box 23.8 Causes of Catatonia Due to a General Medical Condition.

Stuporous catatonia
Associated with epilepsy:
  Ictal catatonia
  Postictal catatonia
  Psychosis of forced normalization
  Chronic interictal psychosis
Medications:
  Antipsychotics
  Disulfiram
  Benzodiazepine withdrawal
Viral encephalitis:
  Herpes simplex encephalitis
  Encephalitis lethargica
Focal lesions, especially of the frontal lobes
Miscellaneous conditions:
  Hepatic encephalopathy
  Limbic encephalitis
  Systemic lupus erythematosus
  Lyme disease, in stage III
  Subacute sclerosing panencephalitis, in stage I
  Tay–Sachs disease
  Thrombotic thrombocytopenic purpura

Excited catatonia
Viral encephalitis

epilepsy. Of medications capable of causing catatonia, antipsychotics are by far the most common. Viral encephalitis is suggested by concurrent fever and headache: herpes simplex.

Excited catatonia manifests with varying degrees of bizarre, frenzied, and purposeless behavior. Such patients typically keep to themselves.

23.8.2 Treatments

Stuporous catatonia must be distinguished from akinetic mutism and from stupor of other causes. Excited catatonia must be distinguished from mania. In addition to treating, if possible, the underlying cause, catatonia may be symptomatically relieved by lorazepam given parenterally in a dose of 2 mg. In severe cases where lorazepam is not sufficiently effective and the patient is at immediate risk, consideration should be given to emergency electroconvulsive therapy, which is typically dramatically effective, generally bringing relief after a few treatments.

23.9 Personality change

23.9.1 Clinical patterns

The appearance of a significant change in an adult's personality is an ominous clinical sign and indicates the presence of intracranial pathology. An individual may not be aware of the change, but to others who have known the person over time the change is often quite obvious: they often note that the person is "not himself." In most cases the change is nonspecific. There may be either a gross exaggeration of hitherto minor aspects of the person's personality or the appearance of a personality trait quite uncharacteristic for the individual. Traits commonly seen in a personality change, as noted in DSM-IV-TR, include lability, disinhibition, aggressiveness, apathy, and suspiciousness.

Box 23.9 Causes of Personality Change of the Nonspecific or Frontal-Lobe Type.

Secondary to precipitants
Traumatic brain injury
Head trauma with subdural hematoma
Postviral encephalitis
Gunshot wounds
Cerebral infarction

Secondary to cerebral tumors
Frontal lobe*
Corpus callosum* (in its anterior part)
Temporal lobe

Occurring as part of certain neurodegenerative or dementing disorders
Pick's disease*
Frontotemporal dementia*
Alzheimer's disease*
Amyotrophic lateral sclerosis*
Progressive supranuclear palsy*
Corticobasal ganglionic degeneration*
Multiple system atrophy*
Huntington's disease
Wilson's disease
Lacunar syndrome*
Normal-pressure hydrocephalus
AIDS
Neurosyphilis
Creutzfeldt–Jakob disease

Miscellaneous causes
Granulomatous angiitis
Vitamin B_{12} deficiency
Limbic encephalitis
Metachromatic leukodystrophy
Adrenoleukodystrophy
Mercury intoxication
Manganism

* Diseases that are particularly prone to cause a personality change of the frontal lobe type.

Personality change of the nonspecific or of the frontal lobe type, as noted in Box 23.9, may occur *secondary to precipitants* (e.g., traumatic brain injury), *secondary to cerebral tumors* (especially those of the frontal or temporal lobes), or *as part of certain neurodegenerative or dementing disorders*. Finally, there is a group of miscellaneous causes. In Box 23.9, those disorders or diseases that are particularly prone to cause a personality change of the frontal lobe type are indicated by an asterisk. The interictal personality syndrome occurs only in the setting of chronic repeated grand mal or complex partial seizures, and may represent microanatomic changes in the limbic system, which have been "kindled" by the repeated seizures.

In the case of personality change occurring *secondary to precipitants*, the etiology is fairly obvious; an exception might be cerebral infarction, but here the acute onset and the presence of "neighborhood" symptoms are suggestive. In addition to infarction of the frontal lobe, personality change has also been noted with infarction of the caudate nucleus and of the thalamus. Personality change occurring *secondary to cerebral tumors* may not be accompanied by any distinctive features, and indeed a personality change may be the only clinical evidence of a tumor for a long time. Personality change *occurring as part of certain neurodegenerative or dementing disorders* deserves special mention, as in many instances the underlying disorder may present with a personality change; this is particularly the case with Pick's disease, frontotemporal dementia, and Alzheimer's disease. The inclusion of amyotrophic lateral sclerosis here may be surprising to some, but it is very clear that, albeit in a small minority, cerebral symptoms may not only dominate the early course of ALS, but may even constitute the presentation of the disease. In the case of the other neurodegenerative disorders (i.e., progressive supranuclear palsy, corticobasal ganglionic degeneration, multiple system atrophy, Huntington's disease, and Wilson's disease) a personality change, if present, is typically accompanied by abnormal involuntary movements of one sort or other, such as parkinsonism, ataxia, or chorea. The lacunar syndrome, occurring secondary to multiple lacunar infarctions affecting the thalamus, internal capsule, or basal ganglia, deserves special mention as it very commonly causes a personality change of the frontal-lobe type by interrupting the connections between the thalamus or basal ganglia and the frontal lobe. Normal-pressure hydrocephalus is an important diagnosis to keep in mind, as the condition is treatable; other suggestive symptoms include a broad-based shuffling gait and urinary urgency or incontinence.

AIDS should be suspected whenever a personality change is accompanied by clinical phenomena suggestive of immunodeficiency, such as thrush. Neurosyphilis may present with a personality change characterized by slovenliness and disinhibition. Creutzfeldt–Jakob disease may also present with a personality change.

As in the previous diagnostic categories, the *miscellaneous causes* represent the more rare causes in the differential for personality change. Two deserve comment, given their treatability: granulomatous angiitis is suggested by prominent headache, and vitamin B_{12} deficiency by the presence of macrocytosis or a sensory polyneuropathy.

23.9.2 Treatments

Treatment, if possible, is directed at the underlying cause. Mood stabilizers (e.g., carbamazepine) may be helpful for lability and disinhibition. Antipsychotics may be helpful with suspiciousness and may also attenuate disinhibition. Antidepressants may relieve depressive symptoms. Regardless of which agent is chosen, it is prudent, given the general medical condition of many of these patients, to "start low and go slow." In many cases, some degree of supervision will be required.

23.10 Mental disorders not otherwise specified

This is a *residual* category in DSM-IV-TR for those clinical situations in which the mental disorder occurring secondary to a general medical condition does not fall into one of the specific categories described earlier. Of these various disorders, two are worthy of detailed description: pseudobulbar palsy and the Klüver–Bucy syndrome. Both are commonly seen in dementia clinics, and their occurrence often prompts a request for psychiatric consultation.

When fully developed, pseudobulbar palsy is characterized by emotional incontinence (also known as "pathological laughing and crying"), dysarthria, dysphagia, a brisk jaw-jerk and gag reflex, and difficulty in protruding the tongue. The most remarkable aspect of the syndrome is the emotional incontinence. Patients experience uncontrollable paroxysms of laughter or crying, often in response to minor stimuli, such as the approach of the clinician to the bedside. Pseudobulbar palsy is not uncommon: as noted above, it is found in almost half of patients with amyotrophic lateral sclerosis. It may also be seen in a much smaller, but still clinically significant, proportion of patients with vascular lesions, Alzheimer's disease, and multiple sclerosis.

In addition to treating, if possible, the underlying cause, various medications (antidepressants or mood stabilizers) may be used to reduce the severity of the emotional incontinence.

Klüver–Bucy syndrome is a behavior disorder that occurs when both the right and left medial temporal lobes of the brain malfunction. The amygdala has been a particularly implicated brain region in the pathogenesis of this syndrome. Symptoms include hypersexuality, hyperorality and the ingestion of inappropriate substances, docility, diminished fear response, unusually low aggressiveness and an inability to recognize familiar persons or objects. The causes are Picks disease, status epilepticus, lobotomy, Alzheimers disease, heat stroke, and traumatic brain injury. The underlying cause, if possible, is treated. There are no controlled studies regarding symptomatic treatment; anecdotally, overall improvement has been reported with carbamazepine, sertraline, and various antipsychotics.

Clinical Vignette 1

In 2000, Liebson reported the case of a 53-year-old man with a right thalamic hemorrhage, who presented with headache and left-sided hemiparesis and hemianesthesia. Four days later he displayed significant anosognosia for his hemiparesis; more remarkable, however, was the change in his mood. One week after the stroke his "mood was remarkably cheerful and optimistic . . . he was noted to praise extravagantly the hospital food, and the nurses found him 'talkative.' When he arrived on our ward 11 days after the stroke he was flirtatious with female staff and boasted of having fathered 64 children. His girlfriend was surprised when he kissed her in front of the staff because he had never publicly displayed affection before. He reported excellent energy and expansively invited all the staff to his home for Thanksgiving. . . The mania resolved gradually over a 10-week period after [the] stroke."

Clinical Vignette 2

In 1977, Rush and associates described a patient with simple partial seizures that manifested as panic attacks. The patient, at the age of 44 years, began to have "attacks of palpitation accompanied by dizziness, faintness and anxiety. . . [which] occurred during wakefulness and sleep, and, if asleep, the patient was awakened by them." At the age of 49 years he was evaluated and an EEG obtained between attacks "revealed mild slowing with intermittent, low-voltage, sharp waves over the right temporal region. Because of the paroxysmal nature of the attacks and the electroencephalographic abnormality, the patient was reevaluated utilizing telemetry" During telemetry, the patient had an attack: "he was pale and mildly diaphoretic and was tightly gripping his chair. . .no abnormal movements were detected. . . [he] remained fully alert and was not incontinent." Concurrent with the attack, ictal EEG activity was observed on the right. At craniotomy, a glioma was removed from the right frontal lobe and the attacks subsequently did not recur.

KEY POINTS

- One of the first steps of a complete assessment involves reviewing the history, physical examination, and laboratory tests for evidence of a general medical disorder that might be causing the mental symptoms.

- Psychoses and other symptoms of a mental disorder can occur secondary to precipitants, secondary to diseases with distinctive features, and secondary to miscellaneous causes.

- The appearance of a significant change in an adult's personality is an ominous clinical sign and indicates the presence of intracranial pathology.

- Drugs of abuse and medications are among the most common precipitants of psychiatric symptoms that are not due to a primary mental health disorder.

- Treatment of a mental disorder that occurs as a result of a medical condition is directed at the underlying cause.

Further Reading

Andreoli, T. *et al.* (2007) *Andreoli & Carpenter's Cecil Essentials of Medicine*, 7th edn, Elsevier, New York.

Lishman, W.A. (1998) *Organic Psychiatry: The Psychological Consequences of Cerebral Disorder*, Wiley & Sons, New York.

Rundell, J. and Wise, M. (1999) *Essentials of Consultation Liaison Psychiatry*, APA Press, Washington, DC.

Factitious Disorder

24.1 Introduction

Factitious disorder, also called Munchausen's syndrome, refers to the condition in which patients consciously induce or feign illness in order to obtain a psychological benefit from being in the sick role. They usually have little insight into the motivations of their behavior but are still powerfully driven to appear ill to others. In many cases, they endanger their own health and life in their desire to appear sick. Patients with this disorder will often induce serious illness or undergo numerous unnecessary, invasive procedures. This chapter defines the sick role and describes factitious disorder and its etiology and treatment.

24.2 Sick-role behavior

The sick role has been described with four aspects. First, the person is not able to will himself or herself back to health but instead must "be taken care of." Second, the patient in the sick role must regard the sickness as undesirable and want to get better. Third, the sick patient is obliged to seek medical care and cooperate with his or her medical treatment. Finally, the sick patient is exempted from the normal responsibilities of his or her social role.

24.3 Factitious disorder

24.3.1 Diagnostic criteria

For a diagnosis of factitious disorder to be justified, a person must be intentionally producing illness. His or her motivation is to occupy the sick role, and there must not be external incentives for the behavior. While DSM-IV-TR is clear that no external incentives can be present to meet the criteria for the diagnosis, it is rarely the case that there is absolutely no secondary gain for a patient (as the sick role automatically conveys some external benefits such as release from usual duties). In practice, clinicians will often diagnose patients with factitious disorder in the presence of some external gain as long as the external benefits do not appear to be a major motivation for the production of symptoms.

24.3.1.1 Factitious disorder with predominantly physical signs and symptoms

Individuals with this subtype of factitious disorder present with physical signs and symptoms. The three main methods patients use to create illness are (1) giving a false history, (2) faking clinical and laboratory findings, or (3) inducing illness, such as by surreptitious medication use. Particularly common presentations include fever, self-induced infection, gastrointestinal symptoms, impaired

Fundamentals of Psychiatry, First Edition. Allan Tasman and Wanda K. Mohr.
© 2011 John Wiley & Sons, Ltd. Published 2011 by John Wiley & Sons, Ltd.
This chapter is based on Chapter 75 (Anne M. Fleming, Stuart J. Eisendrath) of *Psychiatry, Third Edition*

wound healing, cancer, renal disease (especially hematuria and nephrolithiasis), endocrine diseases, anemia, bleeding disorders, and epilepsy.

True Munchausen's syndrome fits within this subclass and is the most severe form of the illness. According to DSM-IV-TR, patients with Munchausen's syndrome have chronic factitious disorder with physical signs and symptoms, and in addition have a history of recurrent hospitalization, peregrination, and "pseudologia fantastica" – dramatic, untrue, and extremely improbable tales of their past experiences. They are often very familiar with hospital procedures and use this knowledge to present dramatically during times when the factitious nature of their symptoms is least likely to be discovered.

24.3.1.2 Factitious disorder with predominantly psychologic signs and symptoms

This subtype includes patients who present feigning psychological illness. They both report and mimic psychiatric symptoms. There are reports of factitious psychosis, homicidal ideation, and alcohol dependence in the literature and it is likely that patients feign psychiatric disorders across the full spectrum of mental illnesses. There are reports of false claims of being a victim of stalking or rape, and these cases are often diagnosed with a factitious psychological disorder such as post-traumatic stress disorder.

24.3.1.3 Factitious disorder with combined psychologicl and physical signs and symptoms

Some individuals present with simultaneous psychological and physical factitious symptoms, and some move between physical and psychological presentations over time. DSM-IV-TR was revised to account for patients who present with both psychological signs and symptoms, though this category of patients is the least well studied.

24.3.2 Epidemiology

The nature of factitious disorder makes it difficult to determine how common it is within the general population. Patients attempt to conceal themselves, thereby artificially lowering the prevalence. The tendency of patients to present several times at different facilities, however, may artificially raise the prevalence. Most estimates of the prevalence of the disease rely on the number of factitious patients within a given inpatient population. Such attempts have generated estimates that 0.5–3% of medical and psychiatric inpatients suffer from factitious disorder.

Patients with factitious disorder span a broad age range. Reports in the literature show patients ranging from 8 to 85 years. Case series suggest that the majority of people with factitious disorder are women – one case series found 78% of patients to be women while the majority of patients with the more severe Munchausen's variant are men.

24.3.3 Comorbidity

All types of factitious disease show a strong association with substance abuse as well as borderline and narcissistic personality disorders.

24.3.4 Etiology

While factitious disorder appears to run in families, it is not known if this is explainable by genetic factors, environmental factors or both. Patients with factitious disorder are thought to create illness in pursuit of the sick role. For these patients, being in the sick role may allow them to compensate for an underlying psychologic deficit, act out angry impulses, or meet their underlying dependency needs.

Childhood developmental disturbances are thought to contribute to factitious disorder. Predisposing factors are thought to include: (1) serious childhood illness or illness in a family member during childhood, especially if the illness was associated with attention and nurturing in an otherwise distant family; (2) past anger with the medical profession; (3) past significant relationship with a healthcare provider; and (4) factitious disorder (especially factitious disorder by proxy) in a parent. It is thought that factitious disorder is more common in people in the healthcare professions, though it is not known if working in healthcare increases the risk for developing factitious disorder or if people with factitious disorder are drawn to healthcare work.

24.3.5 Course

The course of untreated factitious disorder is variable. Patients commonly suffer a great deal of morbidity, both physical and psychological, and in some cases the condition can be fatal. Patients with psychologic signs and symptoms are reported to have a high rate of suicide and a poor prognosis.

24.3.6 Differential diagnosis

The differential diagnosis of factitious disorder includes rare or complex physical illnesses, somatoform disorders, malingering, other psychiatric disorders, and substance abuse. As in the somatoform disorders (see Chapter 26), it is especially important to rule out genuine physical illness since complex medical illnesses can be mistaken for factitious disorder, and because patients with factitious disorder often induce real physical illness.

The conscious awareness of the production of symptoms differentiates factitious disorder from the somatoform disorders. Patients with somatoform disorders are unaware of the psychological origins of their symptoms, and they genuinely believe themselves to be ill. In contrast, it is the underlying motivation to produce symptoms that separates factitious disorders from malingering. Patients who malinger consciously feign or induce illness in order to obtain some external benefit (such as money, narcotics, or excuse from duties) as opposed to the internal, psychological motivation of a patient with factitious disorder. While the distinctions among these disorders appear satisfyingly clear, patients often blur the boundaries in practice.

24.3.7 Treatments

The goals in treating patients with factitious disorder are twofold: (1) to minimize the damage done by the disorder to both the patient's own health and the healthcare system; and (2) to help patients recover, at least partially, from the disorder. These goals are furthered by treating comorbid medical illnesses, avoiding unnecessary procedures, encouraging patients to seek psychiatric treatment, and providing support for healthcare clinicians. Patients with true Munchausen's syndrome (including antisocial traits, pathological lying, wandering, and poor social support) are felt to be refractory to treatment.

There are no clear data supporting the effectiveness of psychiatric medications in treating factitious disorder. Obviously medical conditions induced by patients should be treated with appropriate pharmacologic agents.

Aggressive confrontation with what the clinician suspects is usually unsuccessful; supportive, nonpunitive confrontation may be helpful for some. While many patients with factitious disorder are hesitant to pursue psychiatric treatment, there are numerous case reports of successful treatment of the disorder with long-term psychotherapy. Managed care and limiting of mental health treatment in many insurance carriers make providing such psychotherapy a challenge.

24.4 Factitious disorder by proxy

Some individuals pursue the sick role not by feigning illness in themselves, but by creating it in another person, usually someone dependent on the perpetrator. They seek the role of caring for an ill individual (the sick role by proxy). In this disorder, there are two patients, the individual with the diagnosis, and his or her victim. While people who suffer from factitious disorder by proxy have a mental illness, they often also commit criminal acts, usually dependant or child abuse, and the criminal justice and child protective systems are often involved.

24.4.1 Diagnosis

In factitious disorder by proxy, one person creates or feigns illness in another person, usually a child, though occasionally the victim is an elder or developmentally delayed adult. The veterinary literature even reports cases of factitious disorder by proxy in which the victim is a pet. Factitious disorder by proxy is not defined as a specific disorder in DSM-IV-TR but instead is listed under the "not otherwise specified" heading with research criteria included. The diagnostic criteria for factitious disorder by proxy are similar to that of factitious disorder itself, with the exception of the victim of the feigned or induced illness.

While numerous symptoms have been reported, common presentations include apnea, seizures, and gastrointestinal problems. The perpetrators appear extremely caring and attentive when observed, but appear indifferent to the child when they are not aware of being observed.

24.4.2 Epidemiology

As in factitious disorder, the exact prevalence of factitious disorder by proxy is unknown.

24.4.3 Comorbidity

There is high psychiatric morbidity in the children – many go on to develop factitious disorder or other psychiatric illnesses themselves. For the adults with factitious by proxy, there is high comorbidity with other psychiatric disorders and a history of abuse. In reported cases, there is an increased rate (up to 30%) of personal factitious disorder in patients with factitious disorder by proxy.

24.4.4 Course

Factitious disorder by proxy appears to have a much higher morbidity and mortality rate (for the victim) than self-inflicted factitious disorder. Rates of long-term disability from repeated induced illnesses are high.

24.4.5 Differential diagnosis

As with factitious disorder, the differential includes complex medical illness. In addition, in an older child, the differential might include personal factitious disorder in the child. As yet, there are no reports of personal factitious disorder in a child aged under 8 years, whereas the victim in factitious by proxy is usually a younger child.

24.4.6 Etiology

The perpetrator in factitious disorder by proxy appears to seek not the "sick role" but the "parent to the sick child" role. This role is similar to the sick role in that it provides structure, attention from others, caring, and relief from usual responsibilities. In addition, the psychological factors that play a role in other forms of child abuse may also be present.

Childhood developmental disturbances are thought to contribute to the development of factitious disorder by proxy. Based on case reports, the perpetrator often has a history of family dysfunction.

24.4.7 Treatments

Owing to the high morbidity and mortality, treatment requires at least temporary separation from the parent and notification of local child protective agencies. The perpetrators often face criminal charges of child abuse. There is high psychiatric morbidity in the children – many go on to develop factitious disorder or other psychiatric illnesses themselves. Psychiatric intervention is necessary to ameliorate this morbidity as much as possible in these children. There are some case reports of successful psychotherapeutic treatments of the parents in this disorder.

Clinical Vignette 1

A 42-year-old man was brought in by ambulance from a public park after complaining of shortness of breath and collapsing. Onlookers called emergency services. In the emergency room the patient complained of shortness of breath and chest pain. He reported that he had a history of multiple pulmonary emboli necessitating Greenfield filter placement. He seemed to be very familiar with the medical terminology and clinical findings in pulmonary emboli. The patient had an extensive workup including a high-resolution CT scan, but all studies were normal. The medical team noted that the patient appeared to be holding his breath when his oxygen saturation was being measured, and was performing a Valsalva maneuver during his ECGs. The medical resident attempted to clarify the patient's history by obtaining collateral information. The hospitals contacted reported that the patient had presented numerous times with the same complaints, and there had been suspicion of a factitious disorder. The medical resident informed the patient of the conflicting information, at which point the patient became very angry and immediately left the hospital. He was lost to follow-up.

Clinical Vignette 2

A 46-year-old man presented complaining of symptoms of post-traumatic stress disorder. He reported intense flashbacks, numbing and avoidance, and irritability resulting from his experience as a combat veteran. He began intensive treatment for PTSD including support groups, individual therapy, and medication management. He was an extremely active participant in the support groups and would recount detailed horrors of his time in combat. A staff member verifying the patient's history learned the patient had served in the military but was not a combat veteran. The patient was confronted in a supportive manner, and he admitted that he had fabricated his history. It was recommended that the patient would continue in psychiatric treatment, and he agreed to do so.

Clinical Vignette 3

In 2000, Owen and associates described how a 6-month-old infant presented to the emergency room after a seizure. The family reported no significant past medical history. The infant was resuscitated. There was no evidence of infection, the patient had a normal blood glucose, and the urine toxicology screen was negative. After 5 hours, the child recovered. The infant presented again 5 days later with another seizure. The infant's blood glucose was low, and continued to fall below normal levels despite administration of dextrose. A blood insulin level was elevated and a c-peptide level suggested endogenous hyperinsulinism. The workup (including CT scan) was otherwise normal. Further history revealed that both grandmothers had Type II diabetes and took oral hypoglycemic agents. A blood test on the infant was positive for sulfonylurea. A case conference was held, and it was discovered that the mother's first child had been removed from the home due to some charges of abuse. It was recommended that the infant be placed in foster care while the police investigated the case.

KEY POINTS

- Factitious disorder, also called Munchausen's syndrome, refers to the condition in which a patient consciously induces or feign illness in order to obtain a psychological benefit from being in the sick role.

- For a diagnosis of factitious disorder to be justified, a person must be intentionally producing illness. His or her motivation is to occupy the sick role, and there must not be external incentives for the behavior.

- Factitious disorder subtypes include those with predominantly physical signs and symptoms, those with predominantly psychologic signs and symptoms, and those with combined signs and symptoms.

- Patients with factitious disorder commonly suffer a great deal of morbidity, both physical and psychological, and some cases the condition can be fatal.

- The goals in treatment are to minimize the damage done by the disorder to both the patient's own health and the healthcare system, and to help patients recover, at least partially, from the disorder.

Further Reading

Phillips, K.A. (2001) *Somatoform and Factitious Disorders*, APA Press, Washington, DC.
Rogers, R. (2008) *Clinical Assessment of Malingering and Deception*, 3rd edn, Guilford, New York.

Schizophrenia and Psychoses

25.1 Introduction

This chapter discusses thought disorders – serious and often persistent mental illnesses characterized by disturbances in reality orientation, thinking, and social involvement. Schizophrenia is the most prevalent of the thought disorders and the discussion will focus primarily on this condition, while touching briefly on psychotic disturbances that are related closely to schizophrenia.

The word *schizophrenia* originally referred to a "splitting off" of one's thoughts from one's emotions. Thus, the word has long been confused in the public's mind with "split personality" or "multiple personality" and the term is still used erroneously. A more accurate interpretation of schizophrenia might be "a disconnected mind." Such disconnection involves a lack of coherence in mental functioning, in which thoughts, feelings, perceptions, behavior, and experience in the absence of the normal connections that make mental life comprehensible, adaptive and effective. Individuals with schizophrenia manifest alterations in their cognitive functioning, which entails the entire gamut of skills necessary for people to process information correctly. Through cognition, people learn about the world and their place in it. Cognition includes such important functions as memory, attention, and judgment. People with schizophrenia often have difficulties with many areas of their cognitive functioning.

25.2 Psychopathology, signs, and symptoms

Signs and symptoms of schizophrenia can be broadly subsumed under a number of dimensions.

25.2.1 The disorganization dimension

The disorganization dimension of schizophrenia involves a formal thought disorder that affects the verbal form in which thoughts are expressed. Individuals with schizophrenia have disturbances in their conceptual thinking that make their ideas difficult to follow. These disturbances are manifested by disorganized speech, disorganized or bizarre behavior, and incongruous affect. Patients with mania or psychotic depressions may also manifest thought disorder.

Disorganized speech as a manifestation of formal thought disorder has historically been considered one of the primary characteristics of schizophrenia. The lack of a logical relationship between thoughts and ideas may be manifested by speech that is vague, diffuse, unfocused (loose associations), or incoherent (e.g., emitting words that are totally unrelated – the "word salad") or by a patient's inability to get to the point of a conversation (tangentiality).

Fundamentals of Psychiatry, First Edition. Allan Tasman and Wanda K. Mohr.
© 2011 John Wiley & Sons, Ltd. Published 2011 by John Wiley & Sons, Ltd.
This chapter is based on Chapter 65 (Jayendra K. Patel, Debra A. Pinals, Alan Breier) of *Psychiatry, Third Edition*

People with schizophrenia also may use words in peculiar ways. They may *perseverate* (repeat themselves), demonstrate *echolalia* (repeat what others say), *clang* (sound associations replace conceptual connections), or manifest *neologisms* (use made-up words whose meaning is known only to the person). They may experience thought blocking which is a sudden derailment of a train of thought with a complete interruption in the flow of ideas.

Another aspect of the disorganization dimension is disorganized motor or social behaviors. People with schizophrenia may have profound psychomotor retardation or excitement, and they may exhibit a bizarre posture (in the catatonic subtype). Their social behavior often deteriorates. Patients may withdraw from others and isolate themselves and may become unkempt, neglect their hygiene, and wear the same clothing for weeks at a time or may exhibit socially inappropriate behaviors, such as defecating or masturbating in public. Their surroundings may become cluttered and unfit for habitation.

The final component of the disorganization dimension is incongruity or inappropriateness of affect. Affect refers to an observable behavior that expresses feeling or emotional tone in response to a certain stimulus. Patients manifesting incongruent affect express themselves in a way that is not congruent to the situation or content of thought. They may smile or giggle in response to no outward stimuli, or they may laugh wildly while recounting tragic or frightening experiences.

25.2.2 *The psychotic dimension*

The psychotic dimension involves delusions and hallucinations. These are phenomena that reflect a patient's confusion about the loss of boundaries between self and the external world. Delusions and hallucinations are very real to patients with schizophrenia.

Delusions involve disturbances in thought content. They are firmly held false beliefs that reasoning cannot correct and for which there is no support in reality. The delusions may have different content and may be persecutory, grandiose, somatic, nihilistic, religious, or referential. Patients with paranoid schizophrenia generally have delusions of persecution, believing, for example, that someone is tormenting them, trying to poison them or spying on them. They may believe that organizations, such as the CIA, may be taking over their mind or body. Patients with grandiose delusions may believe that they are persons of great wealth, talent, influence, power, or beauty or even a different historical figure, such as Moses. Patients with somatic delusions concerning their bodies might believe that they are incredibly ugly and that certain aspects of their appearance (e.g., their nose) disgust others. Those experiencing nihilistic delusions may believe that they are dead or dying or even that they no longer exist. Those with religious delusions may believe that they have a special mission from God or that they are the greatest sinner that ever lived. Those with referential delusions might believe that other people's words, newspaper articles, television shows, or song lyrics are directed specifically at him or her.

Delusional beliefs also are accompanied by thought broadcasting, thought insertion, and thought withdrawal. In *thought broadcasting,* patients believe that others can perceive their thoughts (as though they are being broadcast out loud). Those exhibiting *thought insertion* are convinced that their thoughts are not their own but rather the thoughts of another that have become implanted in their heads. In *thought withdrawal,* patients believe that their thoughts are somehow being removed from their heads.

Hallucinations are sensory perceptions with a compelling sense of reality. During auditory hallucinations, the most common form, the person may hear the voice of God or a close relative, two or more voices that keep up a running commentary about his or her behavior, or a voice that commands the person to commit a certain act. Usually the voices are obscene and condemn, accuse, or insult the person. Auditory hallucinations also may involve the sounds of bells, whistles, whispers, rustlings, and other noises, but most often they are of voices talking.

Visual hallucinations (e.g., monsters or frightening scenes) are less common than auditory hallucinations. They are likely to be threatening experiences and are often accompanied by delusional ideas and other sensory perceptions. For example, a patient with religious delusions may hear and see the image of a deity beckoning. A person with schizophrenia also may have tactile (touch), olfactory (smell), and gustatory (taste) hallucinations, but these are fairly uncommon.

25.2.3 The negative dimension

DSM-IV-TR lists three negative symptoms as characteristic of schizophrenia: alogia, affective blunting, and avolition. Other negative symptoms common in schizophrenia include anhedonia and attentional impairment. Negative symptoms account for the substantial degree of morbidity and impairment associated with schizophrenia. They are the most intractable and difficult to treat, and they reflect a deficiency of mental functioning that is normally present.

Alogia is a poverty of thinking that is inferred from observing the patient's language and speech. People with alogia may have great difficulty producing fluent responses to questions and instead may manifest brief and very concrete replies. Spontaneous speech also may be reduced. Speech content may be empty and impoverished (poverty of speech). Sometimes the words themselves may be adequate or even plentiful, but they convey little information because they are too abstract, repetitive, or stereotypic (poverty of content).

Negative affect disturbances include *flat or blunted affect*. This is a reduced intensity of emotional expression and response. The difference between flat and blunted affect is in degree. A person with flat affect has no or nearly no emotional expression. He or she may not react at all to circumstances that usually evoke strong emotions in others. A person with blunted affect, on the other hand, has a significantly reduced intensity in emotional expression. He or she may react to circumstances, but only slightly.

People with affective flattening or blunting fail to change their facial expressions in response to circumstances. Their movements lack spontaneity, their expressive gestures are slow and infrequent, their voice lacks inflection, and their speech is slow. They may appear wooden and robot-like; a loss of sense of self may accompany affective flattening. For example, a patient may report that he or she has no feelings whatsoever and feels "dead" inside.

Complicating the picture of the reduced intensity in emotional response is that significant depressive symptoms can occur in up to 60% of people with schizophrenia. Depression often is difficult to recognize and diagnose, however, because the symptoms of major depression and schizophrenia often overlap.

Avolition is the inability to start, persist in, and carry through any goal-directed activity to its logical conclusion. In its most severe manifestation avolition severely impairs social and occupational functioning. Patients seem to have lost their will or drive. They cannot sustain work or engage in self-care activities. Some patients may actually initiate a project and then disappear, abandoning it for weeks or even months. They may wander aimlessly or fail to show up to their jobs, if they have them. Others often accuse them of laziness. Avolition, however, is not laziness but a loss of basic drives and capacity to formulate and pursue goals.

Anhedonia is the loss of the capacity to experience pleasure subjectively. Patients may describe themselves as feeling empty and no longer able to enjoy activities, such as hobbies, family, and friends, which once gave them pleasure. This symptom is particularly tragic because patients are very much aware that they have lost the capacity for pleasure. A recent study suggests that anhedonia may result from abnormalities in the complex functional interactions between the mesolimbic and frontal brain regions.

Patients also manifest impairment of *attention*. This can be seen in their inability to concentrate. This attentional impairment may result from having to attend to multiple stimuli. For example, they may be listening to their inner voices and thus be unable to attend to the external world of social interactions.

25.2.4 Other symptoms

Lack of insight is a common symptom of schizophrenia. People with this illness may not believe that they are ill or that their behavior is odd or abnormal. Lack of insight is one of the most difficult aspects of schizophrenia to treat. It may remain even if the other symptoms, such as delusions and hallucinations, are successfully brought under control.

25.3 Diagnostic criteria

In DSM-IV-TR, Criterion A of schizophrenia includes delusions, hallucinations, disorganized speech, disorganized or catatonic behavior, and negative symptoms. Two or more of these symptoms are required during the active phase of the illness. However, if the patient describes bizarre delusions or auditory hallucinations consisting of a voice commenting on the patient's behavior or voices conversing, only one of these symptoms is required to reach the diagnosis.

DSM-IV-TR lists the three negative symptoms as characteristic of schizophrenia: alogia, affective blunting, and avolition. Other negative symptoms common in schizophrenia include anhedonia and attentional impairment. Negative symptoms account for the substantial degree of morbidity and impairment associated with schizophrenia. They are the most intractable and difficult to treat, and they reflect a deficiency of mental functioning that is normally present. Patients with prominent negative symptoms are sadly at a disadvantage in society. The addition of negative symptoms as a separate criterion in DSM-IV recognizes the prominence of these symptoms in patients with schizophrenia.

Criterion B addresses loss of social and occupational functioning, not exclusively because of any one of the items in Criterion A. Patients may have difficulties maintaining employment, relationships, or academic achievements. If the illness presents at an early age, rather than as a degeneration or reversal of function, there may be a break from continued academic and social gains that are developmentally appropriate so that the person never achieves what had been expected.

Criterion C eliminates patients with less than 6 months of continued disturbance and again requires at least 1 month of the symptoms from Criterion A. Criterion C allows prodromal and residual periods to include only negative symptoms or a less severely manifested version of the other symptoms of the A criteria. Criterion D excludes patients who have a more compelling mood aspect of their illness and therefore their symptoms might instead meet criteria for schizoaffective disorder or a mood disorder. Both of these restrictions force a narrower view of the diagnosis of schizophrenia, which lessens the tendency of psychiatrists to overdiagnose schizophrenia.

Criterion E clarifies the fact that patients with schizophrenia are not suffering from other medical illnesses or the physiological effects of substances that might mimic the symptoms of schizophrenia.

Finally, Criterion F acknowledges that schizophrenia can be diagnosed in patients with autistic disorder or developmental disorder, as long as there have been prominent delusions or hallucinations that have lasted at least 1 month.

Table 25-1	Subtypes of schizophrenia
Subtype	**Features**
Paranoid	Existence of hallucinations or delusion in presence of clear sensorium and unchanged cognition
	Disorganized speech or behavior and flat or inappropriate affect not present to a significant degree
	Delusions usually of a persecutory or grandiose nature
	Hallucinations centered around particular themes
	Later onset than other subtypes, with better prognosis
Catatonic	Marked negativism or mutism, profound psychomotor retardation or severe psychomotor agitation, echolalia (repetition of words or phrases in a nonsensical manner), echopraxia (mimicking the behaviors of others), or bizarreness of voluntary movements and mannerisms.
	Some patients demonstrate a waxy flexibility, which is seen when a limb is repositioned on examination and remains in that position as if the patient were made of wax
	May stay in the same position for weeks at a time
Disorganized	Presents with the hallmark symptoms of disorganized speech and/or behavior, along with flat or inappropriate (incongruent) affect
	Any delusions or hallucinations, if present, also tend to be disorganized and are not related to a single theme
	In general have more severe deficits on neuropsychological tests.
	Earlier onset of illness, unremitting course, and poor prognosis
Undifferentiated	No hallmark symptom
	Does not fit criteria for paranoid, disorganized, or catatonic
Residual	Used when past history of acute episode of schizophrenia is present
	Continued evidence of negative symptoms or low grade or minimal form symptoms of Criterion A
	Unpredictable, variable course

25.4 DSM-IV-TR subtypes

In DSM-IV-TR, schizophrenia has been divided into clinical subtypes, based on field trials of the reliability of symptom clusters. The subtypes are divided by the most prominent symptoms, although it is acknowledged that the specific subtype may exist simultaneously with, or change over, the course of the illness. These types are summarized in Table 25.1.

25.5 Epidemiology

The epidemiology of schizophrenia is complex and different models of measurement produce different numbers. Numbers tend to vary over a number of criteria. Based on conservative estimates (i.e., the central 80% of the cumulative distribution), rates for the incidence of schizophrenia fall within a range of 7.7–43.0 per 100 000. The number most frequently cited comes from the World Health Organization, which is 7 per thousand of persons aged 15–35 are affected (24 million worldwide). The main age range of risk for schizophrenia is 15–45 years. The age of onset is earlier in men; men tend to show the first signs of disease during their mid twenties, women during their late twenties. According to WHO, more than 50% of people with schizophrenia are not being appropriately treated. Ninety percent of people with untreated schizophrenia are in developing countries.

25.6 Course and prognosis

The natural course of schizophrenia follows a three-phase model: an early phase marked by deterioration from premorbid levels of functioning; a middle phase characterized by a prolonged period of little change, termed the "stabilization phase"; and the last period called the "improving phase."

There a great deal of evidence from long-term follow-up studies that patients have a higher risk of relapse and exacerbations if not maintained with adequate antipsychotic regimens. Nonadherence to medication, possibly because of intolerable antipsychotic side-effects as well as other factors, may contribute to increased relapse rates.

The outcomes for people with schizophrenia are variable. Among the factors determining course and outcome are level of social development at onset, the disorder itself (e.g., genetic liability, severity of symptoms, and functional deficits), general biologic factors (e.g., estrogen), and sex- and age-specific illness behavior. Earlier treatment yields more favorable outcomes.

Patients with schizophrenia are at high risk for suicide. About 10–15% commit suicide; 50% attempt suicide at least once. Risk factors for suicide in this population include depressive symptoms, young age at the disorder's onset, and a high level of premorbid functioning. Patients with schizophrenia also have a higher mortality rate from accidents and medical illnesses. They generally experience poor health because of unhealthy lifestyles and neglect.

25.7 Etiology

Schizophrenia appears to be a complex genetic disorder that does not show a simple Mandelian pattern of inheritance. The cause(s) of schizophrenia currently remain unknown. Research is progressing rapidly and optimism at unraveling the mystery of this syndrome is increasing.

25.7.1 The double-hit hypothesis

A leading view is that the etiology of schizophrenia may be heterogeneous. Thus, multiple causative mechanisms may give rise to distinct disease subtypes. Moreover, it has been proposed that more than one causative mechanism might interact (the so-called "double-hit" hypothesis) to cause the illness in some individuals. The double-hit hypothesis posits that genetic vulnerability or problems in the womb set the stage for schizophrenia, but that a second event in adolescence or early adulthood leads to the development of schizophrenia. This "second hit" may be a major life event or episode of stress.

Available data strongly indicate that the interactions between genetic and environmental factors may lie at the core of this illness. Thus, the focus has shifted to multiple genes of small to moderate effects which may compound their effects through interactions with each other and with other nongenetic risk factors.

25.7.2 Pathophysiology

The brain processes that give rise to schizophrenia are currently not known. However, rapidly converging bodies of neuroanatomic and neurochemical data appear to be closing in on defining the pathophysiology of this illness. These data are reviewed below.

- **Enlarged ventricles**. The most consistent morphologic finding in the literature of schizophrenia is enlarged ventricles that have been confirmed by a large number of CT and MRI studies. Chronically ill patients are reported to have substantially more ventricular enlargement compared to those who are in their first episode. Increase in ventricular size with the progression of illness has been reported as well. The pathophysiologic significance of larger than normal ventricles is unclear.

- **Limbic system**. The limbic structures that have been implicated in schizophrenia are the hippocampus, entorhinal cortex, anterior cingulate, and amygdala. These structures have important functions for memory (hippocampus), attention (anterior cingulate), and emotional expression and social affiliation (amygdala).

- **Temporal lobe**. The superior temporal gyrus (STG) is involved in auditory processing and, with parts of the inferior parietal cortex, is a heteromodal association area that includes Wernicke's area, a language center. Because of the important role it plays in audition, it was hypothesized to be involved in auditory hallucinations. MRI studies have found the STG to be reduced in size in schizophrenia and have found a significant relationship between these reductions and the presence of auditory hallucinations. Similarly, Wernicke's area, which is involved in the conception and organization of speech, has been hypothesized to mediate the thought disorder of schizophrenia, particularly conceptual disorganization.

- **Prefrontal cortex**. The prefrontal cortex (PFC) is the most anterior portion of the neocortex which has evolved through lower species to become one of the largest regions of the human brain. It is responsible for some of the most sophisticated human functions containing a heteromodal association area that is responsible for integrating information from all other cortical areas as well as from several subcortical regions for the execution of purposeful behavior. Among its specific functions are working memory, which involves the temporary storage (seconds to minutes) of information, attention, and suppression of interference from internal and external sources. The most inferior portion of the PFC, termed the orbital frontal cortex (OFC), is involved in emotional expression. Several lines of evidence have implicated the PFC in schizophrenia. CT studies have provided evidence for prefrontal atrophy, and some, although not all, MRI studies have found evidence for decreased volume of this structure.

- **Other regions**. There are positive as well as negative reports of both parietal and occipital lobes showing differences between patients with schizophrenia and healthy controls. Abnormalities involving cerebellum have been reported too. At present, the significance of these findings is not clear.

Several neuroanatomic and physiologic theories have been proposed dealing with abnormal neuronal circuitry, among others, but are beyond the scope of this chapter. Readers are referred to the readings at the end of this chapter to access more comprehensive literature dealing with these theories and findings that support them.

25.7.3 Neurochemical theories

Readers are reminded as they read the following section that schizophrenia is a syndrome of heterogeneous etiology and pathology. If one neurotransmitter is disturbed, it will inevitably have an impact on other neurotransmitters.

25.7.3.1 Dopamine

Dopamine is the most extensively investigated neurotransmitter system in schizophrenia. In 1973 it was proposed that schizophrenia is related to hyperactivity of dopamine. This proposition became the dominant pathophysiological hypothesis for the next 15 years. Its strongest support came from the fact that all commercially available antipsychotic agents have antagonistic effects on the dopamine D2 receptor in relation to their clinical potencies. In addition, dopamine agonists, such as amphetamine and methylphenidate, exacerbate psychotic symptoms in a subgroup of patients with schizophrenia. Moreover, the most consistently reported postmortem finding in the literature of schizophrenia is elevated D2 receptors in the striatum. The DA hypothesis of schizophrenia has been critical in guiding schizophrenia research for several decades. It is likely that D2 is not the only receptor involved, as five different subtypes of dopamine receptors have been discovered and other neurotransmitters have been implicated in schizophrenia.

25.7.3.2 Serotonin

There has been interest in serotonin's role in schizophrenia because of the action of second-generation antipsychotics that have an affinity for specific serotonin receptors. This has led to the hypothesis that the balance between serotonin and dopamine might be altered in schizophrenia. Several postmortem studies have found elevations of serotonin and its metabolites in the striatum of patients with schizophrenia.

25.7.3.3 Glutamate

Some of the risk genes identified for schizophrenia also affect the glutamatergic system. In animal models of NMDA receptor antagonists, second-generation antipsychotics are more effective in ameliorating symptoms. Thus, hypoglutamatergia in schizophrenia may have very important downstream modulatory effects on catecholaminergic neurotransmission and play a critical role during neurodevelopment. It also plays an important role in synaptic pruning and underlies important aspects of neurocognition.

25.7.3.4 GABA

Alterations in the GABA neurotransmitter system are found in clinical and basic neuroscience schizophrenia studies as well as animal models and may be involved in the pathophysiology of schizophrenia. The interaction of GABA with other well-characterized neurotransmitter abnormalities remains to be understood.

25.7.3.5 Peptides

Neurotensin, somatostatin, dynorphin, substance P, and neuropeptide Y are under consideration for a pathophysiological role in schizophrenia.

25.7.3.6 Norepinephrine

Heightened noradrenergic function has been implicated in psychotic relapse in subgroups of schizophrenia patients.

25.7.4 Neurodevelopmental and neurodegenerative hypotheses

A leading hypothesis for the etiology of schizophrenia is related to disturbance in normal brain development. The principal assumption is that normal brain development is disrupted in specific ways at critical periods and the resulting lesion produces the symptoms of schizophrenia through interaction with the normal maturation processes in the brain, which occur in late adolescence or early adulthood. The neurodegenerative hypothesis suggests an ongoing neurodegenerative processes with loss of neuronal function during the course of the disease, and that neurons degenerate as a consequence of excessive glutamatergic neurotransmission. Most recently researchers have proposed the combined neurodevelopmental and neurodegenerative hypothesis to suggest that schizophrenia may be a neurodegenerative process superimposed on a neurodevelopmental abnormality.

25.8 Differential diagnosis

Making an accurate diagnosis of schizophrenia requires high levels of clinical acumen, extensive knowledge of schizophrenia, and sophisticated application of the principles of differential diagnosis. It is unfortunately common for patients with psychotic disorders to be misdiagnosed and consequently treated inappropriately. The importance of accurate diagnosis is underlined by an emerging database indicating that early detection and prompt pharmacologic intervention may improve the long-term prognosis of the illness. The following are conditions that resemble schizophrenia.

25.8.1 Schizoaffective disorder

A patient with schizoaffective disorder must have an uninterrupted period of illness during which, at some time, he or she has symptoms that meet the diagnostic criteria for a major depressive episode, manic episode, or a mixed episode concurrently with the diagnostic criteria for the active phase of schizophrenia.

25.8.2 Brief psychotic disorder

Brief psychotic disorder is a transient psychotic state, not caused by medical conditions or substance use, that lasts for at least 1 day and up to 1 month.

25.8.3 Schizophreniform disorder

Schizophreniform disorder requires symptoms for at least 1 month and not exceeding 6 months, with no requirement for loss of functioning.

25.8.4 Delusional disorder

Delusional disorder is usually characterized by specific types of false fixed beliefs such as erotomanic, grandiose, jealous, persecutory, or somatic types. Unlike schizophrenia it is not associated with marked social impairment or odd behavior. Patients with delusional disorder do not experience hallucinations or typically have negative symptoms.

25.8.5 Affective disorder with psychotic features

If the patient experiences psychotic symptoms solely during times when affective symptoms are present, the diagnosis is more likely to be mood disorder with psychotic features. If the mood disturbance involves both manic and depressive episodes, the diagnosis is bipolar disorder.

25.8.6 Substance-related conditions

Psychotic disorders, delirium, and dementia that are caused by substance use, in DSM-IV-TR, are distinguished from schizophrenia by virtue of the fact that there is clear-cut evidence of substance use leading to symptoms.

25.8.7 General medical conditions

General medical conditions ranging from vitamin B_{12} deficiency to Cushing's syndrome have been associated with schizophrenia-like symptoms. It is imperative to rule out any general medical condition prior to making a diagnosis of any psychiatric disorder.

25.9 Interdisciplinary goals

Both pharmacologic and psychosocial interventions are necessary to safeguard the patient and promote his or her recovery. Continuity of care, including discharge planning and ongoing care within the community, are essential interventions for patients with schizophrenia. Overall goals of treatment include the following:

- Safety in all settings

- Stabilization on antipsychotic medication

- Patient and family education about schizophrenia and its treatment

- Physical care of patient

- Psychosocial support of patient and family.

The scope and breadth of needs of the person with schizophrenia are too great for any one professional to meet. An interdisciplinary team works together to provide the comprehensive care necessary to achieve these goals. Professionals from psychiatry, nursing, psychology, and social work supply therapeutic services. Case management and rehabilitation services are also essential to recovery. The most effective treatment model to help people with schizophrenia and their families requires coordination of multidisciplinary care by a case manager. An optimal model of interdisciplinary treatment for those with schizophrenia includes elements in Box 25.1.

Box 25.1 Model of Interdisciplinary Treatment for Serious Mental Illness.

Assessment of current functioning
Medication management
Patient and family education
Life and social skills training
Family counseling
Vocational training and rehabilitation
Housing assistance
Crisis intervention and brief inpatient services
Continuity of care providers
Network of ongoing social support including advocacy group involvement

---

25.10 Treatments

25.10.1 Pharmacotherapy

Antipsychotic medications do not cure schizophrenia, but treat the symptoms during both the acute and maintenance phases of the illness. Like every pharmacotherapeutic agent, these drugs have side-effects, some of which are sometimes intolerable to patients and some of which result in undesirable health effects. Nevertheless, early intervention with medication decreases some of the associated long-term comorbid, or coexisting, conditions. Medications also render patients more amenable to social, cognitive, and rehabilitative therapies. Two types of drug are used as the mainstay of treating schizophrenia: first- and second-generation antipsychotics.

First-generation antipsychotics (FGAs) have been used successfully since 1952, and until 1994 (with the exception of clozapine) were the only medications available in the United States. FGAs, which are dopamine antagonists, have associated side-effects (see Chapter 35) that are numerous and distressing, and they often cause the patient to become noncompliant.

Second-generation antipsychotics (SGAs) were developed in response to neurobiologic-based schizophrenia research findings and are serotonin dopamine antagonists. The SGAs can be slightly more effective against both positive and negative symptoms than the FGAs, are less likely to induce extrapyramidal symptoms, and were initially thought to help promote adherence. This is not the case as studies have shown that almost 50–75% of patients will switch or discontinue medications within the first 18 months or less regardless of whether they were taking FGAs or SGAs. One study has suggested that early discontinuation of medication was higher in an FGA (haloperidol) group of patients than in a group taking the SGA risperidone.

Antipsychotic medications are usually taken orally in liquid or tablet form, but intramuscular (IM) injections also can be given for immediate action. For patients who have compliance difficulties, depot preparations of fluphenazine, haloperidol, and risperidone are available and administered every one to six weeks, eliminating the need to monitor daily compliance.

The Texas Medication Algorithm for Schizophrenia is a public–academic collaborative effort to develop, implement, and evaluate medication treatment algorithms for public sector patients. It is a useful tool for choosing antipsychotic treatment, managing treatment-emergent side-effects and associated or coexisting symptoms. For more information or to view the most current version of the algorithm, visit http://www.dshs.state.tx.us/mhprograms/TMAP.shtm.

25.10.2 Nonpharmacologic treatments

Interdisciplinary goals and treatment have already been discussed and the need for a comprehensive approach to treatment has been stressed. These may have to be modified over the life of treatment with modalities changing in response to treatment. Interventions are described below.

25.10.2.1 Psychosocial rehabilitation

The rehabilitation process should appreciate the unique life circumstances of each person and respond to the individual's special needs while promoting both the treatment of the illness and the reduction of its attendant disabilities. The treatment should be provided in the context of the individual's unique environment taking into account social support network, access to transportation, housing, work opportunities, and so on. Rehabilitation should exploit the patient's strengths and improve his or her competencies. Ultimately, rehabilitation should focus on the positive concept of restoring hope to those who have suffered major setbacks in functional capacity and their self-esteem due to major mental illness. To have this hope grounded in reality, it requires promoting acceptance of one's illness and the limitations that come with it.

Psychosocial rehabilitation has to transcend work to encompass medical, social, and recreational themes. Psychosocial treatment's basic principle is to provide comprehensive care through active involvement of the patient in his or her own treatment. Intervention has to be ongoing. Given the chronicity of the illness, the process of rehabilitation must be enduring to encounter future stresses and challenges and goal achievement is built on a stable relationship between patient and counselors/caregivers. Psychosocial rehabilitation is intimately connected to the biologic intervention and forms a core component of the biopsychosocial approach to the treatment of schizophrenia. Too often, the above programs deviate from the aforementioned principles and end up putting excessive and unrealistic expectations on patients, thus achieving exactly the opposite of the intended values of the program.

25.10.2.2 Psychotherapy

Acutely psychotic patients do not benefit from group interaction. Quiet places with decreased social contact is desirable until medications have controlled acute symptoms.

Individual and group therapies that offer support, education, and behavioral and cognitive skills training are recommended to improve functioning and address specific problems, such as medication noncompliance or social isolation. The focus of individual therapy should be on building a therapeutic relationship, helping the client stay oriented to reality, and helping the client improve coping skills. This relationship can help the client experience guidance, support, and reinforcement for his or her health promotion efforts and successes.

Group therapy sessions should focus on social skills, concentrating on appropriate interpersonal interaction and social skills aquisition. Treatment also addresses practical matters such as personal care, living skills, and money management.

25.10.2.3 Family therapy

Family interventions have been shown to reduce relapse rates by one-half over the first year of combined treatment with medications and family therapy. Medications and family therapy augment each other. Psychoeducation is an important component of such therapy, as is identification of family stressors. It also seems that multiple family groups are more efficacious than single family sessions. The National Alliance for the Mentally Ill (NAMI) has such a 12-week comprehensive program called Family to Family, which is free; see http://www.nami.org/Template.cfm?Section=Family-to-Family.

Clinical Vignette

Mrs F, a 35-year-old recently separated immigrant woman, was brought to the emergency room in an acutely agitated state with auditory hallucinations and confusion. She immigrated to the US two years ago to join her husband of five years. They separated 3 months ago. She lost her job a month later and had to bear significant financial hardship. Her father was medically ill and passed away unexpectedly 6 weeks previously.

According to people close to her, Mrs F started having symptoms approximately 7 days before her admission. She was reported to be restless, pacing, and preoccupied with the recent stressors. On various occasions her speech was tangential or incoherent. Her mood was labile and she appeared to be perplexed at times. Her attention and concentration was poor. She was paranoid of her husband (family members denied him being a threat to her) and often felt that her deceased father was communicating with her. She had passive suicidal thoughts.

Mrs F was often upset about being hospitalized and demanded release from the hospital. She would get quite angry and throw tantrums if her request for discharge was denied. There was no history of alcohol or drug use. She was in good physical health. There was no history of similar or other episodes.

Admission work up was essentially normal. The urine toxicology screen, pregnancy test, and EEG were normal. Following admission, she was started on a low dose of benzodiazepine and an atypical antipsychotic agent. Her symptoms of agitation and psychosis responded rapidly within 1 week. Individual and group therapy sessions were very helpful in addressing her recent stressors and providing emotional support. Family therapy was offered but the patient and her family rejected it. With the help of individual and group therapy, she was able to develop some coping skills.

Following discharge, Mrs F continued to respond to the low-dose antipsychotic treatment and other therapies. She was not having any symptoms of psychosis and was able to deal with her stressors better. Approximately 3 weeks after discharge, though her stressors continued, she was responding well to the treatment, reached her baseline functioning, but due to significant weight gain and sedation she decided to discontinue her medication. Six months later she had continued with psychotherapy and group therapy and had maintained her baseline functioning.

KEY POINTS

- Schizophrenia, which manifests during late adolescence and early adulthood, is the most common and severe psychotic disorder, affecting about 1% of the population.

- Proposed etiological theories include genetic, neurochemical, and neuropathologic; viral; immunologic; and structural abnormalities of the brain.

- Other psychotic disorders include schizophreniform disorder, schizoaffective disorder, delusional disorder, brief psychotic disorder, shared psychotic disorder, and psychosis NOS.

- Schizophrenia is a heterogeneous disorder with some common features, including thought disturbances, affect disturbances, and behavioral or social disturbances.

- Three dimensions of psychopathology in schizophrenia include the disorganization dimension, the psychotic dimension, and the negative dimension.

- The five subtypes of schizophrenia are paranoid, disorganized, catatonic, undifferentiated, and residual.

- Antipsychotic medications are the primary treatment for schizophrenia.

- Continuity of care involving discharge planning and aggressive care within the community setting after hospitalization for the patient with schizophrenia is essential.

Further Reading

Castle, D.J. and Buckley, P.F. (2008) *Schizophrenia*, Oxford University Press, New York.
NIMH Clinical Antipsychotic Trial of Intervention Effectiveness (Treatment Choices for Schizophrenia). Available at: http://www.nimh.nih.gov/health/trials/practical/catie/index.shtml.

26.1 Introduction

The somatoform disorders are a group of psychologic disorders in which a patient experiences physical symptoms despite the absence of an underlying medical condition that can fully explain their presence. Symptoms are not intentionally produced and are not attributable to another mental disorder. To warrant the diagnosis, symptoms must be clinically significant in terms of causing distress or impairment in important areas of functioning. The disorders included in this class are somatization disorder, undifferentiated somatoform disorder, conversion disorder, pain disorder, hypochondriasis, body dysmorphic disorder, and a somatoform disorder "not otherwise specified."

26.2 Features of the somatoform disorders

26.2.1 Somatization disorder

Somatization disorder was referred to historically as "hysteria" or Briquet's syndrome. The physical complaints appear before the age of 30 years and persist over several years. Patients living with somatization disorder usually present exaggerated, inconsistent, yet complicated medical histories with individual symptoms that include the following at any time during its course: four pain symptoms, two gastrointenstinal symptoms, one sexual symptom, and one pseudoneurological symptom. Patients often seek treatment from multiple healthcare providers when their physical complaints are not addressed to their satisfaction.

The conceptualization of somatization disorder is diagnostically complex and cumbersome as described in the DSM, hence the category may be underused and the diagnosis under-reported. In addition, the term "somatization" has acquired a pejorative connotation. Clinicians are reluctant to so label a patient, and to diagnose more readily treatable symptoms such as anxiety and depressive syndromes and downplay the underlying illness. Moreover, authorization and reimbursement for treatment of this chronic condition are often challenged or denied. It is relatively easier to obtain approval for an intervention on the basis of major depressive disorder, for example, than on the basis of a disorder that is much more likely to be poorly understood by case reviewers.

Somatization disorder is rare in children younger than 9 years. Characteristic symptoms begin in adolescence, and the full criteria as designated by DSM-IV-TR are met by the mid twenties. The active symptomatic phase of the condition occurs during early adulthood and aging does not appear to lead to remission. The course is chronic and full remission is rarely, if ever achieved.

Fundamentals of Psychiatry, First Edition. Allan Tasman and Wanda K. Mohr.
© 2011 John Wiley & Sons, Ltd. Published 2011 by John Wiley & Sons, Ltd.
This chapter is based on Chapter 74 (Sean H. Yutzy, Brooke S. Parish) of *Psychiatry, Third Edition*

26.2.2 Undifferentiated somatoform disorder

As defined by DSM-IV-TR, the persistent, unexplained physical symptoms that characterize undifferentiated somatoform disorder last for at least 6 months and do not fully meet the criteria for somatization disorder or any other somatoform disorder. Common complaints include fatigue, loss of appetite, and gastrointestinal or urinary symptoms. This category includes one or more unintentional, clinically significant, medically unexplained physical complaints. In a sense it is a residual category, subsuming syndromes with somatic complaints that do not meet criteria for any of the "differentiated" somatoform disorders yet are not better accounted for by any other mental disorder.

People suffering from undifferentiated somatoform disorder experience negative repercussions in interpersonal, occupational, or other aspects of functioning. The patient's history, physical examination, and laboratory tests do not explain or verify the physical symptoms or disruption in life experiences. The course and prognosis of this disorder are exceedingly variable.

26.2.3 Conversion disorder

Conversion disorders are characterized by symptoms or deficits affecting voluntary motor or sensory function that suggest, yet are not fully explained by, a neurologic or other general medical condition or the direct effects of a substance. The diagnosis is not made if the presentation is explained as a culturally sanctioned behavior or experience, such as bizarre behaviors resembling a seizure during a religious ceremony. Symptoms are not intentionally produced or feigned; that is, the person does not consciously contrive a symptom for external rewards, as in malingering, or for the intrapsychic rewards of assuming the sick role, as in factitious disorder. Age at onset is typically from late childhood to early adulthood. Onset is rare before the age of 10 years and after 35 years, but cases with an onset as late as the ninth decade have been reported.

Four subtypes with specific examples of symptoms are defined: (1) with motor symptom or deficit (e.g., impaired coordination or balance, paralysis or localized weakness, difficulty swallowing or lump in throat, aphonia, and urinary retention); (2) with sensory symptom or deficit (e.g., loss of touch or pain sensation, double vision, blindness, deafness, and hallucinations); (3) with seizures or convulsions; and (4) with mixed presentation (i.e., has symptoms of more than one of the other subtypes).

26.2.4 Pain disorder

The diagnosis of pain disorder is new to DSM-IV-TR. The classic symptom is the unexplained presence of physical pain. Psychologic factors have a prominent role in the genesis. Patients suffering from pain disorder experience pain as a major focus in their lives, frequently access healthcare services, and commonly take medications for the symptoms. Pain disorders are expressed in various body areas (e.g., abdomen, back, bone, breast), each of which is coded individually in DSM-IV-TR. In addition, DSM-IV-TR requires that pain be the predominant focus of the clinical presentation and that it cause clinically significant distress or impairment. Specifiers of acute (duration of less than 6 months) and chronic (duration of 6 months or longer) are provided.

Little literature is available on this condition, its onset, or its course. Habituation with drugs is associated with greater chronicity.

26.2.5 Hypochondriasis

The person with hypochondriasis has an unwarranted fear or belief that he or she has a serious disease, without significant pathology. This is in contrast to somatization disorder, conversion disorder, and pain disorder, in which the symptoms themselves are the predominant focus. Much of the patient's psychic energy may be bound in unrealistic fears that healthcare providers are missing diagnoses, such as cancer, cardiac disease, or sexually transmitted diseases.

Data are conflicting but it seems that the most common age at onset of hypochondriasis is early adulthood. About 25% of patients have a poor outcome; 65% have a chronic but fluctuating course, and 10% recover.

When patients do not obtain satisfaction from one care provider, they often will go to another or a series of others in an attempt to find an answer to their symptoms. Preoccupation with bodily distress and the accompanying expectation that others also should focus on the patient's physical well-being may disrupt social relationships and work. In contrast to the lack of anxiety seen in patients with conversion disorder, patients with hypochondriasis often appear anxious about their symptoms. They can sometimes acknowledge that their fear of a dreaded disease is unfounded; however, they are unaware of their anxiety or depression.

26.2.6 Body dysmorphic disorder

The primary feature of body dysmorphic disorder is preoccupation with an imagined defect in appearance when no abnormality or disturbance is present. Patients tend to obsess about imagined facial defects, such as wrinkles, spots on the skin, facial asymmetry, or excessive facial hair. Other body parts, such as the genitals, breasts, buttocks, hands, or feet may be the focus of distress and embarrassment. Thinking that others are noticing the imagined flaw may be an associated feature. Because of extreme self-consciousness about the imagined defect, individuals may retreat from usual activities and resort to social isolation and display decreased academic and occupational functioning.

Age at onset appears to peak in adolescence or early adulthood. Body dysmorphic disorder is generally a chronic condition, with a waxing and waning of intensity but rarely full remission. Research on body dysmorphic disorder is limited and the disorder is often under-recognized.

26.2.7 Somatoform disorder not otherwise specified

This diagnosis is used for disorders that do not meet criteria for other specific somatoform disorders. Physical symptoms must be present for less than 6 months. The NOS category includes conditions such as pseudocyesis (a false belief that one is pregnant) and unexplained physical symptoms of fatigue or body weakness.

26.3 Comorbidities and dual diagnoses

Many somatoform disorders coexist with other psychiatric disorders, such as major depression, anxiety disorders, personality disorders, and panic disorders. Community studies have shown that psychological distress, stressful life events, and depression and anxiety disorders often are associated with medical symptoms for which a physiologic etiology cannot be found, increased use of healthcare services, and increased costs. Conversely, patients who have symptoms of diagnosed medical illnesses that are characterized by lack of well-defined pathology (e.g., irritable bowel syndrome, fibromyalgia) have significantly higher rates of anxiety and depressive disorders than do patients with comparable, well-defined medical diseases and similar symptoms. In the case of hypochondriasis, the dual diagnoses of depression and hypochondriasis are described frequently in the literature; however, some people suffer from hypochondriasis alone.

26.4 Epidemiology

Estimates of the frequency of this group of disorders in the general population as well as in clinical settings are inconsistent. The data seem to indicate that such problems are common and account for a major proportion of clinical services, especially in primary care settings. A World Health Organization study reported ICD-10 diagnoses of hypochondriasis in nearly 1% and of somatization disorder in nearly 3% of patients in primary care clinics in 14 countries.

Generally, somatoform disorders are diagnosed more commonly in women than in men, with somatization disorder being 10 times more common in women than in men. The first symptoms of somatoform disorders usually appear in adolescence; patients may meet the full criteria for the disorders by 30 years of age.

26.5 Differentiation among the somatoform disorders

It is often assumed that the specific disorders in the somatoform grouping are heterogeneous in terms of pathogenesis and pathophysiology, but they are also phenomenologically diverse. In somatization disorder, undifferentiated somatoform disorder, conversion disorder, and pain disorder, the focus is on the physical complaints themselves, and thus on perceptions. In hypochondriasis and body dysmorphic disorder, emphasis is on physically related preoccupations or fears, and thus on cognitions. Somatization disorder and, to a lesser extent, undifferentiated somatoform disorder are characterized by multiple symptoms of different types; conversion disorder, pain disorder, hypochondriasis, and body dysmorphic disorder are defined on the basis of a single symptom or a few symptoms of a certain type. Whereas somatization disorder, undifferentiated somatoform disorder, and hypochondriasis are, by definition, at least 6 months in duration, conversion disorder, pain disorder, body dysmorphic disorder, and somatoform disorder "not otherwise specified" may be of short duration as long as they are associated with clinically significant distress or impairment.

26.6 Cultural considerations

Culture influences the patient's experience and manifestation of symptoms, both physiologic and psychologic. Somatization is ubiquitous culturally and somatic symptoms often serve as cultural symbols of distress for many ethnocultural groups. If the clinician misinterprets these symptoms, unnecessary diagnostic procedures or treatments may result.

26.7 Etiology

The basis for somatoform disorders is often unclear and complicated. Many theories on the causes have been proposed. Most clinicians advocate a multidimensional causal model, including a complex interplay of psychologic, neurobiologic, and familial factors. Somatization disorders have been shown to be familial. Likewise, patients with unexplained pain are more likely than others to have close relatives with chronic pain. People with conversion disorder have been found to be in chaotic domestic and/or occupational situations.

26.8 Differential diagnosis and complications

Diagnosis requires an extensive history of many physical symptoms that cannot be explained fully by a physical disorder. Physicians often conduct many examinations and tests to eliminate a physical disorder, but complications from invasive testing can result. Patients often become frustrated and demand that "something be done," so they may be exposed to unnecessary surgeries and their

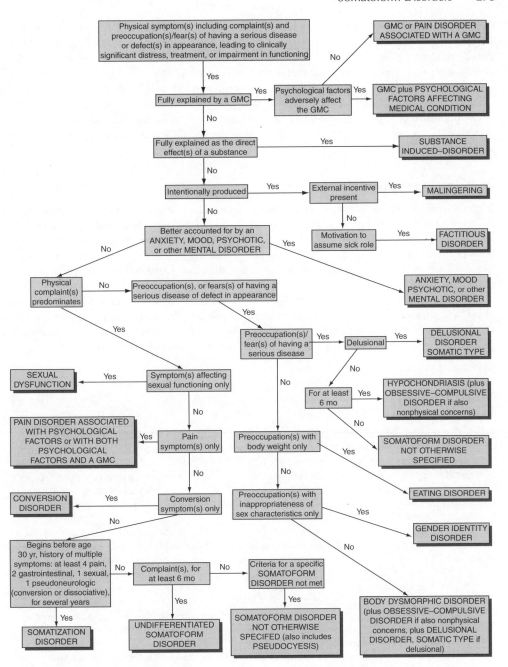

Figure 26-1 *Diagnostic exploration and treatment algorithm.*

attendant complications; or the professional relationship deteriorates and the patient goes on to "doctor shop" – resulting in the same cycle of searching for symptom causation. Multiple care providers may lead to patients being prescribed numerous medications, some of which in combination may produce their own adverse results (e.g., serotonin syndrome from more than one reuptake inhibitor). Patients may become dependent on pain medications, resulting in a comorbid condition complicating treatment. Because patients with somatization disorder may develop concurrent physical disorders, appropriate examinations and tests should also be done when symptoms change or when objective signs develop. Figure 26.1 illustrates the diagnostic exploration and treatment algorithm.

26.9 Treatment principles

Whereas specific somatoform disorders indicate specific treatment approaches, some general guidelines apply. There are three therapeutic goals: (1) as an overriding goal, prevention of the adoption of the sick role and chronic invalidism; (2) minimization of unnecessary costs and complications by avoiding unwarranted hospitalizations, diagnostic and treatment procedures, and medications (especially those of an addictive potential); and (3) effective treatment of comorbid psychiatric disorders, such as depressive and anxiety syndromes.

The general treatment strategies include: (1) consistent treatment, generally by the same physician, with careful coordination if multiple physicians are involved; (2) supportive clinic visits, scheduled at regular intervals rather than in response to symptoms; and (3) a gradual shift in focus from symptoms to an emphasis on personal and interpersonal problems.

Clinical Vignette 1

Ms Q, a 47-year-old divorced woman, was referred for psychiatric consultation by her primary care physician at the recommendation of a neurologist. She had been admitted to the hospital 2 days earlier, after presenting with mild acidosis attributed to poor control of her insulin-dependent diabetes mellitus. She had become concerned that insulin was "making me fat" and had been taking it erratically for several weeks. On admission, she also complained of generalized muscle weakness, more pronounced on the left side, especially in the arm, and reported that she had a "stroke" affecting the right side 1 year before, for which she was not hospitalized.

On examination, the neurologist observed that Ms Q showed no atrophy or spasticity and that deep tendon reflexes were decreased but equal bilaterally. On testing of the left upper extremity, she was observed to show weakness in extending and flexing the arm against resistance, yet more careful examination revealed residual strength inconsistent with that shown in these tests. Her primary care physician reported some question of a stroke 1 year before, which was never clearly ascertained. A "hysterical component to the neurological symptoms" was considered. Nonetheless, diagnostic procedures were instituted, including magnetic resonance imaging which proved negative. Two days later it was concluded that a stroke was improbable, and noting reports of depressed mood, the neurologist recommended psychiatric consultation.

When seen by the psychiatric consultant, Ms Q still complained of the weakness, although it was somewhat improved and not so clearly localized to the left side. She also mentioned that she had been depressed for several weeks before admission and that she had been treated with some success with fluoxetine in the past. She reported multiple conflicts concerning her living situation. She was living with her married son and felt that his wife resented her presence. She felt "trapped" in that she could not afford to live independently. Medical records indicated that diabetes mellitus had been diagnosed at age 36 years and was treated with oral hypoglycemic agents until age 41 years, when insulin became necessary for adequate control. The record also revealed several episodes of transient unexplained weakness as well as occasional problems with headaches and joint pain going back to age 26 years, with several mentions of temporal proximity of such symptoms to marital and occupational difficulties. Yet, criteria for somatization disorder were not fulfilled.

The psychiatrist's provisional diagnoses were: (1) psychological factors affecting medical condition (noncompliance with insulin regimen); (2) conversion disorder, with motor symptoms or deficit; and (3) possible major depressive disorder, recurrent. Treatment with sertraline, 50 mg at bedtime, was recommended. It was also suggested to the patient that her tests were now completed and that it was expected that her weakness would continue to improve. When the psychiatrist visited her the next day, she reported that her weakness was better and that she was also beginning to feel less depressed. Ms Q was encouraged to continue to see her primary care physician and to comply with his recommendations, and she was referred to social work for assistance with her living situation. Referral for outpatient psychiatric care was also recommended.

This clinical vignette illustrates several important aspects concerning the diagnosis, course, and treatment of conversion disorder. As is not uncommon, the patient does suffer from a medical illness to which many symptoms can ordinarily be attributed. However, the extent of her complaints, the lack of neuroanatomical verification, and inconsistencies of her report and the documented history suggested a possibility that her motor symptoms were not fully attributable to a general medical condition. This interpretation was supported by her past history of apparent conversion symptoms as well as some other somatic complaints. Although she was also complaining of depression, her history was vague, and her "response" to one day's treatment with an antidepressant drug was unlikely to be pharmacologic. Her motor symptoms were resolving with reassurance and suggestion, such that the short-term prognosis for her motor symptoms was good. However, her history of noncompliance with medical treatment, and multiple situational and interpersonal problems indicated the advisability of continued psychosocial if not psychiatric intervention.

Clinical Vignette 2

Mr P, a 26-year-old single man, presented for psychiatric evaluation at the insistence of his job supervisor, who was concerned that the patient was not keeping up with his assignments at work. Mr P reported that he could not concentrate on his work because for the past 4 years he had been constantly preoccupied with the thought that there was something seriously wrong with his arms resulting from a "strain" while he moved furniture. Although there was minimal pain associated, he was convinced that the problem would progress and he would lose the use of his arms. Multiple consultations with orthopedic surgeons and neurologists had not identified any underlying physical problem. He rejected physical therapy for fear that it would only aggravate the underlying problem. Physical activity involving his arms was avoided as much as possible. Not able to avoid driving to work, he wore a prosthesis that he had constructed from various elastic bandages "to prevent any strain." He arrived at work early to be sure of a parking space that was easy to enter.

In addition to this preoccupation, Mr P also feared that ulcerative colitis was developing. This began after his father died of a GI hemorrhage when the patient was 16 years old. Initially diagnosed as possible ulcerative colitis, it was found at postmortem to be due to a ruptured abdominal aneurysm. The patient fully accepted this diagnosis, yet he could not stop thinking that he was at risk for ulcerative colitis despite multiple GI evaluations that failed to find any signs of the illness in him. He adhered to a strict diet, avoiding any "roughage," and was concerned about "regularity." He would awaken every day 2 hours earlier than necessary to have enough time for a bowel movement before going to work. The slightest GI sensation would aggravate his concern, and he would carefully examine his stool for any signs of blood or mucus. He reported that his work attendance was excellent but that most of the time he would just sit at his desk and move papers around to look busy while thinking about his health problems. "I have a civil service job and until now I got away with it." The patient had no prior psychiatric evaluations. For both of his health concerns, he was able to consider the possibility that there was no underlying physical cause, "but I can't stop thinking about them. What if all the doctors are wrong?"

The psychiatrist's diagnosis was hypochondriasis, with poor insight. The patient was to be further evaluated for a concurrent major depressive episode and also for nonhealth preoccupations that would suggest an additional diagnosis of obsessive–compulsive disorder. The psychiatrist's recommendations included: (1) a trial of fluoxetine to be increased to 60 mg/day if tolerated; (2) supportive–educative psychotherapy to ensure compliance and for support; and (3) cognitive–behavioral therapy to reinforce use of his arms, to extinguish assumptions that he needed a special diet, and to reassure him that dire consequences would not occur if his bowel movements were not absolutely punctual.

This clinical vignette illustrates several important typical aspects of hypochondriasis. First, the onset of the disorder was early, in the late teens, with consolidation of symptoms by early adulthood. Second, a chronic course was observed, with some fluctuation in severity. The physical complaints themselves were minimal. It was the preoccupation with fears of underlying illness that predominated and led to distress and impairment.

KEY POINTS

- Somatoform disorders are those in which patients present psychosocial distress through physical symptoms that have no organic basis.

- Somatization is ubiquitous culturally and somatic symptoms often serve as cultural symbols of distress for many ethnocultural groups.

- Symptoms of somatoform disorders must be clinically significant in terms of causing distress or impairment in important areas of functioning.

- Disorders included in this class are somatization disorder, undifferentiated somatoform disorder, conversion disorder, pain disorder, hypochondriasis, body dysmorphic disorder, and somatoform disorder not otherwise specified.

- Therapeutic treatment goals include: prevention of the adoption of the sick role and chronic invalidism, avoiding unwarranted hospitalizations, diagnostic and treatment procedures and medications, and effective treatment of comorbid psychiatric disorders, such as depressive and anxiety syndromes.

Further Reading

American Psychiatric Association (2000) *Diagnostic and Statistical Manual of Mental Disorders*, 4th edn, Text Revision. APA, Washington, DC.

Phillips, K.A. (2001) *Somatoform and Factitious Disorders*, APA Press, Washington, DC.

Woolfolk, R.L. and Allen, L.A. (2006) *Treating Somatization: A Cognitive Behavioural Approach*, Guilford, New York.

27 Dissociative Disorders

27.1 Introduction

Dissociative disorders are a group of psychiatric syndromes characterized by disruptions of aspects of consciousness, identity, memory, motor behavior, or environmental awareness. They are not among the more common psychiatric illnesses, and there is a controversy about them, specifically regarding the more dramatic manifestation, dissociative identity disorder (DID). This chapter discusses the phenomenon of dissociation and the disorders subsumed under this DSM category.

The debate over DID arose in the context of the furor over repressed and later recovered memories of childhood sexual abuse, the child sex abuse panic of the 1980s, and associated stories of satanic ritual abuse. It was fueled by the excesses of some mental health clinicians, who began to diagnose and "treat" individuals for DID. In some instances clinicians reported the existence of hundreds of "alter" personalities and claimed that an epidemic of DID was occurring across the United States, Canada, and the United Kingdom. Critics of the disorder assert that the diagnosis was a result of iatrogenesis, where the therapist unintentionally shaped the manifestation of the disorder. Despite an enormous amount of published literature on dissociative disorders, dissociation remains a poorly understood phenomenon and one that is controversial.

Currently, most psychiatric physicians believe that dissociation is a legitimate phenomenon. They also believe that DID, its most dramatic manifestation (formerly known as multiple personality disorder), is a rare condition when it occurs spontaneously but that it is easy to create iatrogenically. Clinicians reading this chapter are urged to keep an open mind and to understand that this area of psychopathology is poorly developed from an empirical standpoint.

27.2 Dissociation

Dissociation refers to the situation of altering one's usual level of self-awareness in an effort to escape an upsetting event or feeling. It is a normal reaction to an emotionally overloaded situation and happens in the service of self-preservation when neither resistance nor escape is possible. This process can include actively pretending to be somewhere or someone else, experiencing amnesia, and having the ability to "cut off" pain perception from parts of the body. The cognitive outcome of dissociation is fragmentation of memory. This fragmentation can result in patchy or disorganized recall, seemingly illogical associations, and seemingly extreme affective reactions such as displaying extreme rage in reaction to relatively minor interpersonal "offenses." All humans have the capacity to dissociate. Acts of daydreaming or amnestic episodes constitute common types of dissociation.

Fundamentals of Psychiatry, First Edition. Allan Tasman and Wanda K. Mohr.
© 2011 John Wiley & Sons, Ltd. Published 2011 by John Wiley & Sons, Ltd.
This chapter is based on Chapter 76 (José R. Maldonado, David Spiegel) of *Psychiatry, Third Edition*

27.3 Dissociation versus repression

Conceptually, dissociation differs from the defense mechanism of repression in several different ways. Repression is hypothesized to result from intrapsychic conflicts. Dissociation, in contrast, is hypothesized to result from external trauma with amnestic barriers presumed to divide subunits of memory. Moreover, in dissociation, the information is kept out of awareness for a sharply delimited period, whereas in repression information is kept out of awareness for a variety of experiences across time. In other words, the memories that are "repressed" in dissociation are specific to events. They are not the result of "forgetting" as a way to avoid anxiety associated with intrapsychic conflicts that may have nothing to do with specific events.

Pathologic dissociation occurs when a person experiences more frequent or "deeper" states of dissociation and everyday functioning deteriorates. Dissociation leading to impaired functioning requires treatment. The degree of disruption of the self and the intensity and types of intervention vary in the dissociative disorders. People may not remember their identity and travel far away from home (dissociative fugue), they may lose their memory (dissociative amnesia), they may assume two or more identities or personalities (DID), or they may feel that they are not in touch with their body (depersonalization disorder).

27.4 Epidemiology

Few good epidemiologic studies have been performed. Some estimate the prevalence at only 1 per 10 000 in the population but some have found people with these disorders to be as high as 1% of the population. Reliable and unbiased statistics are unavailable. Women make up the majority of reported cases, accounting for over 90% of the cases in some studies.

27.5 Cultural considerations

Although dissociative phenomena have occurred around the world, they seem to be more prevalent in the less heavily industrialized, developing countries. Cultural considerations regarding dissociative disorders should bear in mind that trance states are seen in some cultures, including Indonesia, Malaysia, the Arctic, India, and Latin America, and that trance states may be seen or included as part of spiritual belief systems. For diagnostic purposes, however, an individual must be experiencing dysfunction and stress, and the behaviors noted must not be a normal part of a broadly accepted collective cultural or religious practice.

Research shows that DID can be misdiagnosed in the Latino population because "ataque de nervios" is accepted as a diagnosis for this group, yet it has symptoms similar to DID. Amnesia is a predominant symptom of "ataque" and often is a culturally acceptable reaction to stress within the Latino community.

27.6 Etiology

The etiology of dissociative disorders is not known. Results of the few genetic studies examining dissociative disorders have been inconclusive. The ability to dissociate is believed to be partly related to having the capacity to do so when subjected to repeated stress.

27.6.1 Biologic factors

Various substances or medical conditions can induce dissociative symptoms. For example, a seizure disorder or prolonged use of alcohol may cause amnesia. Patients experiencing such symptoms, then, must undergo a thorough medical evaluation before a definitive diagnosis of dissociative disorder is made.

People with dissociative disorders appear to be particularly susceptible to hypnotism when tested for this capacity. They also seem to be highly suggestible and have low sedation thresholds. Physiologic studies suggest that dissociative reactions may be precipitated by excessive cortical arousal, which triggers reactive inhibition of signals in sensorimotor pathways by way of negative-feedback relationships between the cerebral cortex and the brainstem reticular formation.

27.6.2 *Psychological and social factors*

Dissociative disorders are believed to be a way for individuals to defend themselves against painful or distressing circumstances. Based on case study material, some experts in this area contend that abused people are especially likely to dissociate to defend against feeling the pain of remembering what has been done (or is being done) to them. However, there are no studies that provide methodologically sound evidence that dissociative amnesia is more prevalent in victims of abuse than in the general population.

27.7 Signs and symptoms/diagnostic criteria

DSM-IV-TR defines dissociative disorders as "a disruption in the usually integrated functions of consciousness, memory, identity, or perception." The disturbance may be sudden or gradual, transient or chronic. This definition includes four disorders:

1. **Depersonalization disorder** is characterized by a recurring or persistent feeling that one is detached from one's own thinking. Affected patients feel that they are outside their mind or body, much like an observer.

2. **Dissociative amnesia** is characterized by loss of memory that is not organic and involves an inability to recall events or facts too extensive to be labeled as mere forgetfulness.

3. **Dissociative fugue** involves sudden travel away from home coupled with an inability to remember the past and confusion about identity or the adoption of a new identity.

4. **Dissociative identity disorder** involves the person acquiring two or more identities or personality states (alters) who take control over his or her behavior. As with amnesia, DID involves an inability to recall important personal information that is too extensive to be labeled as forgetfulness.

DSM-IV-TR also includes a fifth category, "dissociative disorder not otherwise specified." Most patients determined to have a dissociative disorder will receive this diagnosis. The disorders in this category have a dissociative symptom as a primary feature but do not meet the criteria for any of the four dissociative disorders.

27.8 Comorbidities and dual diagnoses

The most significant comorbid psychiatric conditions include depression, substance abuse, and borderline personality disorder (BPD). Sexual dysfunction, eating, and sleep disorders occur less frequently. Self-mutilative behavior, impulsivity, and labile interpersonal relationships are frequently exhibited by DID patients. Nearly one-third of DID patients also meet diagnostic criteria for BPD. Patients exhibiting this interaction (DID plus BPD) also experience higher levels of depression. Some studies have identified that approximately one-third of DID patients may suffer from complex partial seizures. Newly diagnosed cases with DID should be evaluated for the possibility of a seizure disorder or other medical conditions.

27.9 Treatment approaches

Proponents of DID as a distinct diagnosis with a unique treatment approach assert that treatment must involve fusion of all "alters" into a single personality. The process of integration of "alters" involves unlearning an overreliance on dissociation and acquiring a new set of adaptive coping strategies. Treatment involves breaking down amnestic barriers and integrating altered conscious states. Hypnosis is posited to facilitate psychotherapy in DID patients. There have been no controlled studies of the outcomes of psychotherapy in this population.

There is little evidence that psychoactive drugs are of great help in reversing dissociative symptoms. Research data provide no evidence suggesting that any medication regimen has any significant therapeutic effect on the dissociative process manifested by DID patients. To date, pharmacologic treatment has been limited to symptom control (e.g., insomnia, panic attacks) or the management of comorbid conditions (e.g., depression). Of all available classes of psychotropic agents, antidepressants may be the most useful class for the treatment of patients with DID. Patients suffering from dissociation frequently experience comorbid dysthymic or major depressive disorder.

Benzodiazepines have mostly been used to facilitate recall by controlling secondary anxiety associated with memory recall in psychotherapy. Clinicians who treat patients with dissociateive problems warn that all CNS-depressant agents may cause sudden mental state transitions, which may in turn increase rather than decrease amnesic barriers. Therefore, as useful as they could be on a short-term basis (i.e., acute management of a panic attack), extended use of these agents may contribute rather than treat dissociative episodes. The long-term use of these agents is therefore not indicated.

Anticonvulsant agents may be useful in this patient population. As seizure disorders have a high rate of comorbidity with DID, anticonvulsant agents may help control the dissociation associated with epileptogenic activity. Anticonvulsant agents have also proven effective in the management of mood disorders that are prevalent in DID patients. Additionally, anticonvulsant agents have been found to be effective in the treatment of impulsive behaviors associated with personality disorders. These agents may produce less amnestic side-effects than the benzodiazepines and thus may be preferred in controlling the symptoms of these conditions.

Of all pharmacologic agents available, antipsychotics may be the least desirable. There is no evidence that they are useful in reducing dissociative symptoms. In fact, there have been reports of increased levels of dissociation and an increased incidence of side-effects when used in patients suffering from dissociative disorders. Therefore, the use of these agents in DID is not recommended.

Clinical Vignette 1

In 2004, Spiegel and Spiegel described how a woman in hospital had lost all memory for the preceding 10 months and insisted that she was in another hospital where she had been the previous December. She proved on testing with the Hypnotic Induction Profile (HIP; developed in the 1970s by Herbert Spiegel) to be highly hypnotizable (10 of 10 on the induction score). She was hypnotized with a simple rapid induction technique involving the following instruction: "On 1, do one thing, look up. On 2, do two things, slowly close your eyes and take a deep breath. On 3, do three things, let the breath out, let your eyes relax but keep them closed, and let your body float. Then let one hand or the other float up into the air like a balloon and that is your signal to yourself to that you are ready to concentrate."

When the woman had done this, she was told that the therapist and her would be changing times, counting backward in years, and that when her eyes opened she would be at an earlier time in her life. Then, when the therapist touched her forehead, she would close her eyes and they would change times again. They counted several years back. When she opened her eyes, she spoke as though she were in a different location earlier in her life. She was reoriented to the time when she really was in the other psychiatric hospital in a different city, and she talked about that experience. She was then instructed to close her eyes again and count forward in months to the present month. She opened her eyes and was then properly oriented and had episodic memory for what had transpired in her life in recent months.

Clinical Vignette 2

Mrs J, a 54-year-old businesswoman, was referred for evaluation of lifelong depersonalization symptoms, episodes characterized by a feeling of detachment, alternating with eruptions of uncharacteristic anger, or childlike behavior. The episodes occurred more frequently after relationship problems or losses, dismissive or controlling treatment by others, and especially around important family holidays, such as Thanksgiving and her birthday. She had a history of parental physical abuse early in life.

Mrs J was tested with the Hypnotic Induction Profile (see Clinical Vignette 1) and scored 8.5/10 points, indicating moderate-to-high hypnotizability. She was taught a self-hypnosis exercise in which she felt her body to be floating comfortably while she pictured herself in a pleasant outdoor scene. She was then able to experience an emotion of anger as she thought about her last episode of depersonalization, and made an association to an earlier episode of parental mistreatment. She was instructed to practice this self-hypnosis exercise three times a day, and observe if she felt a depersonalization episode coming on.

Follow-up 3 weeks later indicated that there was a decrease in the number of spontaneous depersonalization episodes, and Mrs J found that she could use the self-hypnosis to identify and work through feelings that she had previously been unaware of, or that had created difficulties for her. She was, for example, able to recognize a feeling of hurt and rejection at the close of a prior therapy, cry over it, and "move beyond it." She saw the hypnosis exercise as a means of understanding previously alien feelings and working through them, while increasing her ability to induce relaxation and handle stress.

KEY POINTS

- Dissociative disorders are controversial; they seem to be more prevalent in the less heavily industrialized, developing countries.

- They are characterized by disruptions of aspects of consciousness, identity, memory, motor behavior, or environmental awareness.

- They include depersonalization disorder, dissociative amnesia, dissociative fugue, dissociative identity disorder, and dissociative disorder NOS.

- Dissociative identity disorder, formerly known as multiple personality disorder, is a rare condition when it occurs spontaneously and is easily created iatrogenically.

- People with dissociative disorders appear to be particularly susceptible to hypnotism and to be highly suggestible.

- Treatment involves breaking down amnestic barriers and integrating altered conscious states, but there have been no controlled studies of the outcomes of psychotherapy in this population.

Further Reading

Acocella, J. (1999) *Creating Hysteria*, Jossey-Bass, New York.

Hunter, M.E. (2004) *Understanding Dissociative Disorders: A Manual for Family Physicians and Health Professionals*, Crown House Publishing, Williston, VT.

Icon Health Publishing (2004) *Dissociative Identity Disorder: Medical Dictionary, Bibliography, and Annotated Research Guide*, Icon Group International, San Diego, CA.

Maldonado, J.R.and Spiegel, D. (2005) Dissociative states in personality disorders, in *Textbook of Personality Disorders* (eds J.M. Oldham, A.E. Skodol,and D.S. Bender), American Psychiatric Publishing, Washington, DC, pp. 493–521.

McHugh, P.R. (1995) Dissociative identity disorder as a socially constructed artifact. *Journal of Practical Psychiatry and Behavioral Health*, **1**, 158–166.

Psychological Factors Affecting a Medical Condition

28.1 Introduction

Psychological factors affecting a medical condition (PFAMC) is a diagnostic category that recognizes the variety of ways in which specific psychological or behavioral factors can adversely affect medical illnesses. The diagnosis of PFAMC differs from most other psychiatric diagnoses in its focus on the interaction between the mental and medical realms.

The overall category of PFAMC includes situations in which psychological factors interfer with medical treatment, pose health risks, or cause stress-related pathophysiological changes. Such factors may contribute to the initiation or the exacerbation of the illness, interfere with treatment and rehabilitation, or contribute to morbidity and mortality. Psychological factors may themselves constitute risks for medical diseases, or they may magnify the effects of non-psychological risk factors. The effects may be mediated directly at a pathophysiologic level (e.g., stress inducing cardiac arrhythmias) or through the patient's behavior (e.g., nonadherence with treatment).

28.2 Diagnosis

The diagnosis is structured in DSM-IV-TR so that both the psychological factor and the general medical condition are to be specified. The psychological factor can be an Axis I or Axis II mental disorder (e.g., major depressive disorder aggravating coronary artery disease), a psychological symptom (e.g., anxiety exacerbating asthma), a personality trait or coping style (e.g., type A behavior contributing to the development of coronary artery disease), maladaptive health behaviors (e.g., unsafe sex in a person with HIV infection), a stress-related physiological response (e.g., tension headache), or other or unspecified psychological factors.

PFAMC requires that the patient have both a medical illness and contemporaneous psychological factors, because their coexistence does not always include significant interactions between them. To make the diagnosis of PFAMC, the factors must have either influenced the course of the medical condition, interfered with its treatment, contributed to health risks, or physiologically aggravated the medical condition. PFAMC has descriptive names for subcategories, described in Table 28.1.

Fundamentals of Psychiatry, First Edition. Allan Tasman and Wanda K. Mohr.
© 2011 John Wiley & Sons, Ltd. Published 2011 by John Wiley & Sons, Ltd.
This chapter is based on Chapter 83 (James L. Levenson) of *Psychiatry, Third Edition*

Table 28-1 PFAMC subcategories	
Subcategory	**Comment**
Mental disorder affecting a general medical condition	If the patient has a mental disorder meeting criteria for an Axis I or Axis II diagnosis, the diagnostic name is mental disorder affecting medical condition, with the particular medical condition specified
Psychological symptoms affecting a general medical condition	Patients who have psychological symptoms that do not meet the threshold for an Axis I diagnosis may still experience important effects on their medical illness, and the diagnosis would be psychological symptoms affecting a medical condition
Personality traits or coping style affecting a general medical condition	This may include personality traits or coping styles that do not meet criteria for an Axis II disorder and other patterns of response considered to be maladaptive because they may pose a risk for particular medical illnesses
Maladaptive health behaviors affecting a general medical condition	This refers to maladaptive health behaviors that have significant effects on the course and treatment of medical conditions
Stress-related physiologic response affecting a general medical condition	Used for cases in which stress is not the cause of the illness or symptoms; the patient has an underlying medical condition, and the stressor instead represents a precipitating or aggravating factor
Other or unspecified psychological factors affecting a general medical condition	Residual category referring to psychological phenomena that may not fit within one of the above subcategories, such as cultural or religious issues, family dysfunction, among others

28.3 Differential diagnosis

The close temporal association between psychiatric symptoms and a medical condition does not always reflect PFAMC. If the two are considered merely coincidental, then separate psychiatric and medical diagnoses should be made.

When a medical condition is judged to be pathophysiologically causing the mental disorder (e.g., hypothyroidism causing depression), the correct diagnosis is the appropriate mental disorder due to a general medical condition (e.g., mood disorder due to hypothyroidism, with depressive features). In PFAMC, the psychological or behavioral factors are judged to precipitate or aggravate the medical condition.

Substance use disorders may adversely affect many medical conditions, and this can be described through PFAMC. However, in some patients, all of the psychiatric and medical symptoms are direct consequences of substance abuse, and it is usually parsimonious to use just the substance use disorder diagnosis.

Patients with somatoform disorders (e.g., somatization disorder, hypochondriasis) present with physical complaints which may mimic a medical illness, but the somatic symptoms are actually accounted for by the psychiatric disorder.

28.4 Epidemiology

Because this diagnosis describes a variety of possible interactions between the full range of psychiatric disorders as well as symptoms and behaviors, on the one hand, and the full range of medical diseases, on the other, it is impossible to estimate overall rates of prevalence or incidence.

28.5 Course

Given the wide range of psychiatric disorders and psychological factors that may affect medical illness and the large number of different medical disorders that may be influenced, there are no general rules about the course of the PFAMC interaction. Psychological factors may have minor or major effects at a particular point or throughout the course of a medical illness.

28.6 Etiology

It has been recognized for many years that psychological factors seem to affect medical illnesses, and research elucidating the intervening causal mechanisms is now rapidly growing. Psychological factors may promote other known risks for medical illness. Smoking is a risk factor for heart disease, cancer, and pulmonary and many other diseases, and individuals with schizophrenia or depression are much more likely to smoke than the general population. A wide variety of psychiatric illnesses are associated with an increased likelihood of abuse of other substances. Depression and schizophrenia also are associated with a sedentary lifestyle. Patients with affective disorders often have chronic pain and chronically tend to overuse analgesics. Individuals with some Axis I and Axis II conditions are more likely to engage in unsafe sex, which in turn increases the risk of sexually transmitted diseases, including HIV infection and hepatitis B. Depression, eating disorders, and other emotional and behavioral factors affect the pattern and content of diet.

In addition to promoting known risk factors for medical illness, psychological factors also have an impact on the course of illness by influencing how patients respond to their symptoms, including whether and how they seek care. For example, anxiety is a common cause of avoidance or delay of healthcare; phobic fears of needles, sight of blood, surgery, and other healthcare phobias are common. Patients may also neglect their symptoms and fail to promptly seek medical care because of depression, psychosis, or personality traits.

Psychological factors also affect the course of illness through their effects on the provider–patient relationship, since they influence both patients' health behaviors and diagnostic and treatment decisions. A substantial proportion of the excess mortality experienced by individuals with mental disorders is explained by their receiving poor-quality medical care. One explanation for the poorer quality and outcomes of medical care in patients with both serious medical and mental illnesses is the lack of integration between their medical and mental care.

Psychological factors can also reduce a patient's adherence to diagnostic recommendations, treatment, and lifestyle change, and can interfere with rehabilitation through impairment of motivation, understanding, optimism, or tolerance. In addition, many of the effects of psychological factors on medical illness appear to be mediated through a wide array of social factors, including social support, job strain, disadvantaged socioeconomic and educational status, and marital stress.

28.7 Treatment principles

Management of psychological factors affecting the patient's medical condition should be tailored both to the particular factor of relevance and to the medical outcome of concern. Some general guidelines, however, can be helpful.

The physician, whether in primary care or a specialty, should not ignore apparent psychiatric illness. Unfortunately, this occurs too often because of discomfort, stigma, lack of training, or disinterest. Referring the patient to a mental health specialist for evaluation is certainly better than ignoring the psychological problem but should not be regarded as "disposing" of it, because the clinician must still attend to its potential impact on the patient's medical illness. Similarly, mental health practitioners should not ignore coincident medical disease and should not assume that referral to a nonpsychiatric care provider absolves them of all responsibility for the patient's medical problem.

28.7.1 Mental disorder affecting a medical condition

If the patient has a treatable Axis I disorder, treatment for it should be provided. Whereas this is obviously justified on the basis of providing relief from the Axis I disorder, psychiatric treatment is further supported by the myriad ways in which the psychiatric disorder may currently or in the future adversely affect the medical illness. The same psychopharmacologic and psychotherapeutic treatments used for Axis I mental disorders are normally appropriate when an affected medical condition is also present. However, even well-established psychiatric treatments supported by randomized controlled trials have seldom been validated in the medically ill, who are typically excluded from the controlled trials. Thus, psychiatric treatments may not always be directly generalizable to, and often must be modified for, the medically ill.

If the patient has an Axis II personality disorder or other prominent personality or coping style, the psychiatrist should modify the patient's treatment accordingly, which is usually more easily accomplished than trying to change the patient's personality. For example, patients who tend to be paranoid or mistrustful should receive more careful explanations, particularly before invasive or anxiety-provoking procedures.

28.7.2 Psychiatric symptoms affecting a general medical condition

In some instances, psychiatric symptoms not meeting the threshold for an Axis I diagnosis will response positively to the same treatments used for the analogous Axis I psychiatric disorder, with appropriate modifications. There is not a great amount of treatment research on subsyndromal psychiatric symptoms, and even less in patients with comorbid medical illness, so this area of practice remains less evidence-based. Some psychiatric symptoms affecting a medical condition may be amenable to stress management and other behavioral techniques as well as appropriate reassurance.

28.7.3 Personality traits or coping style affecting a general medical condition

As with Axis II disorders affecting a medical condition, clinicians should be aware of the personality style's effects on the practitioner–patient relationship and modify management to better fit the patient. For example, with type A "time urgent" patients, psychiatrists may need to be more sensitive to issues of appointment scheduling and waiting times. Group therapy interventions can enhance active coping with serious medical illnesses like cancer, heart disease, and renal failure but to date have usually been designed to be broadly generalizable rather than targeted to one particular trait or style (with the exception of type A behavior). Another general guideline is not to attack or interfere with a patient's defensive style unless the defense is having an adverse impact on the medical illness or its management.

28.7.4 Maladaptive health behavior affecting a general medical condition

This is an area of research with many promising approaches. To achieve smoking cessation, bupropion, varenicline, nicotine replacement, behavioral therapies, and other pharmacologic strategies all warrant consideration. Behavioral strategies are also useful in promoting better dietary practices, sleep hygiene, safe sex, and exercise. For some patients, change can be achieved efficiently through support groups, whereas others change more effectively through a one-on-one relationship with a healthcare professional.

28.7.5 Stress-related physiologic response affecting a medical condition

Biofeedback, relaxation techniques, hypnosis, and other stress management interventions have been helpful in reducing stress-induced exacerbations of medical illness, including cardiac, gastrointestinal, headache, and other symptoms. Pharmacologic interventions have also been useful (e.g., the widespread practice of prescribing benzodiazepines during acute myocardial infarction to prevent stress-induced increase in myocardial work).

28.7.6 Psychological factors in specific medical disorders

A specific discussion on the effects of psychological factors on selected medical disorders are beyond the scope of this book. Readers are encouraged to avail themselves of the readings provided at the end of this chapter. The primary focus is on those effects for which there is reasonable evidence from controlled studies. Most of the early research suffers from serious methodologic flaws, including use of small biased samples, limited or no statistical analysis, poor (if any) controls, and retrospective designs subject to recall and other biases. This early work generated excitement and interest in psychosomatic medicine but also produced ideas that in retrospect were intellectually appealing but erroneous and simplistic regarding the special designation of certain diseases as psychosomatic.

Clinical Vignette

Mrs A, a 46-year-old married attorney, was referred for psychiatric evaluation by her gastroenterologist, who was following her for longstanding irritable bowel syndrome. She had had IBS since the age of 20, with complaints of intermittent constipation, diarrhea, crampy abdominal pain, and bloating. She felt that these symptoms had gradually worsened, particularly in the previous month.

Mrs A described a highly pressured job and a stressful marriage. She has specifically noticed a precipitous increase in intestinal symptoms immediately after arguments with her husband and when facing deadlines at work. Three months ago, she developed depressed mood, early morning awakening, anorexia, fatigue, crying spells, impaired concentration, irritability, and preoccupation with thoughts of ill-health. Her family physician diagnosed major depression and prescribed amitriptyline, which was discontinued after it caused worsening of her constipation.

The psychiatrist tried fluoxetine (discontinued because of diarrhea) and trazodone (too sedating). Mrs A then responded well to nortriptyline with disappearance of the symptoms of depression and improvement in her IBS. However, severe IBS symptoms continued to follow the frequent marital arguments. The psychiatrist asked the patient to invite her husband to join one of their sessions so that marital issues could be further explored. He did so, resulting in the discovery that her husband was himself significantly depressed. He was referred to another psychiatrist for treatment, the marital discord abated, and her IBS symptoms returned to a manageable level.

In this case the patient had features of both mental disorder (major depressive disorder) affecting a general medical condition and stress-related physiologic response affecting a general medical condition. Treatment included individual psychotherapy and antidepressant medication as well as marital assessment and intervention. Pharmacotherapy required modification because of gastrointestinal sensitivity to side-effects.

KEY POINTS

- For PFAMC to be determined, a general medical condition (coded on Axis III) should be present.

- Psychological factors adversely affect the general medical condition in one of several ways that include influence on the course of the medical condition, interference with the treatment of the medical condition, increasing the health risks for the individual, or exacterbating the symtoms of the general medical condition.

- Management of psychological factors affecting the patient's medical condition should be tailored both to the particular psychological factor of relevance and to the medical outcome of concern.

Further Reading

Ayres, A., Hoon, P.W., Franzoni, J.B. *et al.* (1994) Influence of mood and adjustment to cancer on compliance with chemotherapy among breast cancer patients. *Journal of Psychosomatic Research*, **38**, 393–402.

Bakshi, R., Shaikh, Z.A., Miletich, R.S. *et al.* (2000) Fatigue in multiple sclerosis and its relationship to depression and neurologic disability. *Multiple Sclerosis*, **6**, 181–185.

Barger, S.D. and Sydeman, S.J. (2005) Does generalized anxiety disorder predict coronary heart disease risk factors independently of major depressive disorder? *Journal of Affective Disorders*, **88**, 87–91.

Blumenfield, M. and Tiamson-Kassab, M. (2008) *Psychosomatic Medicine: A Practical Guide*, Lippincott, Williams & Wilkins, Philadelphia, PA.

Covic, T., Adamson, B., and Hough, M. (2000) The impact of passive coping on rheumatoid arthritis pain. *Rheumatology*, **39**, 1027–1030.

Cwikel, J., Gidron, Y., and Sheiner, E. (2004) Psychological interactions with infertility among women. *European Journal of Obstetrics, Gynecology, and Reproductive Biology*, **117**, 126–131.

Farinpour, R., Miller, E.N., Satz, P. *et al.* (2003) Psychosocial risk factors of HIV morbidity and mortality: findings from the Multicenter AIDS Cohort Study (MACS). *Journal of Clinical and Experimental Neuropsychology*, **25**, 654–670.

Herschbach, P., Henrich, G., and von Rad, M. (1999) Psychological factors in functional gastrointestinal disorders: characteristics of the disorder or of the illness behavior? *Psychosomatic Medicine*, **61**, 148–153.

Neggers, Y., Goldenberg, R., Cliver, S. *et al.* (2006) The relationship between psychosocial profile, health practices, and pregnancy outcomes. *Acta Obstetricia et Gynecologica Scandinavica*, **85**, 277–285.

Porcelli, P. and Sonino, N. (2007) *Psychological Factors Affecting Medical Conditions: A New Classification for DSM-V*, Karger Publishers, Basel, Switzerland.

Yoshiuchi, K., Kumano, H., Nomura, S. *et al.* (1998) Psychological factors influencing the short-term outcome of antithyroid drug therapy in Graves' disease. *Psychosomatic Medicine*, **60**, 592–596.

29 ⬤ Sexual Disorders

29.1 Introduction

Often people believe that their psychiatric care provider is best equipped to help then when they are have difficulties in the area of sexuality. However, the field of mental health has been remarkably quiet regarding the issue of sexual disorders, despite sex being a ubiquitous activity and an essential part of human life. Disorders in sexuality and gender identity are some of the most intimate concerns that human beings can have. These dysfunctions have significant consequences for self-concept, self-esteem, and overall quality of life.

This chapter presents a short discussion of normal sexuality, followed by sexual and gender disorders. The three subgroups of sexual and gender disorders are sexual dysfunction, paraphilias, and gender identity disorders. Sexual dysfunction is the most common subgroup and thus receives special focus in this chapter.

29.2 Components of sexuality

An adult's sexuality has seven components: gender identity, orientation, intention (what one wants to do with a partner's body and have done with one's body during sexual behavior), desire, arousal, orgasm, and emotional satisfaction. The first three components constitute our sexual identity. The next three comprise our sexual function. The seventh, emotional satisfaction, is based on our personal reflections on the first six.

DSM-IV-TR designates impairments of five of these components as pathologies. Concerns about orientation and the failure to find sexual behaviors emotionally satisfying are not officially considered to be sexual disorders.

29.3 Dsm-IV-TR diagnoses

DSM-IV-TR specifies three criteria for each sexual dysfunction. The first criterion describes the psychophysiologic impairment; for example, absence of sexual desire, arousal, or orgasm. The second requires that the patient have marked distress or interpersonal difficulty as a result, while the third asks the clinician to ascertain that some other Axis I diagnosis, medical illness, medication, or substances of abuse does not best explain the problem.

29.4 Sexual desire

The diverse and changeable sexual desire manifestations are produced by the intersection of three mental forces: drive (biology), motive (psychology), and values (culture).

Fundamentals of Psychiatry, First Edition. Allan Tasman and Wanda K. Mohr.
© 2011 John Wiley & Sons, Ltd. Published 2011 by John Wiley & Sons, Ltd.
This chapter is based on Chapter 77 (Stephen B. Levine) of *Psychiatry, Third Edition*

Sexual drive is recognized by genital tingling, heightened responsivness to erotic environmental cues, plans for self or partner sexual behavior, nocturnal orgasm, and increased erotic preoccupations. These are spontaneous particularly among adolescents and young adults. Without drive, the sexual response system is less efficient. While men as a group seem to have significantly more drive than women as a group, in both sexes, drive requires at least the presence of a modest amount of testosterone. Drive is frequently dampened by medications, substances of abuse, psychiatric illness, systemic physical illness, despair, and aging.

The psychological aspect of desire is referred to as *motive* and is recognized by willingness to bring one's body to the partner for sexual behavior either through initiation or receptivity. Motive often directly stems from the person's perception of the context of the nonsexual and sexual relationship. Sexual desire diagnoses are made in people who have adequate drive manifestations and those who apparently have none. Most sexual desire problems in physically healthy adults are generated by one partner's unwillingness to engage in sexual behavior. This is often kept secret from the partner.

Sexual motives are originally programmed by social and cultural experiences. Children and adolescents acquire values – beliefs, expectations, and rules – for sexual expression. Young people have to negotiate their way through the fact that their early motives to behave sexually frequently coexist with their motives *not* to engage in sexual behavior. Conflicting motives often persist throughout life but the reasons for the conflict evolve.

29.5 Sexual dysfunction disorders

Sexual dysfunction refers to sexual expression that is distinguished by a disturbance in the processes that typify the sexual response cycle or by pain associated with sexual intercourse. In other words, disruption of any of the phases of human sexual response results in a sexual dysfunction disorder. These disorders are broken into the following subgroups:

- Desire disorders

- Arousal disorders

- Orgasmic disorders

- Pain disorders.

These disorders can be classified also as either lifelong or acquired, generalized or situational, and caused by psychological factors or combined factors.

29.5.1 Sexual desire diagnoses

Two official diagnoses are given to men and women whose desires for partner sexual behavior are deficient: hypoactive sexual desire disorder (HSDD) and sexual aversion disorder (SAD). The differences between the two revolve around the emotional intensity with which the patient avoids sexual behavior. When visceral anxiety, fear, or disgust is routinely felt as sexual behavior becomes a possibility, sexual aversion is diagnosed. HSDD is far more frequently encountered. It is present in at least twice as many women as men; female-to-male ratio for aversion is far higher.

As with all sexual dysfunctions, the desire diagnoses may be lifelong or may have been acquired after a period of ordinary fluctuations of sexual desire. Acquired disorders may be partner-specific ("situational") or may occur with all subsequent partners ("generalized").

29.5.2 Arousal disorders

29.5.2.1 Female sexual arousal disorder

The specificity and validity of female sexual arousal disorder (FSAD) is unclear. In women, it is far more difficult to separate arousal and desire problems than in young men. New desire/arousal problems arise typically in the middle-to-late forties in up to 50% of women as perimenopausal vaginal lubrication diminishes. It is assumed to be endocrine in origin even though estrogen treatment only reliably improves the symptoms relating to vaginal moisture deficiency. The disorder is also seen among regularly menstruating women, who claim that they desire sex but simply do not become aroused with the same efficiency and intensity. Making the diagnosis of FSAD implies that drive and motivation are reasonably intact.

The disorder is typically an *acquired* one. The women focus on the lack of moisture in the vagina or their failure to be excited by the behaviors that previously reliably brought pleasure. Assuming that some mental factor distracts them from excitement during lovemaking, therapy focuses on identifying what this might be. In menopausal women, FSAD is more often focused on the body as a whole rather than just genital moisture deficiencies.

29.5.2.2 Male erectile disorder

Erectile disorder (ED) is characterized by a persistent or recurrent inability to attain, or to maintain until completion of the sexual activity, an erection sufficient for satisfactory sexual performance. While it is widely recognized that young men more commonly have pure psychogenic ED and men over 50 often have significant organic contributants, some younger men have organic factors and some older men have significant psychologic and interpersonal reasons for their inability to sustain potency.

The prevalence of ED rises dramatically in the sixth decade of life from less than 10% to 30%; it increases further during the seventh decade. Aging, medical conditions such as diabetes, prostate cancer, hypertension, and cardiovascular risk factors predict the most common pattern of ED due to a medical condition in this age group. While medication-induced, neurologic, endocrine, metabolic, radiation, and surgical causes of erectile dysfunction also exist, in population studies diabetes, hypertension, smoking, lipid abnormalities, obesity, and lack of exercise are correlated with the progressive deterioration of erectile functioning in the sixth and seventh decades.

29.5.3 Orgasmic disorders

Men and women exhibit a wide variability in the type or intensity of stimulation that triggers orgasm. These diagnoses should take into account the person's age, life circumstances, and the adequacy of intensity and duration of the sexual stimulation because these disorders may be caused by psychologic or medical conditions.

Female orgasmic disorder (FOD) and male orgasmic disorder (MOD) are characterized by a persistent or recurrent delay in, or absence of, orgasm after a normal sexual excitement phase. Orgasm is the reflexive culmination of arousal. When a woman can only readily attain orgasm during masturbation, she is diagnosed as having a *situational* type of FOD. The acquired varieties of this disorder are more common and may present as complete anorgasmia, too-infrequent orgasms, or too-difficult orgasmic attainment. The most common cause of this problem is serotonergic compounds, such as the selective serotonin reuptake inhibitors. The diagnosis of FOD is made when the woman's psychology persistently interferes with her body's natural progression through arousal.

When a man can readily attain a lasting erection with a partner, yet is consistently unable to attain orgasm in the body of the partner, he is diagnosed with MOD. The disorder has three levels of severity. The most common form is characterized by the *ability* to attain orgasm with a partner outside of her or his body, either through oral, manual, or personal masturbation. The more severe form is characterized by the man's inability to ejaculate in his partner's presence. The rarest form is characterized by the inability to ejaculate when awake.

Premature ejaculation is characterized by a persistent or recurrent onset of orgasm and ejaculation with minimal sexual stimulation before, on, or shortly after penetration and before the person wishes it. The range of intravaginal containment times among self-diagnosed patients extends from immediately before or upon vaginal entry (rare), to less than a minute (usual), to less than the man and his partner desire within <5 minutes (not infrequent). Time alone is a misleading indicator. The essence of the self-diagnosis is an emotionally unsatisfying sexual equilibrium apparently due to the man's inability to temper his arousal and choose when he ejaculates. Most men occasionally ejaculate before they wish to, but not persistently.

29.5.4 Pain disorders

Dyspareunia (not from a general medical condition) is characterized by genital pain that is associated with sexual intercourse in either a man or woman. Although it is most commonly experienced during coitus, it also may occur before or after intercourse. The intensity of symptoms may range from mild discomfort to sharp pain.

DSM-IV-TR presents dyspareunia and vaginismus as distinct entities. However, they have been viewed as inextricably connected in much of the modern sexuality literature; vaginismus is known to create dyspareunia and dyspareunia has been known to create vaginismus. Vaginismus (not resulting from a general medical condition) is characterized by the recurrent or persistent involuntary spasm of the musculature of the outer third of the vagina that interferes with sexual intercourse. The physical obstruction caused by muscle contraction usually prevents coitus. These conditions tend to be chronic unless treated.

In lifelong vaginismus, the anticipation of pain at the first intercourse causes muscle spasm. Pain reinforces the fear and on occasion the partner's response gives her good reason to dread a second opportunity to have intercourse. Early episodic vaginismus may be common among women, but most of the cases that are brought to medical attention are chronic. Lifelong vaginismus is relatively rare. The clinician should focus attention on what may have made the idea of intercourse so overwhelming negative to her: parental intrusiveness, sexual trauma, childhood genital injury, illnesses whose therapy involved orifice penetration, and surgery. The woman with lifelong vaginismus not only has a history of unsuccessful attempts at penetration but also displays an avoidance of finger, tampon, or speculum penetration.

Male dyspareunia is usually due to a medical condition. Herpes, gonorrhea, prostatitis, and Peyronie's disease cause pain during intercourse. Remote trauma to the penis may cause penile chordee or bowing, which makes intercourse mechanically difficult and sometimes painful. Pain experienced upon ejaculation can be a side-effect of trazodone.

29.5.5 Sexual dysfunction not otherwise specified

This diagnosis is reserved for circumstances that leave the clinician uncertain as to how to diagnose the patient. This may occur when the patient has too many fluctuating dysfunctional symptoms without a clear pattern of prominence of any one of them. It is usually possible to find a better dysfunction diagnosis after therapy begins.

29.6 General goals and treatment of sexual dysfunction

Some typical areas that need to be addressed in treatment of sexual disorders include the following:

- Complete psychological and physical ssessment of the couple affected by the sexual disorder

- Medication management as needed to improve sexual functioning or to provide symptom management or relief

- Education regarding "normal" sexual functioning

- Training in couple communication and sexual skills

- Couple's counseling to address other issues that may exist in the couple's relationship.

Treatment of specific sexual dysfunctions focuses mainly on targeting the individual and contributing causal factors (which could be psychologic, physical, or pharmacologic) related to the particular disorder. Treatment of desire disorders might include determining and treating the cause of hypoactive sexual desire disorder, which could be childhood sexual abuse, hormonal imbalances, depression, and other sexual disorders. Treatment for aversion disorder focuses on managing the anxiety symptoms, using medication, behavioral desensitization, and relaxation techniques, and uncovering and working through the dynamic issue that may underlie the disorder (e.g., sexual abuse or related trauma).

When the cause of the dysfunction is determined to be drug-related, these drugs should be discontinued when possible, and a drug without these side-effects should be administered. If this is not possible, the cause of the problem should be explained to the patient, with encouragement to alter sexual activity as necessary.

Antianxiety medications sometimes are used with patients whose anxiety and tension interfere with their ability to engage in sexual relations. The SSRIs have been used to prolong sexual activity in men with premature ejaculation.

Several medications are approved by the US Food and Drug Administration for the treatment of male ED. Sildenafil, vardenafil, and tadalafil work by blocking the action of phosphodiesterase type-5 inhibitor (PDE5) which is involved in the erectile response, achieving smooth muscle relaxation in the corpus cavernosum of the penis, and allowing for the inflow of blood to the penis.

Another treatment modality for sexual dysfunction is sex therapy. This is a particular approach to sexual counseling practiced by clinicians with specialized training in this mental health specialty. Most of sex therapy currently consists of a combination of cognitive and behavioral interventions, teaching communication skills, and education about sexuality.

29.7 Gender identity disorders

Gender identity disorders (GIDs) are characterized by a strong and persistent cross-gender identification and persistent discomfort with one's assigned sex. In addition, there must be evidence of clinically significant distress or impaired social, occupational, or other important areas of functioning.

People who identify with and live as if they are of the opposite sex are called "transsexuals." The number of transsexuals in the United States is unknown. Data from smaller countries in Europe with access to total population statistics and referrals suggest that roughly 1 per 30 000 adult men and 1 per 100 000 adult women seek sex-reassignment surgery. In child clinic samples, approximately five boys for each girl are referred with this disorder. In adult clinic samples, men outnumber women by a ratio of between 2 : 1 and 3 : 1.

Advocates of transsexuals suggest that the psychiatric diagnosis of gender identify disorder stigmatizes them as mentally disordered rather than recognizing that cross-gender identity is a serious condition that is treatable with medical procedures. Gender identity disorder is also thought to be an over-inclusive diagnosis that pathologizes ordinary behaviors. These views are more fully described by the Gender Identity Disorder Reform Organization on their web site: http://www. GIDreform.org.

There is no psychotherapy technique to cure an adult's gender problem. People who have long lived with profound cross-gender identifications do not simply obtain insight, get behaviorally modified, or get medicated into a conventional gender identity. Psychotherapy can be useful, nonetheless. If the patient is able to trust a therapist, there can be much to talk about – family relationships are often painful, barriers to relationship intimacy are profound, work poses many difficult issues, and there is the matter of psychic reality.

Hormones should be administered by endocrinologists who have a working relationship with a mental health team dealing with gender problems.

Surgical techniques for the creation of a vaginal barrel or penis are limited, expensive, and may have unpleasant side-effects. At least 35% of patients complain of inadequate vaginal depth in the years after re-assignment surgery, and as many as 30% regret having undergone the procedure. In male-to-female hormone treatment in which breast enlargement is inadequate, surgical breast implants may be an option. Because of the expense and limitations of sophisticated surgeries, many patients seeking female-to-male re-assignment undergo a double mastectomy with cosmetic chest resculpting and no attempt to create a penis.

29.8 The paraphilias

A paraphilia is a disorder of intention that is characterized by unusual eroticism (images) and often socially destructive behaviors such as sex with children, rape, exhibitionism, voyeurism, masochism, obscene phone calling, or sexual touching of strangers. DSM-IV-TR stipulates that these should have occurred over a period of at least 6 months. Also, to be considered a paraphilia, the urges, fantasies, and behaviors must cause clinically significant distress or impair social, occupational, or other important areas of functioning.

For some patients the paraphiliac behaviors are necessary for erotic arousal and sexual release (orgasm). For others, paraphiliac behaviors occur episodically (e.g., during periods of stress). Although the frequency and intensity of the sexual urges, fantasies, and behaviors may vary, these disorders tend to be lifelong and chronic. Only about 5% of the diagnoses of paraphilia are given to women.

29.8.1 Specific paraphilias (criminal types)

29.8.1.1 Exhibitionism
Exhibitionism generally involves a teenager or man displaying his penis so that the witness will be shocked or (in the paraphilic's fantasy) sexually interested. They may or may not masturbate during or immediately following this act of victimization.

29.8.1.2 Voyeurism
Men whose sexual life consists of watching homosexual or heterosexual videos occasionally come to psychiatric attention after being charged with a crime following a police raid. The voyeurs who are more problematic for society are those who watch women through windows or break into their dwellings for this purpose. Some of these crimes result in rape or nonsexual violence, but many are motivated by pure voyeuristic intent (which is subtly aggressive).

29.8.1.3 Pedophilia

Pedophilia is the most widely and intensely socially repudiated of the paraphilias. Pedophiles are men who erotically and romantically prefer children or prepubertal adolescents. They are grouped into categories depending upon their erotic preferences for boys or girls and for infant, young, or pubertal children.

29.8.1.4 Sexual sadism

While rape is an extreme type of sadism, paraphilic sadism is present only in a minority of rapists. It is defined by the rapist's prior use of erotic scripts that involve a partner's fear, pain, humiliation, and suffering. Rapists, whether paraphilic or not, are highly dangerous men whose antisocial behaviors are generally thought to be unresponsive to ordinary psychiatric methods.

29.8.1.5 Frotteurism

Frotteurism, the need to touch and rub against nonconsenting persons, although delineated as a criminal act, is probably better understood as the most socially benign form of paraphilic sadism. Frotteurism often occurs in socially isolated men who become sexually driven to act out.

29.8.1.6 Stalking

Stalking is the latest erotic preoccupation to be criminalized. Forensic psychiatry has defined various motivations for arrested stalkers, including those who have made the transition from romantic to violent preoccupation with the victim. Stalking is particularly frightening because murder occasionally results. It is likely that stalking as a behavior is the product of further deterioration of an already compromised mind, although not necessarily a paraphilic one. Some stalkers are found to be sexual sadists.

29.8.2 Specific paraphilias (noncriminal types)

29.8.2.1 Fetishism

Fetishism, the pairing of arousal with wearing or holding an article of clothing or inanimate object such as an inflatable doll, has a range of manifestations, from infantilism in which a person dresses up in diapers to pretend he is a baby, to the far more common use of a female undergarment for arousal purposes.

29.8.2.2 Sexual masochism

Sexual masochism is diagnosed over a range of behaviors from the sometimes fatal need to nearly asphyxiate oneself to the request to be spanked by the partner in order to be excited. Masochism may be the most commonly reported or acknowledged form of female paraphilia, although it is more common among men.

29.8.3 Paraphilia not otherwise specifi ed

Paraphilia not otherwise specified is a DSM-IV-TR category for other endpoints of abnormal sexual development that lead to preoccupations with other paraphilic stimuli, including amputees, feces, urine, sexualized enemas, sex with animals, sex with the dead, to name a few.

29.8.4 Treatments for paraphilic disorders

Frequently, involvement in treatment is not voluntary but is court-ordered. Sometimes a patient will enter treatment at the insistence of the sexual partner.

Treatment for paraphilic disorders often is a difficult and lifelong process. Patients who engage in paraphilic behavior, especially those whose behavior endangers the safety of others (pedophiles, violent sadists), may be treated with drugs that reduce their sexual desire, arousal, and paraphilic fantasies. Cyproterone acetate and medroxyprogesterone acetate reduce testosterone levels, which results in decreased levels of deviant sexual behavior. Sertraline and fluoxetine and other SSRIs have been useful in reducing depressive symptoms in patients with paraphilias and decreasing some paraphilic behaviors.

Other treatments include *satiation* (a boredom technique in which sex offenders use their most erotic fantasies after orgasm in a boring, repetitive manner to extinguish their erotic quality); *signaled punishment* (a combination of aversion therapy and biofeedback of erections to deviant stimuli); and treatments aimed at the paraphiliac's deficits (e.g., deficits in arousal to adult partners, deficits in assertive skills, deficits in ability to relate socially to adult partners, treatment to reduce distorted cognitions regarding their paraphilic behavior). For example, child molesters may describe themselves as victims of children's seductive behavior toward them, blaming children for their behavior. These and other personality deficits are treated using a variety of treatment modalities and approaches.

Clinical Vignette

A couple married for 32 years sought help immediately after the wife unexpectedly returned home and discovered that her husband had been out in public dressed as a woman. She was certain that this behavior represented a worsening of his judgment. Thirty years before, he had revealed that he was sexually aroused by women's clothing and wanted to cross-dress for lovemaking. She adamantly refused to consider it. Since that incident, she never mentioned it again trying to act as though she was unaware of his "secret." Privately, she periodically worried that he was putting on her underwear to masturbate. Their sexual frequency declined after his initial request and, over the ensuing 20 years, she slowly developed an aversion to being touched by him. Sexual behavior ceased 10 years ago.

The 55-year-old masculine-appearing physical education teacher husband elected to enter individual therapy where he expressed his dilemma. He wanted to spare his wife pain. She believed that his "prurient" interest would go away if only he had more faith and prayed more, but he knew that nothing, including his fundamentalist religious patterns, diminished his periodic need to wear women's clothing. "If I tell her about my cross-dressing, she withdraws in anger. If I do not tell her about it, her imagination about how often I am doing it runs wild and she punishes me for cross-dressing that I don't do. If I stop cross-dressing, I deprive myself of unparalleled comfort and sumptuous pleasure and the desire eventually overtakes me. I lose either way. Should I honor my wife or my own identity?" His daily rate of masturbation had not changed much. He said he masturbated to cope with her refusal to have sexual behavior together. "My cross-dressing has actually kept me from having affairs with other women, thankfully."

Three factors point to the paraphilia "fetishistic transvestism" as a diagnosis. His arousal to female clothing was reported to have increased over time, he cross-dressed without a well-developed feminine identity, and he masturbated daily.

Now add to this description his wife's new diagnosis of advanced ovarian cancer. As he copes with this bad news and helps her with the painful process of dying, within his privacy is stirring his need to increase his social presentation as a woman, his fantasies of having genital reconstruction, and his recognition that his grief is balanced by his opportunity to live as a woman soon. If the psychiatrist sees him after his wife's death, "GID not otherwise specified" might appear to be the new diagnosis. Fetishistic transvestism, GIDNOS, and GID can be evolutionary points in a person's life.

KEY POINTS

- The scope of human sexual expression is diverse and influenced by many factors such as genetics, individual preferences, culture, life experiences, and health.

- Sexual dysfunction disorders can be primary (caused by various psychological and emotional conditions) or secondary (caused by a general medical condition or substance use).

- General medical conditions that may affect sexual interest and abilities include injury, disease, or consequences of surgery. Substance use consists of drug and alcohol abuse or use of some prescribed medications, including antihypertensives, antidepressants, and neuroleptics.

- Dyspareunia (not from a general medical condition) is characterized by genital pain that is associated with sexual intercourse in either a man or woman.

- Paraphilias refer to those sexual expressions characterized by recurrent, intense sexually arousing fantasies, urges, or behaviors. They include exhibitionism, fetishism, frotteurism, pedophilia, sexual masochism, sexual sadism, transvestic fetishism, and voyeurism.

- Gender identity manifests differently across the lifespan.

- Evaluation of patients seeking help for sexual dysfunction includes assessment of the identified problem; assessment of physical health, including medication and substance use; and psychological functioning.

- Treatment of specific sexual dysfunctions focuses mainly on targeting the patient and contributing causal factors related to the particular disorder. Frequently, involvement in treatment is not voluntary.

Further Reading

Seftel, A.D., Padma-Nathan, H., Althof, S.E., Giuliano, F., and McMahon, C.G. (2004) *Male and Female Sexual Dysfunction*, Elsevier Health Science, Oxford, UK.

Unit 4
Assessment and Therapeutics

Psychiatric Assessment, Treatment Planning, and the Medical Record

30.1 Introduction

This chapter presents an outline of a thorough approach to psychiatric assessment. This includes the psychiatric interview, physical examination, and laboratory testing, as well as a brief discussion of the diagnostic process, case formulation, treatment planning, and documentation. Clearly the length, detail, and order of the examination will be different across different treatment settings, and much will depend on the patient's tolerance for questioning and the goals of the interview.

Assessment is an *ongoing* set of processes used by clinicians for developing impressions and images, making decisions and checking hypotheses about patients presenting for evaluation and treatment. This happens by way of gathering, classifying, categorizing, analyzing, and documenting information about them and their ecology. The purposes of assessment are to develop descriptions about a patient, to help make decisions about their relation to their environment, and to develop a meaningful plan of care. A comprehensive psychosocial assessment is performed with the understanding that all aspects of the patient's life – spiritual, biological, psychological, social, cultural, cognitive, and behavioral – affect his or her well-being.

Institutions and organizations may often specify, through assessment forms, which data clinicians are to collect. However, all mental health clinicians should know the elements of a comprehensive assessment and should use their judgment to determine the amount of data to collect based on the setting in which the assessment will take place. For instance, on an inpatient unit where a professional is one of several treatment team members, the clinician might triangulate or combine assessment data gathered by different team members to form a complete picture of the patient's functioning. In an office outpatient setting, where the clinician may be the sole practitioner, he/she will conduct a more extensive, autonomous patient and family assessment to develop the plan of care. Regardless of the setting, quality care requires that the clinician conduct a comprehensive *psychosocial assessment*.

30.2 Components of the psychosocial assessment

The clinician obtains assessment data from several sources:

- Interview with the patient and his or her family
- History and physical examination

Fundamentals of Psychiatry, First Edition. Allan Tasman and Wanda K. Mohr.
© 2011 John Wiley & Sons, Ltd. Published 2011 by John Wiley & Sons, Ltd.

- Records from other healthcare facilities or prior treatment
- Laboratory and psychological tests
- Assessments by other professionals and paraprofessionals.

Other assessment techniques that are useful in diagnosis and treatment planning are discussed in Chapter 31.

30.3 The interview

The single most important source of information is the interview with the patient and family, which includes initial and ongoing conversations. Listening carefully to the patient and his or her family is a high-level skill that is essential to quality care across all settings.

Astute observation and attentive listening are hallmarks of the effective interviewer. During the interview, the clinician should be sensitive to both verbal and nonverbal cues that can be used to focus the interview. An effective interviewer lays the groundwork for a therapeutic relationship by building rapport through active listening (see Chapter 2). The interview should be adjusted to fit the needs and understanding levels of the individual patient and family and should proceed in an orderly fashion, letting the patient's answers guide subsequent questions and finishing discussion on one topic before moving to another.

Before beginning the interview the clinician should introduce himself or herself, explain the purpose of the interview, and try to make the patient and family as comfortable as possible. If the clinician and patient are not fluent in the same language, a translator may be needed, but subtleties of patient communication may be sacrificed in the process of translation and interpretation.

The key elements of the interview are the identifying information, the chief complaint, the history of the present illness, the past psychiatric history, the personal history, family history, medical history, substance abuse history, and the Mental Status Examination (MSE).

30.3.1 Identifying information

This information establishes the patient's identity. His or her name should be recorded, along with any nickname or alternative names he/she may have been known by in the past (e.g., maiden name). Date of birth, or at least age, and race are other essential parts of every person's record. If a patient is a member of a particular subculture based on ethnicity, country of origin, or religious affiliation, it may be noted here (e.g., Conservative/observant Jew). A traditional part of the identifying data is a reference to the patient's civil status: single, married, separated, divorced, or widowed. If none of these traditional categories apply, and the person is in a committed relationship (hetero- or homosexual) this should be noted. If the patient is not the sole supplier of information this should be noted in this section.

30.3.2 Chief complaint

The chief complaint is the patient's responses to the question, "What brings you to see me/to the hospital today?" or some variant. The answer is usually quoted verbatim, placed within quotation marks, and should be no more than one or two sentences. Even if patients are very disorganized or hostile, quoting their response can give an immediate sense of where they are as the interview begins and provides information as to the accuracy of the information being provided to the clinician. In such cases, or if patients give no response, a brief statement of how the patient came to be evaluated should be made and enclosed in parentheses.

30.3.3 History of the present illness

The present illness history should begin with a brief description of the major symptoms that brought the patient to psychiatric attention. The most troubling symptoms should be detailed initially and a more thorough review can be subsequent. At a minimum, the approximate time since the patient was last at his/her baseline level of functioning, and in what way he/she is different from that now, should be described, along with any known stressors, the sequence of symptom development, and the beneficial or deleterious effects of interventions. How far back in a patient's history to go, especially when he/she has chronic psychiatric illness, is sometimes problematic. In patients who have required repeated hospitalization, a summary of events since last discharge (if within 6 months) or last stable baseline is indicated. It is rare for more than 6 months of history to be included in this section; it is usually limited to the past month.

Extended elements in the history of the present illness would include events in a patient's life at the onset of symptoms, as well as exactly how the symptoms have affected the patient's occupational functioning and important relationships. Any concurrent medical illness symptoms, medication usage (and particularly changes), alterations in the sleep–wake cycle, appetite disturbances, and eating patterns should be noted. Significant negative findings should also be included.

30.3.4 Past psychiatric history

Most of the major psychiatric illnesses are chronic in nature. Hence, patients may have had previous episodes of illness with or without treatment. New onset of symptoms, without any previous psychiatric history, becomes increasingly important with advancing age in terms of diagnostic categories to be considered. At a minimum, the presence or absence of past psychiatric symptom-atology should be recorded, along with psychiatric interventions taken and the result of such interventions. An explicit statement about past suicide and homicide attempts should be included.

A more detailed history would include names and places of psychiatric treatment, dosages of medications used, and time course of response. The type of psychotherapy, the patient's feelings about former therapists, adherence to treatment as well as circumstances of termination are important. It is also relevant to note what the patient has learned about the biologic and psychologic factors predisposing him/her to illness, signs and symptoms of relapse, and whether there were precipitating events.

30.3.5 Past medical history

In any clinical assessment it is important to know about the patient's general health status. Any current medical illness and treatment should be noted along with any major past illness requiring hospitalization. Previous endocrine or neurologic illness are of particular pertinence. Information should include significant illnesses throughout the lifespan. A careful past medical history can also at times bring to light a suicide attempt, substance abuse, or dangerously careless or risk-taking behavior, which might not be obtained any other way.

30.3.6 Family history

Given the evidence for familial, genetic factors in so many psychiatric conditions, noting the presence of mental illness in biologic relatives of the patient is a necessary part of any database. It is important to specify during questioning the degree of family to be considered –usually to the second degree: aunts, uncles, cousins, and grandparents, as well as parents, siblings, and children.

A history of familial medical illness including a genogram (pedigree), including known family members with dates and causes of death and other known chronic illnesses, is helpful. Questioning about causes of death will also occasionally bring out hidden psychiatric illness, for example sudden unexpected deaths that were likely suicides or illness secondary to substance abuse.

30.3.7 Personal history

At a minimum, this part of the history should include where a patient was born and raised, and in what circumstances – intact family, number of siblings, and degree of material comfort. Note how far the patient went in school. What were his/her experiences and challenges? What has been his/her occupational functioning? If patients are not working, why not? Has there been any involvement in criminal activity, and with what consequences? Has the patient ever married or been involved in a committed relationship? Are there any children? What is his/her current source of support? Does he/she live alone? Has he/she ever used alcohol or other drugs to excess and is there current use? Has he/she ever been physically or sexually abused or been the victim of some other trauma?

A great deal more material can be elicited in this section. An outline of this is included in Table 30.1.

30.3.8 Mental status examination

The Mental Status Examination is used to determine whether a patient is experiencing abnormalities in thinking and reasoning ability, feelings, or behavior. It is part of the clinician's "toolkit" for gathering objective and observational data. The MSE includes observations and questions in the following categories:

- Appearance

- Behavior and speech

- Thoughts

- Mood and affect

- Ability to perform abstract reasoning

- Memory

- Intelligence

- Concentration

- Orientation

- Judgment and insight.

The MSE is particularly useful in identifying cognitive disruptions in such domains as memory, attention, and concentration. Congruence or discrepancies between sections may reveal important information and may be as important as idiosyncratic answers in response to questioning. Table 30.2 contains the elements of an MSE, their definitions, and possible descriptors associated with those elements.

As with other assessments, the MSE is a focused assessment. After determining the patient's general level of functioning and problem areas, the clinician may focus in greater depth on specific areas causing difficulty for the patient.

Table 30-1   Additional elements of the personal history

Aspect	Possible Questions
Family of origin	• Were parents married or in committed relationships? • Personality and significant events in life of mother, father, or other significant caregiver? • Siblings: How many? Their ages, significant life events, personality, and relationship to patient? • Who else shared the household with the family?
Prenatal and perinatal	• Was the pregnancy planned? Quality of prenatal care; mother's and father's response to pregnancy? • Illness, medication or substance abuse, smoking, and trauma during pregnancy; labor – induced or spontaneous? • Week's gestation, difficulty of delivery, vaginal or cesarean section? • Presence of jaundice at birth, birth weight, and Apgar score? • Baby went home with mother or stayed on in hospital?
Early childhood	• Developmental milestones: smiling, sitting, standing, walking, talking, and type of feeding – food allergies? • Consistency of caregiving: interruptions by illness and birth of siblings? • Reaction to weaning, toilet training, and maternal separation? • Earliest memories: any problematic behavior? • Temperament (shy, overactive, outgoing, fussy)? • Sleep problems: insomnia, nightmares, enuresis, parasomnias?
Later childhood	• Early school experiences: evidence of separation anxiety? • Bullied? • Behavioral problems at home or school: fire-setting, bed-wetting, aggressiveness toward others, cruelty to animals, nightmares? • Developmental milestones: learning to read and write? • Relationships with other children and family: any loss or trauma? • Reaction to illness?
Adolescence	• School performance: ever in special classes? • Extra-curricular activities? • Evidence of gender identity concerns: overly "feminine" or "masculine" in appearance/behavior, or perception by peers? • Ever run away? Able to be left alone and assume responsibility? • Age onset of puberty (menarche or nocturnal emissions) and reaction to puberty?
Identity	• Sexual preference and gender identity and religious affiliation? Same as parents? • Career goals: ethnic identification?
Sexual history	• Early sexual teaching: earliest sexual experiences, experience of being sexually abused, and attitudes toward sexual behavior? • Dating history and precautions taken to prevent sexually transmitted diseases and/or pregnancy? • Sexual practices and/or problems? • Sexual preoccupations, current sexual functioning, characteristics of significant relationships?
Adulthood	• Age at which left home and level of educational attainments? • Employment history, relationships with supervisors and peers at work, and reasons for job change? • History of significant relationships, including duration, typical roles in relationships, and patterns of conflict; marital history? • Legal entanglements and criminal history, both covert and detected, ever victim or perpetrator of violence? • Major medical illness as adult? • Participation in community affairs? • Financial status: own or rent home and stability of living situation? • Ever on disability or public assistance? • Current family structure, reaction to losses of missing members (parents and siblings), if applicable? • Substance abuse history?

Table 30-2	The mental status examination	
Category	**Definition**	**Possible Descriptor**
Appearance, behavior, speech	Detailed description of patient as he/she appears during the clinical encounter. Motor behavior, rate, volume and modulation of speech should be described as well	Neat, disheveled, good/poor eye contact, coherent/incoherent, loud/quiet or subdued, rapid speech/slow and hesitant
Mood	Subjective feeling sate of patient sustained over most of interview	Euthymic, dysthymic, sad, irritable, nervous, angry, euphoric
Affect	Objective description of patient's emotional state	Blunted, constricted, appropriate or inappropriate, labile, flat
Thought processes	Organization of the patient's thoughts as reflected in verbal pronouncements	Tangential, loose associations, flight of ideas, blocking, organized, goal-directed
Thought content	Themes of patient's thoughts during the interview, including preoccupations and ruminations, as well as overt signs and symptoms of psychopathology.	Presence or absence of delusions, suicidal or homicidal ideation, paucity of thought (give examples)
Perception	Assessment of the perceptual symptoms: hallucinations, illusions, depersonalization	Absent or describe and specify type
Cognitive	Assessment of the patient's abilities with regard to attention and orientation, as well as intellectual functioning, memory, fund of knowledge and capacity for abstract thought	Alert, attentive and oriented x3 Describe findings of each test done
Insight	Patient's understanding of himself or herself in the context of wanting or needing help	Intact and excellent, fair or impaired
Judgment	Closely related to insight but refers specifically to the actions patients will take based on insight; may reflect impulse control	Intact and excellent, fair or impaired

30.4 Medical history and physical examination

A complete medical history and physical examination is an important part of the comprehensive assessment of a psychiatric patient, for a number of reasons. First, numerous physical disorders produce symptoms mimicking specific mental disorders, and they can also cause changes in mood and energy levels. It is crucial for developing a differential diagnosis and ruling out "physical" causes for the patient's condition, especially when new-onset mental symptoms occur in an otherwise healthy patient, or when atypical symptoms occur in a patient who has a known or stable mental disorder.

The medical assessment looks at new or changed doses of medications or drug use/abuse (both legal and illicit), signs and symptoms (e.g., fever, dyspnea, morning headache, diarrhea) and family and personal history of medical disorders.

A second reason for a comprehensive medical history and physical examination is to provide information about the patient's physical capacity to tolerate certain psychiatric medications, such as lithium or clozaril, and to rule out any conditions that may place the patient in a risky situation should a physical restraint become necessary to contain violent behavior. In addition it is important to have a baseline laboratory screening in order to monitor the patient's physiological changes with reagrd to side-effects.

A third reason for a comprehensive evaluation is that many patients who present to a psychiatrist have had inadequate medical care and should be routinely examined to assess their general level of physical health. This is especially true for patients with chronic mental illness or substance abuse.

30.5 Laboratory testing

Generally testing is based on routine orders, guided by symptoms, and includes those listed in Table 30.3 with their rationales. In certain acute situations it may be necessary to obtain a CT scan if there is history of headache or recent trauma, or if delirium or focal neurologic findings are present. Lumbar puncture is performed in patients with meningeal signs (Kernig's sign or Brudzinki's sign), or a normal head CT with fever, headache, or delirium.

30.6 Risk assessment

Assessment of risk is always a crucial part of a comprehensive evaluation because patients' safety and the safety of those with whom they come in contact should be of foremost concern. While comprehensive and accurate documentation is always a goal for mental health professionals, it is of particular importance in the area of risk assessment.

Table 30-3 Laboratory assessments and rationale	
Whole blood count	Help to detect a wide variety of illnesses or signs of infection or anemias
	If mean corpuscular volume indicates macrocytic anemia (or if alcoholism suspected), procure vitamin B_{12} and folate levels; low levels can present as irritability and forgetfulness
	Monitoring white blood counts with clozaril therapy and certain mood stabilizers
Blood culture	Indicated when high fever and delirium are present; may indicate sepsis
Blood glucose	Hypoglycemia may mimic depression
	Hyperglycemia may mimic anxiety and present as delirium
	Atypical antipsychotics may precipitate diabetes
Kidney function	Kidney failure can cause mental status change
	Important to determine before starting lithium therapy
Liver function	Most medications are metabolized by liver and doses may need to be adjusted when liver function impaired.
	Rule out hepatic dysfunction secondary to alcoholism, hepatitis, and biliary tract disease
Thyroid function	Hyper- and hypothyroidism can both mimic symptoms of psychiatric disorders
	Should also be tested regularly when patients take lithium, as it may cause hypothyroidism
Syphilis and HIV screening	Both associated with psychiatric symptoms
Pregnancy testing	Necessary in all women of childbearing age before conducting imaging studies or initiating psychotropic therapy
Urine testing	Necessary for pregnancy testing and to detect presence of diabetic ketoacidosis and urinary tract infection
	Toxicology testing important if drug abuse is suspected
Electrocardiogram	Screening for conduction disturbances and cardiac arrhythmias before initiating therapy with psychotropics, especially those known to produce ECG changes
Electoenchephalography	History of brain trauma or head injury
	Obtain with new-onset psychosis which may be due to partial complex seizures
	Other seizure disorders and neurological dysfunction may present with hallucinations
CT and MRI	Useful in detecting central nervous system neoplasms, certain infections and hemorrhages

Risk should be viewed on a continuum from very high to very low, as opposed to being present or absent. Four areas are important: suicide risk, assault risk, life-threatening medical conditions, and external threat. Readers are directed to Chapter 38 for a more comprehensive discussion on these risk assessment areas.

30.7 Case formulation

After gathering data, a formulation is necessary to sift, prioritize and integrate data for treatment planning. The case formulation is the summary statement of the immediate problem, the context in which the problem has arisen, the assessment of risk, and the tentative diagnosis. It serves as the basis for intervention and treatment.

30.7.1 The diagnostic process

Diagnosis involves forming and revising hypotheses about what might be wrong with a patient. The steps are not carried out in a rigid sequence and, even when a firm diagnosis has been made, it is possible for this to be corrected. Sometimes, no firm diagnosis is made; in DSM terminology this is coded as "provisional" or "deferred."

There are specific guidelines taught to all physicians in terms of steps to be followed in diagnosing particular conditions and distinguishing between conditions with similar presentations (differential diagnosis). Differential diagnosis is a list of all diagnoses possible for any given patient, and traditionally they are arranged in order of likelihood with the most probable diagnosis listed first. DSM-IV-TR contains criteria for each diagnosis as well as differential diagnoses for each condition.

The act of forming a diagnosis is one of problem-solving. The clinician uses his or her knowledge of disease processes and logical inference to deduce what medical condition(s) may underlie a set of symptoms and what conditions may be ruled out. The system of "if–then" rules that guide this process are sometimes called "production rules." These can be all-or-nothing type rules (assuming that the causal chain between the psychiatric condition and the signs or symptoms is either present or absent), or they can be "probabilistic" (recognizing that the process is often variable and one thing does not always lead to another).

Competent clinicians keep in mind several principles in formulating a diagnosis. These include the principle that an excellent and careful history, taken from a patient and augmented by collateral information, is more useful than cross-sectional observations.

Another principle concerns signs and symptoms. Signs are what the clinician observes, whereas symptoms are patient complaints. While symptoms are important, discrete observations with clinician's clarification and description of his or her observations are more valid in making a diagnosis. Symptoms can often be distorted by patient and clinician interpretation. For example, a patient may deny having auditory hallucinations, but during the interview he may pause, cock his head and appear to be listening to something.

30.7.2 The prognosis

The prognosis is a prediction of the course an illness will take. It is the clinician's best educated guess as to how an illness with play itself out in a particular patient. The prediction is based on the clinician's knowledge of the person, his or her resources, and general knowledge of the condition in question.

30.8 Treatment planning

30.8.1 Initial treatment plan and immediate intervention

The initial treatment plan follows the case formulation, which has already established the nature of the current problem and a tentative diagnosis. The plan should distinguish what must be accomplished now and what may reasonably be postponed for the future. Treatment planning works best when it follows the biopsychosocial model and takes into account the treatment time frame.

The treatment plan should be feasible, both at this point and in the longer term. Perhaps because of the sheer volume of problems and challenges faced by people who have psychiatric illnesses, clinician's too often use a "kitchen sink" approach and develop exhaustive lists of interventions. Interventions should be attainable both by the treatment team and the patient and family. One seemingly obvious fact should be stated here because it is too often neglected: patients' and family goals must be given prime importance when a treatment plan is being developed. Treatment that does not take into consideration patients' wishes and preferences, and lacks the element of their engagement in the treatment process, is doomed to failure.

30.8.2 Comprehensive treatment planning

The comprehensive treatment plan usually includes more definitive diagnoses and a well formulated management plan with central goals and objectives. The comprehensive treatment plan guides and coordinates the direction of treatment and it should be reviewed on a regular and ongoing basis and modified as needed.

30.9 The medical record: from diagnosis to discharge

According to *A Patient's Bill of Rights* of the American Hospital Association and healthcare accrediting agencies in the US, such as the Joint Commission, each patient has a right to a written record that enhances care. Documentation may be in the form of narrative notes, SOAP notes (recording information by Subjective data, Objective data, Assessment, and Plan), or clinical pathways. Records may be kept manually or electronically. Records are legal documents that can be used in court; therefore, all notes and progress records should reflect descriptive, nonjudgmental, and objective statements. Examples of significant data include here-and-now observations of the patient through the use of the critical assessment, an accurate report of verbal exchanges with patients, and a description of the outcomes of the care provided. Verbal communication should be straightforward, forthright, descriptive, without opinion, and limited to those involved in the client's care and treatment.

All comprehensive diagnostic formulation that incorporates the information obtained through the standardized and idiographic diagnostic processes should be recorded. The clinical chart should include a systematic treatment plan, based on the comprehensive diagnostic formulation. Treatment planning should reflect that it is individually developed and include measurable objectives that are connected to signs and symptoms, as well as when it was updated and/or modified.

Tying interventions to signs and symptoms is an indication that thoughtful and precise treatment planning has taken place, in that interventions and treatments are bound to fail when they are not developed on the basis of individuals' development and sensitive to their various cognitive, social and emotional domains and needs. The reality of individual assessment, and individual treatment, is often an unrealized ideal. The use of checklists, structured interviews, and standardized treatment plans and evaluation instruments, though efficient, runs the risk of practitioners building assessments and asking questions that are devoid of context, thereby omitting many important portions of clinical reality. These are not optimal data recording devices. For example, checklists tend to be filled out with expediency as opposed to expertise and thoughtful reflection, and many staff members do not know the definitions of psychiatric terminology. Also, because of their acontextual nature, checklists make it that much more difficult to reconstruct the events of a person's hospitalization, especially given the unreliability of memories.

Various forms (electronic, computer, and paper) and methods (narrative and problem-oriented) are used in charting and progress notes. In most institutions all disciplines use the same progress notes, although some still maintain the physician's progress notes separate from those of the rest of the treatment team. The medical record and what it contains has one primary purpose: communication. The medical record is the single most important communication tool in the healthcare and treatment of patients. Types of information that should be communicated can include medical and nursing assessments, specialty consultations, treatment modalities, the basis for their use and their outcomes, patient responses to treatment modalities, laboratory and other diagnostic testing results, physician orders, and care plans, discharge plans, and summaries.

Most charting systems also permit a narrative entry for the practitioner to include information that may be unique to the patient, shift, or event. An example of this might be a violent episode leading to a patient's being placed in seclusion or restraints.

Regardless of the type or system of documentation, consistency, completeness, and accuracy are key components of a complete medical record. Insofar as the medical record is a roadmap of decisions, rationales, treatments, and patient outcomes, for it to be maximally informative as a treatment planning tool it must contain accurate and complete information. In its optimal form, the medical record relates patient management in sufficient detail for all members of the healthcare team to substantively evaluate those decisions in a critical fashion.

The medical record is a *legal document* designed to provide an overview of the patient's state of health before, during, and after a particular therapy. This overview is normally compiled by different steps: (1) handwritten notes are made during daily rounds; (2) particular events or changes in health condition are subsequently entered into the hospital database and coded according to the DSM system; and (3) the entire body of information is summarized in a cumulative report at the time of patient discharge from the hospital. Each step depends on the physician's and other professionals' time resources, experience, and routine with paperwork and may be susceptible to neglect and data loss if documentation cannot be carried out immediately.

KEY POINTS

- Assessment is an ongoing set of processes used by clinicians for developing impressions and images, making decisions, and checking hypotheses about patients presenting for evaluation and treatment.

- Components of the psychiatric assessment include the interview with the patient and his or her family, history and physical examination, records from other healthcare facilities or prior treatment, laboratory and psychological tests, evaluations of other professionals and paraprofessionals.

- The single most important source of information is the interview with the patient and family, which includes initial and ongoing conversations.

- The key elements of the interview are the identifying information, the chief complaint, the history of the present illness, the past psychiatric history, the personal history, family history, medical history, substance abuse history, and the Mental Status Examination.

- Assessment of risk to patients is always a crucial part of a comprehensive evaluation.

- The case formulation is the summary statement of the immediate problem, the context in which the problem has arisen, the assessment of risk, and the tentative diagnosis.

- The well formulated treatment plan includes diagnoses and a well-formulated management plan with central goals and objectives.

- Medical records are legal documents. All notes and progress records should reflect descriptive, nonjudgmental, and objective statements.

This chapter contains material from the following chapters in *Psychiatry, Third Edition*: Chapter 30 (Francine Cournos, David A. Lowenthal, Deborah L. Cabaniss); Chapter 31 (Christina G. Weston, William M. Klykylo); Chapter 32 (Larry J. Seidman, Gerard E. Bruder, Anthony J. Giuliano); and Chapter 33 (Douglas S. Lehrer, Darin D. Dougherty, Scott L. Rauch).

Further Reading

Cipani, E. and Schock, K.M. (2007) *Functional Behavioral Assessment, Diagnosis, and Treatment: A Complete System for Education and Mental Health Settings*, Springer, New York.

Morrison, J. (2006) *Diagnosis Made Easier: Principles and Techniques for Mental Health Clinicians*, Guilford, New York.

Persons, J.B. (2008) *The Case Formulation Approach to Cognitive Behavior Therapy*, Guilford, New York.

Shea, S.C. (1998) *Psychiatric Interviewing: The Art of Understanding*, 2nd edn, Elsevier Health Sciences, New York.

Zuckerman, E.L. (2005) *Clinician's Thesaurus: The Guide to Conducting Interviews and Writing Psychological Reports*, 6th edn, Guilford, New York.

31 Psychological Testing and Rating Scales

31.1 Introduction

Psychological testing is a single part of the total assessment process. Normally psychological tests are the domain of clinical psychologists who receive many hours of theoretical and practical education in psychometrics. This chapter is not intended as a tutorial in psychological testing or assessment. It aims to acquaint the clinician with some of the more commonly used tests and their purposes. Major psychological testing, such as IQ testing and achievement testing, require clinical or educational psychologists to administer as they require skillful administration and an in-depth knowledge of how to place the results of these tests into proper context. But there are rating scales that can, and often should, be used by clinicians in order to augment other assessment findings. Hence this chapter is also intended to familiarize the practitioner with the utility of some of these tests and rating scales for their own practice, both as part of assessment and as part of ongoing evaluation of patient progress throughout the treatment process.

The goal of testing is to develop a working image or model of the patient. This model/image is a set of hypotheses about the person and his or her life situation or situations. Based on multiple sources of data that include history, interviewing, and testing, clinicians try to develop as accurate a picture of patients as possible prior to considering various plans for intervening and working with them.

31.2 Major assessment approaches

All assessment in the psychological domain is assessment of behavior and/or cognitive or affective states. These involve verbal reports of thoughts and feelings, or the checking of answers on a questionnaire, as well as evaluation of motor performance or actions that are observable. There are three broad techniques involved in personality assessment, behavioral, objective and projective. A comparison of these is contained in Table 31.1.

31.3 Functional analysis of behavior

Functional (behavioral) assessment (FBA) is a systematic process for gathering information in order to determine the relationships between a person's problem behavior and aspects of the environment (see Chapter 32). Through FBA, it is possible to identify specific events that predict and maintain behavior and design a plan that effectively addresses those variables. FBA methods can, and should, vary across circumstances, but typically include record reviews, interviews, and direct observation.

Fundamentals of Psychiatry, First Edition. Allan Tasman and Wanda K. Mohr.
© 2011 John Wiley & Sons, Ltd. Published 2011 by John Wiley & Sons, Ltd.

Table 31-1   Assessment approaches

	Behavioral	Objective	Projective
Aim	Determine antecedents and consequences of target behaviors	Obtain test scores that relate to criteria of a phenomenon	Elicit material for inferring inner dynamics
Level of subjective interpretation	Low	Medium	High
Typical data	Observation, behavioral counts	Scores, profiles	Narrative, observations, scores
Typical format	Natural or contrived situations, report form/checklist	Paper and pencil	Presentation of open-ended stimuli
Theoretical underpinning	Operant theory, learning theory, functional analysis	Psychometrics, trait theory, attitude theory, factor theory	Psychodynamic theory
Examples	Behavioral coding system	Beck inventory, MMPI	Rorschach, sentence completion

FBA methods range from highly precise and systematic to relatively informal. Particular tools and strategies should be selected based on the circumstances, individuals involved, and goals of intervention.

The goal of FBA, regardless of which methods are used, is to answer certain questions.

1. Under what circumstances is the behavior most/least likely to occur (e.g., when, where, with whom)?

2. What outcomes does the behavior produce (i.e., what does the person get or avoid through his or her behavior)?

To answer these questions, the information gathered must be analyzed and summarized. Hypothesis (or summary) statements describe the specific patterns identified through the FBA and, if supported by the data, provide a foundation for intervention. A hypothesis statement must describe the behavior and the conditions under which it occurs. Interventions are designed accordingly, and if the hypothesis is not supported the assessment is conducted again with alternate hypotheses generated from data that may have been overlooked in the first assessment. There are tools available in the public domain that can be downloaded from the internet; see http://www.lessons4all.org/downloads/FAST.pdf. Also, Table 31.2 describes three methods of conducting a functional analysis and the sources clinicians might employ. Table 31.3 lists some commonly used psychiatric rating scales.

Table 31-2   Functional analysis of behavior

Method	Sample Sources
Direct observation	Observations conducted across a variety of settings, times, circumstances and ideally by more than one person Yield frequency measures across conditions
Structured interviews	Family and teachers, other service providers, people who know the patient well and have observed them across a variety of settings
Record review	Diagnostic and medical records, history, incident reports, previous treatment plans and IEPs from educational settings

Table 31-3 Common psychiatric rating scales	
Type of Scale	**Examples**
Observer rating	Mini Mental State Examination (MMSE)
	Brief Psychiatric Rating Scale
	Positive and Negative Syndrome Scale
	Hamilton Depression Inventory
	Hamilton Anxiety Scale
	Yale–Brown Obsessive Compulsive Scale
Self rating	Major Depression Inventory
	Beck Depression Inventory
	Hopkins Symptom Checklist
	Hospital Anxiety Depression Scale
Side-effects	Abnormal Involuntary Movement Scale
	Extrapyramidal symptom rating scale
Global assessment of functioning	Covers Axis V of the DSM

31.4 Objective tests

31.4.1 Intelligence testing

There are numerous controversies regarding the definition, use, and interpretation of the various measures of intelligence, and theories of intelligence abound. Traditionally intelligence is quantified as the global capacity of the individual to act purposefully, to think rationally, and to deal effectively with the environment.

An intelligence quotient (IQ) is a score derived from a set of standardized tests developed to measure a person's cognitive abilities ("intelligence") in relation to his or her age group. Although the intelligence quotient itself seems subject to little variation over a person's lifetime, it is worth keeping in mind that intelligence is neither unitary, nor fixed. IQ is generally predictive for academic, social, and occupational success, but not in all instances. Its most useful quality is a measurement of an individual's strengths and weaknesses in certain areas of ability. The two most commonly used in the United States are the Wechsler series and the Stanford–Binet. Both have been criticized for an over-emphasis on verbal skills and for being culturally biased. These instruments are described below.

31.4.1.1 Wechsler preschool and primary scale of intelligence – revised

The WPPSI-R can be used for children ranging in age from 3 to 7.25 years. Though separate and distinct from the WISC-III (discussed below), it is similar in form and content. The WPPSI-R is considered a downward extension of the WISC-III. These two tests overlap between the ages of 6 and 7.25 years.

The WPPSI-R has a mean of 100 and standard deviation of 15, with scaled scores for each subtest having a mean of 10 and a standard deviation of 3. It contains 12 subtests organized into one of two major areas. The Verbal Scale includes information, similarities, arithmetic, vocabulary, comprehension, and sentences (optional) subtests. The Performance Scale includes picture completion, geometric design, block design, mazes, object assembly, and animal pegs (optional) subtests. The WPPSI-R contains nine subtests similar to those included in the WISC-III (information, vocabulary, arithmetic, similarities, comprehension, picture completion, mazes, block design, and object assembly) and three unique subtests (sentences, animal Pegs, and geometric design). Three separate IQ scores can be obtained: Verbal Scale IQ, Performance Scale IQ, and Full Scale IQ.

The WPPSI-R was standardized on 1700 children equally divided by gender and stratified to match the 1986 US census data. This instrument cannot be used with severely disabled children (IQs below 40) and, with younger children, may need to be administered over two sessions owing to the length of time required to complete the assessment.

31.4.1.2 Wechsler intelligence scale for children – III

The WISC-III can be used for children ranging in age from 6 to 16 years. It is the middle childhood to middle adolescence version of the Wechsler Scale series. It contains 13 subtests organized into two major areas. The Verbal Scale includes information, similarities, arithmetic, vocabulary, comprehension, and digit span (optional) subtests. The Performance Scale includes picture completion, picture arrangement, block design, object assembly, coding, and the optional subtests of mazes and symbol search.

Three separate IQ scores can be obtained: Verbal Scale IQ, Performance Scale IQ, and Full Scale IQ. Each of these separate IQs are standard scores with a mean of 100 and a standard deviation of 15, with scaled scores for each subtest having a mean of 10 and a standard deviation of 3.

31.4.1.3 Wechsler adult intelligence scale – revised

The WAIS-R covers an age range of 16 to 74 years and 11 months. The revised version contains about 80% of the original WAIS and was modified mainly due to cultural considerations. There are 11 subtests: Verbal Scale (information, similarities, arithmetic, vocabulary, comprehension, and digit span) and Performance Scale (picture completion, picture arrangement, block design, object assembly, and digit symbol).

The WAIS-R has a mean of 100 and a standard deviation of 15 with the scaled scores for each subtest having a mean of 10 and a standard deviation of 3.

31.4.1.4 Stanford–binet: fourth edition

The SB: FE is appropriate for use on individuals ranging in age from 2 to 23 years. It comprises 15 subtests, though only six are used in all age groups (i.e., vocabulary, comprehension, pattern analysis, quantitative, bead memory, and memory for sentences). The other nine subtests are administered on the basis of age (picture absurdities, paper folding and cutting, copying, repeating digits, similarities, form-board items, memory for objects, number series, and equation building).

31.4.1.5 Comment

The SB: FE and the Wechsler scales are useful instruments in assessing *mild* mental retardation; however, neither is designed to test individuals with severe/profound mental retardation. In addition, owing to the high floor on the Wechsler scales, the publisher recommends that a child should obtain raw score credit in at least three subtests of the Verbal Scale and the Performance Scale before assuming they provide useful information. Raw score for six subtests (three Verbal and three Performance) are recommended for a valid Full Scale IQ.

31.4.2 Neuropsychological tests

Neuropsychological tests attempt to measure deficits in cognitive functioning (i.e., ability to think, speak, reason, etc.) including memory and perceptual skills that may result from some sort of brain damage, such as a stroke or a brain injury. They are used in targeting areas for rehabilitation. A battery of these may include the IQ tests described above, but also may include tests that target a number of domains of global brain functioning. An example is the Halstead–Reitan Neuropsychological Battery (HRNB) Tactual Performance.

31.4.3 Assessing adaptive behavior

Adaptive behavior is an important and necessary part of the definition and diagnosis of mental retardation. It is the ability to perform daily activities required for personal and social sufficiency. Assessment of adaptive behavior focuses on how well individuals can function and maintain themselves independently and how well they meet the personal and social demands imposed on them by their cultures. There are more than 200 adaptive behavior measures and scales. The most common is the VABS.

31.4.3.1 Vineland adaptive behavior scales

The Vineland Adaptive Behavior Scales (VABS) are a revision of the Vineland Social Maturity Scale and assess the social competence of individuals with and without disabilities from birth to age 19 years. It is an indirect assessment in that the respondent is not the individual in question but someone familiar with the individual's behavior.

The VABS measure four domains: communication, daily living skills, socialization, and motor skills. An adaptive behavior composite is a combination of the scores from the four domains. A maladaptive behavior domain is also available with two of the three forms of administration.

Caution is advised when using this scale with children under the age of 2 years because children with more significant delays frequently attain standard scores that appear to be in the low average range of ability. In this case more weight should be placed on the age equivalents that can be derived.

31.4.3.2 AMMR adaptive behavior scale

The American Association on Mental Retardation's Adaptive Behavior Scale (ABS) has two forms that address survival skills and maladaptive behaviors in individuals living in residential and community settings. The results of this assessment can be readily translated into objectives for intervention.

31.4.4 Achievement tests

Achievement tests are standardized inventories that examine various skills or knowledge learned at a certain grade level. They are commonly employed by educational psychologists (or in educational settings) to determine a child's academic strengths and weaknesses. They are scored according to guidelines required by the tests' developers and the results are calculated into standard scores using tables appropriate for age or time of school year. The standard score provides data that compares a student's achievement and ability to others of the age group.

Achievement tests (such as reading and mathematics) are heavily dependent on formal learning, are more culturally bound, and tend to sample more specific skills than do intelligence tests. Intelligence tests measure one's ability to apply information in new and different ways, whereas achievement tests measure mastery of factual information. Intelligence tests are better predictors of scholastic achievement contributing to the decision-making processes in schools and clinics, and they are a better predictor of educability and trainability than other achievement tests because they sample the reasoning capacities developed outside school which should also be applied in school.

To determine whether learning potential is being fully realized, results from an IQ test and standardized tests of academic achievement can be compared. If there is a significant difference between IQ and achievement, the child may benefit from special assistance in the academic area identified.

A number of achievement tests are described below. A variety of other achievement tests are available for assessing academic performance. These include, but are not limited to, the Kaufman Test of Educational Achievement and the Wechsler Individual Achievement Test.

31.4.4.1 Differential ability scale

The Differential Ability Scale (DAS) consists of a battery of individually administered cognitive and achievement tests subdivided into three age brackets: lower preschool (2 years + 6 months to 3 years + 5 months), upper preschool (3 years + 6 months to 5 years + 11 months), and school age (6 years to 17 years + 11 months). The cognitive battery focuses on reasoning and conceptual abilities and provides a composite standard score.

The DAS has several advantages over other similar measures. It has a built-in mechanism for assessing significantly delayed children who are over the age of 3.5 years. It can also provide information comparable to other similar instruments in about half the time. It is very well standardized and correlates highly with other cognitive measures (e.g., the Wechsler scales).

31.4.4.2 Mccarthy scales of children's abilities

The McCarthy scales can be used with children between the ages of 2.5 and 8.5 years. It contains six scales: verbal, perceptual–performance, quantitative, memory, motor, and general cognitive. In addition to yielding a General Cognitive Index (GCI), the McCarthy scales provide several ability profiles (verbal, nonverbal reasoning, number aptitude, short-term memory, and coordination).

The overall GCI has a mean of 100 and a standard deviation of 16 and is an estimate of the child's ability to apply accumulated knowledge to the tasks in the scales. The ability profiles, in particular, make the McCarthy scales useful for assessing young children with learning problems.

31.4.4.3 Woodcock–johnson psycho-educational battery – revised

The Woodcock–Johnson Psycho-Educational Battery – Revised (WJPEB-R) comprises 35 tests assessing cognitive ability (vocabulary, memory, concept formation, spacial relations, and quantitative concepts) and achievement (reading, spelling, math, capitalization, punctuation, and knowledge of science, humanities, and social studies). The achievement battery can be used with preschool children (4- or 5-year-olds) through to adults. By comparing the tests of cognitive ability and the tests of achievement, the Woodcock–Johnson battery allows for the assessment of an aptitude/achievment discrepancy. The discrepancy reflects disparity between cognitive and achievement capabilities.

31.4.4.4 Wide range achievement test – revised

The Wide Range Achievement Test – Revised (WRAT-R) is a brief achievement test and contains three subtests: reading, spelling, and arithmetic. The WRAT-R is divided into two levels: Level 1 (ages 5 years to 11 years + 11 months) and Level 2 (ages 12 years to 74 years + 11 months).

31.5 Personality assessments

Personality tests attempt to measure an individual's personality style and are used to assist in clinical diagnosis, and sometimes in forensic settings, although they have come under criticism for lack of validity and reliability in a number of countries that once employed them in these settings.

The Minnesota Multiphasic Personality Inventory (MMPI) comprises several hundred forced-choice ("yes" or "no") questions. It is the most widely administered personality inventory. The MMPI was developed in the 1930s as a comprehensive test meant to detect psychiatric problems. It remained unchanged until 1989 when the MMPI-2 was developed. There is a version for adolescents and an abbreviated version (MMPI-3). It has ten clinical scales to indicate different psychiatric conditions, although these are not "pure" and hence the scales are often referred to by their number. There are three "validity" scales to guard against faking. The MMPI is classified as an "objective test" owing to its paper and pencil format.

The Rorschach test is composed of several cards of inkblots (ambiguous stimuli) which are meant to elicit patients' inner dynamics as inferred by the tester. This makes the Rorschach a "projective" test.

31.6 Clinical rating scales

Psychiatric rating scales are measures that consist of a number of questionnaires, interview outcome assessments, and checklists and are among the most versatile of assessment techniques. Rating scales typically present users with an item and ask them to select from a number of choices. The rating scale is similar in some respects to a multiple-choice test, but its options represent degrees of a particular characteristic.

Rating scales are used with increasing frequency as part of an initial assessment, and in a semi-structured interview their use offers some degree of certitude that items will be addressed consistently in subsequent interviews. Moreover, when rating scales are employed regularly, they can provide valuable information about the course of a patient's illness. When there is improvement, they can provide an important and concrete visual feedback mechanism to patients, as well as make them feel better engaged in the therapeutic process.

Most rating scales come with directions on how to score each item. Many scales are copyrighted by their developers and sold for a fee, but there are numerous scales that can be downloaded from the internet free of charge. Some major pharmaceutical companies have provided very useful websites for clinicians which contain comprehensive lists of rating scales, discussing their use, utility, facility, time to administer, inter-rater reliability, benefits and challenges. See http://www.seroquel.info/ assessment-tools/.

The content of psychiatric rating scales are normally derived from the DSM or the ICD-10, but sometimes differ in how symptoms are clustered or quantified due to the structure of the scale. Symptom rating scales are constructed using a Likert-type scale, with 0 (not present), 1 (mild), 2 (moderate), 3 (marked), and 4 (severe). In contrast, the diagnostic symptoms are scored 0 (not present) or 1 (present); that is, checklist-oriented. Moreover, the total score is often the sufficient or appropriate statistic for a symptom rating scale, while an algorithm is used in the diagnostic systems.

31.7 Developmental measures

Several standardized measurement tools have been developed that are used primarily to assess the motor (fine and gross), language (receptive and expressive), and cognitive development of infants and toddlers. One of the most widely used is described below.

The Bayley Scales of Infant Development (Second Edition) are an individually administered instrument for assessing the development of infants and very young children. It is appropriate for children from 2 months to 3.5 years. It comprises three scales: Mental, Motor, and Behavior Rating. The Mental scale assesses the following areas: recognition memory, object permanence, shape discrimination, sustained attention, purposeful manipulation of objects, imitation (vocal/verbal and gestural), verbal comprehension, vocalization, early language skills, short-term memory, problem-solving, numbers, counting, and expressive vocabulary. The Motor scale addresses the areas of gross and fine motor abilities in a relatively traditional manner. The Behavior Rating scale is used to rate the child's behavioral and emotional status during the assessment.

The Bayley Scales are one of the most popular infant assessment tools. The instrument can also be used to obtain the developmental status of children older than 3.5 years who have very significant delays in development and cannot be evaluated using more age- appropriate cognitive measures.

31.8 Advantages and drawbacks of instrumentation and rating scales

Rating scales have certain advantages. It may be faster and easier to elicit certain information, which can be followed up by the clinician in the face-to-face assessment. Moreover they can be valuable "visuals" for patients (and clinicians) as an ongoing evaluation of their progress in treatment. They may also be useful in eliciting information about potentially sensitive areas such as sexual functioning, domestic abuse, suicidal ideation, and cognitive decline, which patients and families may be reluctant to discuss. Finally, in an arena of evidence-based practice and cost containment, they provide useful information for third- party payers who desire "objective" information about patient progress.

There are some important drawbacks as well. Rating scales are not a substitute for face-to-face evaluation. Even those that require clinician administration can become rote and impersonal. They can provide a false sense of security to clinicians, who may assume that, because an item is endorsed in a certain way, there is no need to elicit the information in an interview. Moreover, clinicians are cautioned that words do not necessarily mean the same thing to different administrators or to patients. Many rating scales use "descriptive" or "evaluative" language, rather than "data" or operational language. This may introduce ambiguity into the assessment situation when people are not understanding words in the same way. Hence, tests and psychiatric rating scales are valuable and important tools, but they are only one part of the overall assessment process.

KEY POINTS

- There are multiple ways in which people can be assessed that include observation and testing.

- Achievement tests are usually seen in educational settings. They attempt to measure achieved knowledge about a certain topic.

- Intelligence tests attempt to measure basic ability to understand the world, assimilate its functioning, and apply this knowledge.

- The challenge of IQ testing is to design a test that can actually be culture-free. Most intelligence tests fail in this area to some extent.

- Neuropsychological tests attempt to measure deficits in cognitive functioning (the ability to think, speak, reason, etc.) that may result from some sort of brain damage, such as a stroke or a brain injury.

- Personality tests attempt to measure basic personality style and are used to help with clinical diagnoses. They can be objective or projective. A projective test is a type of personality test in which the individual offers responses to ambiguous scenes, words or images.

- Specific clinical tests attempt to measure specific clinical matters, such as current level of anxiety or depression.

Further Reading

Dawes, R.M. (1994) *House of Cards: Psychology and Psychotherapy Built on Myth*, Free Press, New York.

Haderlie, Michael M. (2007) "The Treatment Utility of the MMPI-2 in Treatment Planning". School of Professional Psychology, Paper 32. Available at: http://commons.pacificu.edu/spp/32.

Hilsenroth, M.J., Segal, D.L., and Hersen, M. (2003) *Comprehensive Handbook of Psychological Assessment*, vol. **2**, Personality Assessment, John Wiley, New York.

Hunsley, J. and Bailey, J.M. (1999) The clinical utility of the Rorschach: unfulfilled promises and an uncertain future. *Psychological Assessment*, **2** (3), 266–277.

Wood, T.N., Nezworski, T., Lilienfeld, S.O., and Garb, H.N. (2003) *What's Wrong with the Rorschach? Science Confronts the Controversial Inkblot Test*, John Wiley, New York.

32 Psychotherapeutic Approaches

32.1 Introduction

Conceptual frameworks and theories are *world views*. In psychiatry, various theories represent world views and are a means of thinking about people and the world. All have different explanations to account for human behavior, as well as propose interventions consistent with their tenets. Major world views having to do with the human condition can be conceptualized broadly as those in which the formation of the "self" happens via feedback from other people, and those that are more ontogenically oriented to a more individual, organic unfolding of consciousness and development.

A common mistake that clinicians make is espousing an overzealous commitment to one theoretical framework, believing that one particular way of understanding the human condition or method of therapeutic intervention is the single most effective option for all people. While commitment and fidelity to a theory is sometimes necessary, a single-minded adherence to one school of thought is not helpful, making it impossible to treat people holistically and to adhere to the principles of an integrated approach to care. Furthermore, forcing one type of approach and its related treatment interventions may make it impossible to reach and help many people who would respond better to another point of view or approach.

No one theory adequately accounts for human behavior or for psychiatric disorders; nor can one theoretical approach adequately shape interventions for the range of problems that we encounter with patients. Alternative and competing theories have dominated the field of mental health at one time or another, sometimes to the detriment of both the field and patients. For example, for decades psychoanalytic therapy was considered the gold standard, then came cognitive therapy. Then it was found that for many adolescents and others interpersonal psychotherapy was more effective. This should have come as no surprise given the importance of relationships. The take-home point is that therapeutic approaches should be tailored to the individual needs and problems of individuals. There is a great deal of data to support the position that various therapies are effective in a range of psychiatric disorders. There is almost no evidence that suggests one type of therapy is superior to another.

This chapter discusses several theories with which clinicians working in the psychiatric–mental health field should be familiar. The complexity of different approaches may not be addressed, and the approach may seem oversimplified, but it is one taken for the sake of systematic discussion. The chapter is not intended to be a tutorial on psychotherapy. It reviews a limited number of theoretical approaches that can be subsumed generally under social (environmental) and individual (internal) psychotherapeutic world views.

Fundamentals of Psychiatry, First Edition. Allan Tasman and Wanda K. Mohr.
© 2011 John Wiley & Sons, Ltd. Published 2011 by John Wiley & Sons, Ltd.

32.2 Behavior theory and therapy

32.2.1 The behaviorist movement

The behaviorist movement emerged in the early twentieth century as a challenge to the supremacy of psychodynamic approaches. Behavioral psychologists believed that the study of subjective experience did not provide acceptable scientific data because observations and interpretations made by psychoanalysts were not open to verification by others. In their view only the study of directly observable behavior and the stimuli and reinforcing conditions that control it could serve as a basis for formulating scientific principles of human behavior. They argued that achieving insight by way of psychoanalysis did not equate to changing behavior.

As with psychodynamics, there are many schools of thought within this perspective. All are organized around a single central theme: the *role of learning* in human behavior. They also all operate on the assumption that behavior is lawful.

32.2.2 General principles and terminology

Because behavior theory maintains that all human behavior is learned, its major scholars have concerned themselves with explaining and researching how learning occurs and focus on the question of how environmental conditions result in the acquisition, modification, maintenance, and elimination of adaptive and maladaptive behaviors. Behavior theory (or learning theory) has strong empirical support and a solid research base, although it has been criticized for neglecting the cognitive component (beliefs, assumptions) underlying people's behaviors.

Several concepts are important within the behavioral perspective. The first is the idea of *conditioning*, which is a basic form of learning. There are two forms of conditioning: respondent ("classical") and operant. Respondent conditioning happens when a response and a stimulus become connected. Unconditioned responses develop before learning and may be innate to all humans. Conditioned responses develop through the repeated pairing of stimuli and responses.

In operant conditioning, individuals respond in order to achieve a certain goal. They "operate" on their environment to achieve something that is rewarding or to avoid something that is aversive. In operant conditioning, the response precedes the stimulus. An example can be observed when patients learn that behaving in a certain way leads to certain positive events, such as praise from staff or family, more freedom, and better privileges. Thus, they increase that behavior to subsequently increase those positive events. Likewise, they also may learn that behaving in certain ways may lead to negative events and, thus, avoid behaving in those ways to prevent the negative circumstances.

A second important but frequently misunderstood concept in behavior theory is *reinforcement*. Contrary to what many professionals believe, a reinforcer is not a reward. A reinforcer is a stimulus that strengthens a new response by its repeated association with that response. That stimulus may be either pleasant (positive) or aversive (negative). Thus, a person may learn a certain response (behavior) either to receive a reward or to avoid a punishment. In both positive and negative reinforcement, the person is rewarded for making an appropriate response.

When positive reinforcement is used, the response happens by *adding* something to increase the probability of the response. Negative reinforcement involves the *termination* or *removal* of a consequence. In negative reinforcement something is *removed* following a desired response to increase the probability of a behavior.

Negative reinforcers are generally unpleasant or aversive so that the person is motivated to exhibit a desired target behavior to escape from the unpleasant condition. The nature of the positive or negative reinforcer can differ from person to person.

High rates of reinforcement are necessary in early learning, with gradual tapering to maintain the response. Responses are particularly persistent when reinforcement is intermittent and therefore unpredictable. The person continually keeps responding based on past reinforcement and hoping for future reinforcement. This is why such activities as habitual gambling may be so difficult to overcome. Gamblers win intermittently and unpredictably. When gambling becomes habitual, it is extremely difficult to overcome precisely because of the intermittent and unpredictable nature of the winnings.

Punishment is a special kind of stimulus that operates in an opposite way from reinforcement. A punishing stimulus is any aversive stimulus that, when introduced after a response, decreases the future likelihood of that response. Punishing stimuli are introduced with the hope of stopping certain behaviors. Punishment is almost always ineffective. It sometimes may result in short-term compliance but is not effective in terms of long-term behavior change. Moreover, punishment can be unpredictable and self-defeating, as most people tend to react to punishment by fighting back, withdrawing into passive apathy, and avoiding the person with whom the punishment is associated.

Generalization happens when a conditioned response becomes associated with similar stimuli. For example, if a child's response happens at home repeatedly, the child is very likely to display that behavior in other circumstances outside the home given similar conditions. Closely allied with generalization is *discrimination*, which occurs when a person learns to distinguish between and respond differently to similar stimuli. An example is when a child learns that he or she is expected to act a certain way within the family but that expectations for the same child may be very different within his or her peer group, because the reinforcers are different. According to behavior theory, generalization and discrimination have many important implications for the development of maladaptive behaviors. An example can be seen in people who become frightened in a given social situation who may gradually develop a social phobia in which they avoid all social situations.

Modeling involves the demonstration of desired behavior patterns to a learner. Therapists model behaviors when they teach social skills, such as assertiveness. The therapist models assertive behavior with the expectation that the learner will copy that behavior. The assertive behavior is then reinforced. Given sufficient practice of the assertive behavior paired with its reinforcement, the assertive behavior gradually becomes part of the patient's behavioral inventory.

Shaping is a procedure that is employed when a person lacks certain behavior in his or her inventory, so that reinforcement of that behavior might take place. The fact that a behavior must occur before it can be reinforced places a therapist in something of a conundrum. In such cases it might be possible to shape behaviors in the desired direction by reinforcing very small incremental successive approximations of those behaviors.

32.2.3 *Applied behavioral analysis*

Psychotherapy and treatment based on behavior theory rests on applied behavior analysis, a systematic way of examining and analyzing the behaviors of patients as they relate to their environments and basing appropriate interventions on this analysis. The central processes of applied behavioral analysis are operationalization of behavior, functional analysis, selection of socially appropriate goals for change, and selection of appropriate behavioral change procedures. While an exhaustive description of these concepts is beyond the scope of this chapter, students should be acquainted with the ideas of operationalization of behavior and functional analysis.

Operationalization of behavior refers to precisely defining behaviors in concrete observations. Thus, a patient who uses the term "depressed" to describe how he or she feels has provided a useless description to a behavior therapist. Depression is a construct with a wide variety of meanings that may differ from person to person. Far more useful are the specific behaviors, events, actions, and stimuli associated with what the patient describes as depression. The goal of operationalization is to change vague words into observable and concrete actions that can serve as the basis for modification. Such specific actions might include withdrawing from family and friends or neglecting one's appearance.

Functional analysis is based on the notion that a person's behavior is directly related to environmental events and stimuli. It involves a systematic and sequential operationalization of behaviors that seek to determine the specific circumstances under which behavior occurs. Functional analysis involves examining the conditions before the behavior and the consequences that follow

32.2.4 The evidence for behavior theory

Behavior theory has been praised for its precision and objectivity and for the enormous amount of empirical research that it has generated, demonstrating therapeutic efficacy in changing behavior. These are too numerous to summarize. Most recently, meta-analysis investigating the effectiveness of functional analysis of behavior-based behavioral interventions when targeting problem behaviors in various populations, especially in school-aged children, demonstrates overall very positive results for these therapeutic interventions. Behavior therapy has also been shown to be highly successful in the treatment of a variety of conditions, such as smoking cessation and insomnia, showing greater reduction in sleep latency than pharmacologic agents.

32.3 Interpersonal psychotherapy

32.3.1 General principles

Interpersonal psychotherapy (IPT) focuses on interpersonal rather than intrapsychic or cognitive aspects of depression. IPT uses a biopsychosocial model framing psychiatric conditions as illness occurring in a social context. IPT is grounded in interpersonal theory and the work of Sullivan and Bowlby.

The core of IPT is the central importance of relationships for human survival and adaptation. IPT integrates biologic and psychosocial approaches into a practical, patient-oriented treatment. IPT emphasizes the relational aspects of individual experience. Proponents of IPT posit that psychologic problems occur, and interpersonal relationships break down, when people's needs for attachment are not being met. This can occur both when individuals cannot effectively communicate their needs to others and when their social support network is incapable of responding adequately to those needs.

32.3.2 Phases of therapy

Interpersonal psychotherapy has three phases. In the beginning (sessions 1 to 3), a psychiatric assessment focuses on interpersonal relationships to assess suitability and establish the focus of the therapy. The need for medication is evaluated and the patient's condition is explained as an illness in a social context, with interpersonal antecedents and sequelae. The focus of therapy is determined according to the current interpersonal problems that appear to be most related to the onset and perpetuation of the individual's current psychiatric episode. Therapeutic goals are then explained to the patient.

During the second or middle phase of treatment, the four IPT focal areas guide therapeutic interventions linking symptoms to interpersonal events, losses, changes or isolation. IPT focal areas are inter personal disputes, role transitions, bereavement, and interpersonal deficits. These are elaborated in Table 32.1.

Table 32-1   Focal areas of interpersonal therapy

Problem area	Features of Therapy
Interpersonal disputes	Non-reciprocal role expectations with significant others
	Accompanied by poor communication or misaligned interpersonal expectations
Role transitions	Involve life events that lead to significant interpersonal changes (e.g., divorce, birth of child)
Bereavement	Grief accompanying the loss of a relationship to death or divorce, recognizing that ambivalence is typical in the experience of bereavement
	Patients are encouraged to grieve, examine positive and negative aspects of the loss and to replace aspects of what was lost and begin moving forward
Interpersonal deficits	Specific focus on difficulty forming and/or sustaining relationships

In addition to focusing on specific goals, throughout its course IPT highlights interpersonal patterns and how they are linked to symptoms. Relationship expectations and communication are examined to develop social supports and a more effective interpersonal behavioral repertoire, in which empathic responsiveness and clearer expression of emotions and needs are encouraged.

In the concluding, or termination, phase of IPT, therapeutic gains are reviewed and consolidated along with contingency planning in the event of a recurrence of symptoms. If the therapy has failed to achieve the goals of remission, one might contract to extend the course of treatment or re-evaluate it and suggest sequencing with a different form of treatment.

In research protocols for acute major depression, the course of treatment is usually 12 to 16 once-weekly sessions. Some experts suggest a tapering schedule and maintenance monthly sessions, especially for individuals with chronic or recurrent conditions.

32.3.3 The evidence for IPT

Most randomized controlled trials of IPT focus on its efficacy as a treatment for depression. Research focusing on its effectiveness and applicability to other psychiatric conditions is still in its infancy, as is research examining the mechanisms underlying this approach.

In a comprehensive review of IPT, the National Institute of Mental Health Treatment of Depression Collaborative Research Program (NIMHTDCRP) compared IPT, CBT, imipramine and a placebo–clinical management arm for the treatment of patients with major depression. IPT was found to be superior to placebo and equal to CBT and imipramine for mild-to-moderate depression. There was some evidence that IPT was superior to CBT for individuals with severe depression.

IPT has been found to be an effective treatment for depression in patients from adolescence to late life, for women with postpartum depression, and for patients with medical comorbidity. IPT has been adapted for other populations, including patients with eating disorders, social anxiety, and bipolar disorder.

32.4 Individual (internally oriented) approaches

32.4.1 Psychodynamic theory

Psychodynamic theory is derived from the ideas of Sigmund Freud who developed it for the treatment of neuroses. The theory has been revised and modified by Freud's descendants, including Karen Horney, Melanie Klein, Alfred Adler, Ernest Jones, Erik Erikson, Carl Jung, Erich Fromm, Harry Stack Sullivan, Otto Kernberg, and Henry Kohut.

There is considerable disagreement about what constitutes the contemporary psychodynamic orientation. Practitioners of psychoanalysis and psychodynamic therapy range from the more orthodox Freudians, who adhere strictly to the original theory, to those who combine psychodynamic theory with techniques from other schools of psychotherapy.

32.4.2 General principles and terminology

Psychodynamic thought has been very influential, especially in Europe and the Western hemisphere. Central to psychodynamic theory is the idea of the *unconscious*. Freud thought that the conscious part of the mind represents a very small area, while the unconscious part, like the submerged part of an iceberg, is much larger. The unconscious contains the hurtful memories, forbidden desires, and other experiences that have been *repressed* – that is, pushed out of consciousness. Although the person is unaware of such unconscious material, the repressed thoughts and feelings seek expression, which may be reflected in dreams and fantasies and may lead to irrational and maladaptive behavior. A goal of psychodynamic therapy is to expand awareness of unconscious functioning and its relation to everyday living in order that the individual can exert more conscious influence over emotional, cognitive, and behavioral responses.

Freud was one of the first theorists to view personality development as a succession of stages, as outlined in Table 32.2. Essentially, he believed that appropriate gratification during each stage is important if the person is not to become *fixated* (stuck) in relying on the typical responses of that period of development at that stage.

One enduring set of constructs is Freud's notions of what set of functions constitutes the human mental life. Basically a person's behavior is assumed to result from the interplay of three subsystems: id, ego, and superego.

- The *id* is the original system of the personality and consists of everything psychologic that a person inherits at birth, including the instincts. It is the reservoir of psychic energy, and it

Table 32-2 Characteristics of Freud's stages of development	
Stage	**Characteristics**
Oral (birth to 18 months)	Urgency of needs Dependency No consideration of others Low frustration tolerance Separation anxiety
Anal (18 months to 3 years)	Need for control and autonomy Orderliness, obstinacy, punctuality Beginning dyadic relationships Conflict over autonomy and compliance Guilt
Genital (3–6 yr)	Emergence of genital sexuality Concern about self image Shift from dyadic to triadic relationships
Latency (6 years to puberty)	Decreased emphasis on sexual gratification Focus on same-sex relationships Emphasis on development of autonomous ego functions
Adolescence (puberty)	Recapitulates early phases Separation from family Important peer bonds Revival of sexual interest Identity formation

furnishes all the power for the other two systems. The id is concerned with immediate gratification of desires and needs, regardless of reality and the external world.

- The second system, the *ego*, mediates between the id and the external world. The function of the ego is to meet the needs of the id, but in a way that ensures the person's well-being.

- The third system, the *superego*, is what might be construed as the conscience. The superego is concerned with matters of right and wrong. Freud viewed the interplay among these systems as crucial in determining behavior.

The theoretical construct of the *ego defense mechanism* is among Freud's most enduring contributions to psychodynamic theory. Freud articulated the function of defense mechanisms as the ego's way of fulfilling its task to avoid danger, anxiety, and "unpleasure." Now, DSM-IV-TR defines defense mechanisms as "automatic psychological processes that protect the individual against anxiety (stress) and from awareness of the internal or external dangers or stressors."

Anna Freud and others elaborated and refined Sigmund Freud's earlier formulations, stating that the analyst's first order of business is to recognize the defense mechanism. She listed and defined 12 of them. Since that time the number of defense mechanisms that has been proposed has increased dramatically: DSM-IV-TR lists 31 and defines 27 of them. Blackman (2004), in the longest compilation to date, lists and defines 101 defense mechanisms, and claims that there is potentially an infinite number. For reasons of space this chapter will not provide an exhaustive list of all the defense mechanisms that have been proposed. Readers are encouraged to access DSM-IV-TR for those that are commonly accepted, and other sources in the recommended readings at the end of the chapter.

32.4.3 Transference and counter-transference

No discussion of psychodynamic thought would be complete without two useful constructs known as *transference* and *counter-transference*. Transference refers to feelings and thoughts that clients have toward the nurse, psychiatrist, or other service provider. In transference, the client is thought to project an imagined image about the provider. That image may be positive or negative and may hamper or move forward the process of therapy. Counter-transference refers to the feelings and thoughts that service providers have toward the client. In counter-transference the provider may harbor certain images of the client that result in "blind spots," which can be destructive or disruptive to the therapeutic process.

Transference and counter-transference are useful conceptualizations and provide a shortcut for discussing and exploring what may happen between service providers and clients that may be destructive to the relationship.

32.4.4 Goals of psychodynamic therapy

The primary objective in psychodynamic therapy is to enhance the patient's understanding, awareness, and insight about repetitive conflicts (intrapsychic and intrapersonal), or psychologic developmental deficits or delays. An assumption in psychodynamic therapy is that a patient's childhood and later experiences, past unresolved conflicts, and historical relationships significantly affect the person's present life situation. In this form of treatment, the therapist concentrates on helping understand how the patient's past, unresolved conflicts, and historical relationships effect his or her present functioning. In psychodynamic therapy the therapist explores a patient's wishes, dreams, and fantasies to gain further understanding of the origins of present-day maladaptive response patterns. Time limitations and the focal explorations of the patient's life and emotions distinguish psychodynamic therapy from actual psychoanalysis.

32.4.5 The evidence for the psychodynamic approach

Several effectiveness studies have provided evidence that long-term psychoanalytic psychotherapy yielded statistically and clinically significant improvements in patients with complex (i.e., multimorbid) mental disorders. Recent meta-analysis of 23 studies of long-term psychodynamic psychotherapy yielded large and stable effect sizes in the treatment of patients with personality disorders, a variety of mental disorders, including depression and chronic mental disorders.

32.5 Cognitive theories

Two major schools of thought are guided by cognitive theory. The first is Albert Ellis's rational–emotive theory. The second is Aaron Beck's cognitive theory. Both emphasize the centrality of the role that cognitions (thoughts) have in how people feel and act.

32.5.1 Rational–emotive theory

The essence of Ellis's theory of psychopathology is that activating events do not directly cause emotional or behavioral consequences. Rather beliefs about these activating events are the most direct and important causes of how we feel and act. Rational–emotive therapy (RET) emphasizes the disputation of certain irrational beliefs. Beliefs are considered irrational when they are unlikely to find empirical support in a person's environment and do not promote survival and enjoyment (Box 32.1).

Cognitions, then, help to determine a person's response to stimuli. The idea behind RET is that patients engage in certain self-statements based on distorted sets of cognitions. These self-statements contribute to maladaptation and related behaviors.

RET therapists teach patients to do a kind of functional analysis of their own behaviors in which they examine the *antecedent condition*, or the cognition that precedes their behaviors and results in

---

Box 32.1 Irrational Beliefs According to Ellis.

- It is a dire necessity for adult humans to be loved or approved by virtually every significant other person in their community.
- One absolutely must be competent, adequate and achieving in all important respects or else one is an inadequate, worthless person.
- People absolutely must act considerately and fairly and they are damnable villains if they do not. They *are* their bad acts.
- It is awful and terrible when things are not the way one would very much like them to be.
- Emotional disturbance is mainly externally caused and people have little or no ability to increase or decrease their dysfunctional feelings and behaviors.
- If something is or may be dangerous or fearsome, then one should be constantly and excessively concerned about it and should keep dwelling on the possibility of it occurring.
- One cannot and must not face life's responsibilities and difficulties and it is easier to avoid them.
- One must be quite dependent on others and need them and you cannot mainly run one's own life.
- One's past history is an all-important determiner of one's present behavior and because something once strongly affected one's life, it should indefinitely have a similar effect.
- Other people's disturbances are horrible and one must feel upset about them.
- There is invariably a right, precise and perfect solution to human problems and it is awful if this perfect solution is not found.

self-statements. Patients then examine the consequences related to those antecedents and self-statements. In RET this approach is known as the "ABCD" approach.

- A is the antecedent behavior (an experience or event)

- B is the irrational or maladaptive belief(s) about the experience or event

- C is the consequence (of the belief).

- D is the disputation of those maladaptive beliefs.

The goals of therapy are for patients to monitor their maladaptive thoughts and beliefs, look for evidence that their beliefs are true, dispute their maladaptive self-statements, substitute more adaptive thoughts, and thus change their pattern of distorted thinking and, consequently, their behavior. This is part of a technique known as *cognitive restructuring*.

The patient describes his or her thoughts systematically, links those self-defeating thoughts to the present discomfort, and then disputes them. The disputation of what Ellis calls "irrational" beliefs is one way for people to change their self-defeating thoughts, which lead to self-defeating behaviors.

32.5.2 Beck's cognitive theory

Aaron Beck, a psychodynamically oriented psychiatrist, initially developed his cognitive model to help explain depression. It is now used to treat any number of psychiatric conditions, such as anxiety and phobias, as well as depression.

Beck's model holds that conditions such as depression result primarily from pervasive, negative misinterpretations of experience. Beck postulates that psychological problems result from faulty learning and making incorrect inferences based on inadequate or incorrect information (Box 32.2). Cognitive therapy uses an information processing model directed toward identifying and modifying incorrect cognitions. In collaboration with the therapist, patients address their biased selection of information and distorted beliefs, and learn to invalidate those beliefs. Cognitive therapy and RET have much in common.

32.5.3 Cognitive–behavior theory: a synthesis

In the 1970s, learning theorists such as Donald Meichenbaum enhanced behavior theory by introducing the role of *cognitions*, or mediating processes between a stimulus and a response. This led to the development of cognitive–behavior therapy;. Subsumed under the heading of CBT is a host of different techniques that incorporate techniques from RET and Beck's cognitive therapy, problem-solving training, behavior therapy, skills training, and self-instructional training.

Box 32.2 Cognitive Distortions According to Beck.

- *Selective abstraction*: Picking out from a complex situation only certain features and ignoring aspects that could lead to a different conclusion
- *Overgeneralization*: Coming to a general conclusion based on a single incident or piece of evidence
- *Fallacy of change*: Expecting that other people will change to suit the patient if they just pressure or cajole them enough
- *Personalization*: thinking that everything people do or say is some kind of reaction to us
- *Dichotomous thinking*: things are either "black" or they are "white," there is no middle ground
- *Heaven's reward Fallacy*: sacrifice and self-denial to pay off, as if someone is keeping score and feeling bitter when the reward doesn't come

There is some diversity in how CBT is implemented, but in general this therapy is active, directive, highly structured, and time-limited. Therapists are seen as teachers or coaches and expect patients to be actively engaged in their treatment, practicing new thoughts and behaviors through homework exercises developed by the therapist. The field of CBT has grown immensely in the past several decades, and studies demonstrate empirical support for the techniques in the treatment of a large number of conditions.

32.5.4 The evidence for CBT

At this writing there are a total of 16 methodologically rigorous meta-analyses on treatment outcomes of CBT for a wide range of psychiatric disorders. Large effect sizes have been found for CBT for unipolar depression, generalized anxiety disorder, panic disorder with or without agoraphobia, social phobia, post-traumatic stress disorder, and childhood depressive and anxiety disorders.

32.5.5 A note on dialectic behavior therapy

Dialectic behavior therapy (DBT) builds on the CBT foundation. Developed by Marsha Linehan, it was developed to treat individuals with borderline personality disorder (see Chapter 19).

Dialectic behavior therapy is based on the idea that some individuals react abnormally to emotional stimulation with extreme lability owing to some combination of invalidating environments during their upbringing coupled with as yet unidentified biologic factors. These individuals lack adaptive coping mechanisms for dealing with their sudden, intense surges of emotion. The overarching goal of DBT is reducing parasuicidal (self-injuring) and life-threatening behaviors. This is followed by the goals of reducing behaviors that interfere with the therapy/treatment process, and reducing behaviors that impede the patient's quality of life. These are accomplished by teaching the skills that will help the person in centering in the moment (mindfulness), making him or her aware of dichotomous thinking, and modulating intense responses to distress.

Across studies, DBT seems to reduce severe dysfunctional behaviors that are targeted for intervention (e.g., parasuicide, substance abuse, and binge-eating), enhance treatment retention, and reduce psychiatric hospitalization. Additional research is warranted to examine which components of DBT contribute to outcomes.

KEY POINTS

- No one theory adequately accounts for human behavior or for psychiatric disorders. Nor can one theoretical approach adequately shape interventions for the range of problems encountered by patients.

- In the behaviorist view, only the study of directly observable behavior and the stimuli and reinforcing conditions that control it could serve as a basis for formulating scientific principles of human behavior.

- Interpersonal therapy is grounded in interpersonal theory and the work of Sullivan and Bowlby. The core of IPT is the central importance of relationships for human survival and adaptation.

- Psychodynamic theory is derived from the ideas of Sigmund Freud who developed it for the treatment of neuroses. Central to psychodynamic theory is the idea of the unconscious.

- Two useful constructs in psychodynamic therapy are transference and counter-transference.

- Cognitive–behavioral therapies are represented by Beck's cognitive therapy and Ellis' rational–emotive therapy. Both emphasize the centrality of the role that cognitions (thoughts) have in how people feel and act.

- A relatively newer development within the CBT framework, dialectic behavior therapy seems to reduce severe dysfunctional behaviors that are targeted for intervention (e.g., parasuicide, substance abuse, and binge eating), enhance treatment retention, and reduce psychiatric hospitalization.

Further Reading

American Psychiatric Association (2000) *Diagnostic and Statistical Manual Of Mental Disorders*, 4th edn, Text Revision, APA, Washington, DC.

Beck, A.T. (1976) *Cognitive Therapy and the Emotional Disorders*, International Universities Press, New York.

Blackman, J.S. (2004) *101 Defenses: How the Mind Shields Itself*, Brunner–Routledge, New York.

Ellis, A. (1962) *Reason and Emotion in Psychotherapy*, Lyle Stuart & Citadel Press, New York.

Freud, A. (1966) *The Ego and the Mechanisms of Defense*, International Universities Press, New York (originally published in 1936).

Meichenbaum, D.H. (1977) *Cognitive Behavior Modification: An Integrative Approach*, Plenum, New York.

Klein, D.F. and Ross, D.C. (1993) Reanalysis of the National Institute of Mental Health Treatment of Depression Collaborative Research Program: general effectiveness report. *Neuropsychopharmacology*, **8**, 241–251.

Leichsenring, F. and Rabung, S. (2008) Effectiveness of long-term psychodynamic psychotherapy: a meta-analysis. *JAMA*, **300** (13), 1551–1565.

Linehan, M.M., Armstrong, H.E., Suarez, A. *et al.* (1991) Cognitive–behavioral treatment of chronically parasuicidal borderline patients. *Archives of General Psychiatry*, **48**, 1060–1064.

Shedler, J. (2010) The efficacy of psychodynamic psychotherapy. *American Psychologist*, **65** (2), 98–109.

Stuart, S. and Robertson, M. (2003) *Interpersonal Psychotherapy: A Clinician's Guide*, Arnold, London.

Weissman, M.M., Markowitz, J.W., and Klerman, G.L. (2000) *Comprehensive Guide to Interpersonal Psychotherapy*, Basic Books, New York.

33 · Pharmacotherapeutic Interventions

33.1 Introduction

This chapter discusses the use of psychoactive medications that alter synaptic transmission and result in a cascade of physiologic reactions that can affect and alleviate the symptoms of mental illnesses. It is important for clinicians who read this chapter to understand the benefits as well as the inexactitude of current psychopharmacologic treatment. Psychotropic medications are powerful therapeutic agents, but much research and development still needs to happen before our patients can have the quality of life afforded by many medications that have been developed in other branches of medicine.

This chapter discusses the basic fundamentals of psychopharmacology, as well as factors that can influence the course of patients' treatment, and talks about actions, therapeutic doses, side-effects, potential toxicity, administration, contraindications, and implications of the most important psychotropic medications in current use. The chapter presents special issues related to the use of these drugs, such as developmental and lifespan considerations and concomitant use with alternative therapies.

Readers are advised that the field of psychopharmacology changes rapidly, and new medications and therapeutics are introduced constantly. It is wise to foster a habit of reading the research literature on a regular basis so as to have as current as possible repertoire of interventions in service of patients and their families.

33.2 Principles of pharmacokinetics and pharmacodynamics

The actions of drugs in the human body involve many biochemical and physiologic responses affecting multiple body systems. Medications alter physiology in a way that results in a biochemical change. This change becomes the drug response. This section reviews important concepts of pharmacodynamics necessary to understand pharmacotherapeutics as interventions in the toolkit in treating psychiatric illnesses.

33.2.1 Definitions

The intensity of a biologic response produced by a drug is related to the concentration of the drug at the site of action, which is in turn affected by a variety of factors grouped together under the heading *pharmacokinetics*. There are four pharmacokinetic phases that all affect drug concentration at the site of action.

Fundamentals of Psychiatry, First Edition. Allan Tasman and Wanda K. Mohr.
© 2011 John Wiley & Sons, Ltd. Published 2011 by John Wiley & Sons, Ltd.
This chapter is based on Chapter 99 (Zahinoor Ismail, Bruce G. Pollock) and Chapter 100 (Keh-Ming Lin, Chia-Hui Chen, Shu-Han Yu, Margaret T. Lin, Michael W. Smith) of *Psychiatry, Third Edition*

1. **Absorption** refers to the ability of a drug to enter the blood stream. It is expressed as a rate (amount per unit of time, such as g/min or mL/h) and indicates the speed with which the drug leaves its site of administration and the degree to which this occurs. Some factors that influence absorption include the type of transport, the physiochemical properties of the drug, and the route of administration.

2. **Distribution** is defined as the movement of a drug throughout the body to various tissue sites. Distribution is affected by the physiochemical properties of the drug, cardiac output and blood flow, the blood–brain barrier, and drug reservoirs.

3. **Biotransformation** reactions alter the chemical structure of a drug. Biotransformation occurs primarily in the liver and involves the enzymatic breakdown of drugs.

4. **Excretion** is the removal of drugs and biotransformation products from the body. This occurs primarily in the kidneys.

"Pharmacodynamics" refers to the study of biochemical and physiologic effects of drugs and their mechanisms of action. Foundational to treatment with psychopharmacologic agents is the idea that the symptoms of psychiatric illnesses result from errors of neurotransmission which affect the patient's ability to accurately perceive incoming information.

Receptors are specific protein-binding sites inside or on the surface of a cell. The receptor is the component of the cell with which the chemical is presumed to interact. When chemicals bind to receptors, various cellular functions are either activated or inhibited.

Drugs generally affect receptors in two ways: they may bind to them, or may change their behavior towards the host cell system. *Binding* is influenced by the chemical property of affinity. *Affinity* is a pharmacological concept that describes the degree of attractiveness between a drug and a specific receptor. It is the product of the mutual attractiveness of the molecular structures of the drug and the receptor.

Axons and dendrites have their own receptors. Axon receptors are called *presynaptic*, while dendrite receptors are called *postsynaptic*. Both are sensitive to the smallest fluctuation of chemicals and have the ability to self-regulate. Other receptors, *autoreceptors*, act like light switches, helping individual neurons to down-regulate, up-regulate, or both (see later).

33.2.2 Agonists and antagonists

- **Agonists** are drugs or endogenous substances that trigger actions from a cell or another drug. A drug that is an agonist has attraction to bind to a given receptor. It will activate that receptor and subsequently lead to a change in the function of the cell.

- **Partial agonists** are drugs that exert a similar but weaker effect than a full agonist.

- **Inverse agonists** do the opposite of agonists.

- **Antagonists** block the actions of everything in the agonist spectrum. They are chemicals that bind to a receptor and block it, producing no response, and prevent agonists from binding, or attaching, to the receptor.

33.2.3 Efficacy and potency

The concept of *efficacy* has to do with how well a treatment, therapy or procedure under ideal conditions produces a desired health outcome (cure, alleviation of pain, return of functional abilities). *Maximal efficacy* refers to the maximal effect that a drug can produce. In clinical use, the maximal efficacy of a medication may be limited by its undesired side-effects, and true maximal efficacy may not be achievable.

Potency refers to the measure of a drug's effectiveness as a medication. Potency may be related to the concentration of a drug in plasma, as well as other factors (i.e., transport across cell membranes, competitive antagonists).

33.2.4 Target symptoms

Symptoms, rather than specific illnesses, are the foci for treatment in psychiatry. Target symptoms are the specific symptoms that a medication aims to alter. Clinicians must identify and understand patients' target symptoms before starting them on a medication regimen. Patients should also be helped to understand their target symptoms and participate in identifying and monitoring changes in symptoms. Instruments are available to systematically rate symptoms before and after drug administration and to augment clinician impressions (see Chapter 31).

33.2.5 Refractoriness

Refractoriness (also called *down-regulation*) occurs when agonists continually stimulate cells. As a result, the cells are repeatedly exposed to the same concentration of the drug, which causes the cells to become desensitized and the drug to have diminished effectiveness (efficacy). Understanding the phenomenon of refractoriness is important in caring for psychiatric patients in that they must take the same medication for months to years. Over time, the efficacy of a medication may diminish, causing the symptoms that first required treatment to reappear. This should not be confused with non-adherence or noncompliance with a medication regimen. Early identification of refractoriness and the resulting changes in medication type or dose could prevent a relapse of symptoms.

33.2.6 Steady state and medication half-life

Steady state is a condition during which a fairly constant level of medication is affecting neurons continuously and a desirable response is beginning to happen. It may take four or more weeks for neurons to make consistent changes in electrical charge, release of neurotransmitters, and responses from receptors.

The "rule of 5s" refers to a principle of pharmacology which states that it takes a drug five half-lives to build to a steady state in the body. Half-life refers to the time required for half the dose of a drug to be metabolized or eliminated by normal biologic processes. The half-life is dependent upon many factors, including the health of the individual, diet, and individual differences among patients.

33.2.7 Enzymes

Enzymes are a class of proteins that are involved in multiple aspects of chemical neurotransmission. Enzymes increase the rate of chemical reactions without being consumed or permanently altered by the reaction. They also increase reaction rates without altering the chemical equilibrium between products and reactants. Substrates result when an enzyme acts on a molecule. The substrates for each enzyme are unique and selective. Both are involved in the inhibition and binding of drug receptors and determine selectivity of drug action, the relation between the dose of a drug and its effects, and its therapeutic effectiveness. *Inhibitors* are drugs that block a specific enzyme system, while *inducers* are drugs that increase the amount of enzyme production.

33.2.8 Metabolism

Drug metabolism occurs via two phases, referred to as I and II. Phase I involves primarily oxidation reactions including dealkylation, hydroxylation, oxidation, deamination, desulfuration, and sulf-oxide formation; this is mediated by the cytochrome P450 (CYP450) system. Phase II metabolism involves conjugation or synthetic reactions that render the molecule more water-soluble and hence available for renal excretion.

The CYP450 system is a generic name describing a super-family of oxidative enzymes important in plant, animal, and human physiology. They metabolize not only endogenous compounds but also xenobiotics including environmental compounds and drugs. This super-family contains over 30 related enzymes, and five human CYP450 proteins metabolize more than 90% of drugs used today. These include CYP 1A2, 2D6, 2C9, 2C19, and 3A4. CYP450 enzymes are found primarily in the liver but also in the gastrointestinal tract, kidneys, and lungs. An up-to-date website highlighting the CYP450 system can be found and downloaded in PDF format at from http://medicine.iupui.edu/clinpharm/ddis/.

Pharmacokinetic drug interactions are well described and result from one drug affecting the metabolism of another. Substrate drugs or xenobiotics for CYP450 can be inducers (increasing enzyme activity) or inhibitors (decreasing enzyme activity) of various CYP450 isoenzymes. Competitive or noncompetitive inhibition by one drug on the relevant hepatic enzyme can result in slowed or decreased metabolism of another drug metabolized by the same enzyme. The increase in plasma concentration of the affected drug is immediate, and this second drug reaches a new steady state.

A high index of suspicion is recommended for identifying pharmacokinetic drug interactions. This is especially true if a drug is highly toxic or has a narrow therapeutic window, or if two or more inhibitors of the same system are used, or if a substrate or inhibitor is suddenly discontinued, or if there is a sudden change in clinical picture.

Variability in the CYP450 system exists owing to genetic polymorphisms in coding genes. Differences in copy number, activity, or substrate affinity of the isoenzymes can result in enzymes with inactive, decreased, normal, or increased activity. These interindividual and interethnic differences can result in variable response to drugs.

It is not possible to commit to memory all potential drug interactions. The use of computer devices, such as smart phones or personal digital assistants, loaded with software containing medications and potential interactions, therapeutic doses, adverse effects, toxicities, and side-effects is a prudent tool to employ, especially when polypharmacy becomes necessary.

33.2.9 Ethnicity and pharmacogenetics

The term "pharmacogenetics" refers to the study of genetic *polymorphisms* that code for enzymes involved in drug metabolism and their ability to affect a medication's efficacy and toxicity. Genetic polymorphisms appear to be responsible for much of the interpatient heterogeneity of responses to many medications. Emerging data now convincingly demonstrate that, for the majority of genes, polymorphism is the rule rather than the exception. Furthermore, the frequency and distribution of alleles responsible for such polymorphisms often vary substantially across ethnic groups, effectively requiring that ethnicity always be considered in genetic studies.

Cross-cultural psychopharmacology is a relatively young, but important, field and a comprehensive discussion is beyond the scope of this book. Clinicians are advised that there are important pharmacokinetic variations among ethnic groups of which they should be aware, and avail themselves of more in-depth discussion provided in further readings at the end of this chapter.

33.3 Principles of prescribing medications

33.3.1 General principles

Most expert psychiatric clinicians have a list of principles or pearls of wisdom that help to guide them in the art and science of prescribing interventions for patients. A number of important ones are contained in Box 33.1.

Box 33.1 Some General Principles of Prescribing Medications.

- A careful assessment and diagnosis is essential prior to any pharmacological intervention.
- Simplicity enhances adherence: fewer drugs is better.
- Pharmacotherapy alone is usually not sufficient treatment to achieve recovery.
- Risk to benefit ratios should be considered when developing any plan of treatment.
- Teaching is an essential part of prescribing.
- Personal history of response should guide prescriptions for subsequent episodes.
- Family history of response may predict patient response.
- Engage families if possible as they may positively influence adherence to medication regimens, act as the first line of assessment for adverse side-effects, and supervise administration of the medication and refill of prescriptions.
- Target symptoms should be monitored on a regular basis and progress should be shared with patients and families.
- Adverse reactions and side-effects should be monitored throughout treatment.
- Clinicians should medicate for remission, not simply for partial response.

33.3.2 Special considerations with children

The state of knowledge regarding medication treatments for children and adolescents lags substantially behind that for adults, yet there are some special aspects to medicating children that are well accepted. Few drugs used for psychiatric treatments have been approved for use in children under age 18 years. Children may require larger doses of psychoactive medications per unit of body weight in order to elicit therapeutic efficacy and comparable blood levels. This is thought to be a result of more rapid hepatic metabolism and more efficient glomerular flitration rate in children compared to adults.

Cognitive, developmental, and communicative differences exist between adults and children that can have a great deal of impact on assessment of drug effects, as well as on adherence to medication regimens. Many problems with children which were first assumed to require medication treatment may turn out to be issues with family discord.

33.3.3 Special considerations with older adults

Pharmacologic actions of medications in people over 60 years of age may result from normal age-related changes in body composition, lean body mass, and muscle mass or increased fatty tissue, differences in drug absorption secondary to diminished gastrointestinal motility, decreased plasma proteins, decreased kidney function, or congestive heart failure. As with children, clinicians should be aware that these adults may respond differently from their younger adult counterparts to psychotropic medications. In addition, because many older adults take several medications simultaneously for various physical ailments, clinicians should be aware and observe for effects resulting from drug interactions. Coordination between medical and psychiatric providers is essential, so it is always optimal prior to meeting with a patient to ask him or her to bring all prescription and nonprescription medications and supplements being taken, so that it is not necessary to rely on the patient's memory about this.

Psychiatric syndromes in older adults produce suffering, disability, and a loss of independence. These problems also increase burdens for caregivers. Nevertheless, psychotropic medications can dramatically improve functioning in older clients when the drugs are administered cautiously. Atypical antipsychotic medications have increased safety and efficacy. Older people still present particular challenges to caregivers because of their propensity for chronic medical conditions.

33.3.4 Special concerns with pregnancy and nursing mothers

Pregnancy and lactation pose challenges to pharmacotherapy owing to the reluctance to expose the fetus or infant to a toxic substance. Teratogenicity of a medication or the chance that it can result in a birth defect is a significant concern. The US Food and Drug Administration's system assigns one of five "pregnancy categories" to the agent in question to balance risk against the potential benefits to the patient. The rating system is contained in Box 33.2.

Box 33.2 US FDA Pharmaceutical Pregnancy Categories.

- **Category A.** Adequate and well-controlled studies have failed to demonstrate a risk to the fetus in the first trimester of pregnancy (and there is no evidence of risk in later trimesters).
- **Category B.** Animal reproduction studies have failed to demonstrate a risk to the fetus and there are no adequate and well-controlled studies in pregnant women.
  OR
  Animal studies have shown an adverse effect, but adequate and well-controlled studies in pregnant women have failed to demonstrate a risk to the fetus in any trimester.
- **Category C.** Animal reproduction studies have shown an adverse effect on the fetus and there are no adequate and well-controlled studies in humans, but potential benefits may warrant use of the drug in pregnant women despite potential risks.
- **Category D.** There is positive evidence of human fetal risk based on adverse reaction data from investigational or marketing experience or studies in humans, but potential benefits may warrant use of the drug in pregnant women despite potential risks.
- **Category X.** Studies in animals or humans have demonstrated fetal abnormalities and/or there is positive evidence of human fetal risk based on adverse reaction data from investigational or marketing experience, and the risks involved in use of the drug in pregnant women clearly outweigh potential benefits.

Breast-feeding also poses dilemmas when nursing mothers take psychotropic medications. The postnatal period is a time of increased onset and relapse of mental illness. All major classes of psychotropic medication pass into maternal breast milk, transferring undetermined amounts of medication to the infant. The goal of treatment should be minimizing infant exposure while maintaining maternal emotional health. Clinicians, patients, and families are encouraged to reference sources at the end of this chapter and carefully read the manufacturers' packet inserts.

33.4 Generic prescriptions

The cost of medications is a significant factor in nonadherence to treatment, and one which far too many clinicians ignore. For example, in the United States, retail prices for commonly prescribed antidepressants range from about $20 a month to more than $400 a month. As a result, generic prescription has become more common, especially in HMO (health maintenance organization) plans.

Generic prescribing is the prescribing of a drug by a physician using the generic name. Generic drugs are the original drug chemical compound which is no longer protected by a patent for a brand name. It is common for patients to receive the generic version of a drug because it is less expensive.

The nongeneric and generic formulations are presumed to be bioequivalent. Two products are considered bioequivalent when they produce similar plasma concentrations of the same active ingredient. Bioequivalence is usually assessed in healthy volunteers by administering the two products on separate occasions, and the peak plasma concentration and extent of absorption of the generic medicine and the original brand are compared.

Bioequivalence between the original brand and the generic version of a medicine is the fundamental basis of generic substitution. Surveys have shown that clinicians are undecided about the bioequivalence of generics. Although there may be exceptions (e.g., medicines with narrow therapeutic indices), this lack of confidence in generic medicines is largely unfounded physiologically.

In addition, pressure in the past on clinicians by third-party payers to prescribe generics in lieu of trade medications have resulted in beliefs that finances rather than efficacy is paramount to the insurance industry. The corollary, of course, is the part played by some pharmaceutical manufacturers to pressure and sometimes withold crucial evidence about their medication. The choice should be up to clinicians and patients to make an informed decision in these matters based on data about bioavailability and bioequivalence.

33.5 Off-label use

Off-label prescribing is the practice of prescribing a drug or medical device for a purpose different from one of the indications for which the product is approved by the US Food and Drug Administration. The practice is widespread; although there are no accurate data, estimates run as high as 60% of all drug prescriptions written in the US in a given year. From a legal and ethical standpoint, off-label use represents a delicate balance between the regulatory objective of protecting patients from unsafe or ineffective drugs and medical devices, and the prerogative of clinicians to use their professional judgment in treating patients. It also raises the thorny question of experimentation with an unapproved treatment.

Off-label prescribing is not against the law, and off-label use of a drug does not constitute malpractice (*Femrite* v. *Abbott Northwestern Hospital*, 568 N.W.2d 535, 542 (Minn. Ct. App. 1997)). Nevertheless, case studies or reports upon which decisions are made by some practitioners when engaging in off-label prescribing constitute anecdotal data, and anecdotal data do not hold the same authority as rigorous clinical trials. Off-label prescribing bears some inherent liability risk for the practitioner. In *Richardson* v. *Miller* (44 S.W.3d 1, 13, n.11 (Tenn. Ct. App. 2000)), for example, the court held that the fact that a drug used was off-label could be introduced as evidence that the prescribing physician deviated from the required standard of care.

33.6 Polypharmacy

Polypharmacy is the practice of employing two or more psychotropic drugs, the use of two or more drugs of the same chemical class, or the use of two more drugs with the same or similar pharmacologic actions to treat the same or different conditions (comorbid disorders). The frequency of polypharmacy tends to be high, especially in the treatment of patients with serious psychiatric disorders. While polypharmacy can be critical in the treatment of psychiatric disorders, it can increase the chance of adverse effects, drug interactions, patient nonadherence, and medication errors. It also can result in symptom amelioration in patients with severe psychosis, resistant schizophrenia, and depression.

It is essential for clinicians to evaluate and question the use of several agents to treat a disorder and they should understand the rationale behind the practice of polypharmacy. While certain complex and/or treatment-resistant cases require multiple medications, there are no data to support poly-pharmacy as a routine practice.

The first step should be to arrive at a proper diagnosis, followed by delineating specific target symptoms, drug-to-drug interactions, and the patient's understanding of medication management. Taking more than one agent can confuse a patient, especially if dosing times differ. Health education can assist patients to understand the purpose, side-effects, and efficacy. The goal of medication management always should be optimal treatment with the fewest medications possible. Nurses should understand the philosophy regarding polypharmacy held by the treatment setting where they practice. Although not appropriate for all patients, with careful management, the practice can provide symptom relief to patients with refractory disorders.

33.7 Medication adherence

One of the most difficult aspects of treatment with psychotropic medications involves patient adherence with a recommended medication regimen. Patients may have many reasons for failing to adhere to their medication regimens. The most frequent reason is unacceptable side-effects, many of which are debilitating and difficult to manage. Some patients with chronic psychiatric disturbances believe that they have little control over their life or environment, and may refuse to take medication as a way to exert control over some aspect of their situation.

Building a medication regimen into one's life is not a straightforward task. Just as habits may be difficult to break, they can be difficult to establish, especially when one's life has the overlay of chaos that frequently characterizes much of the daily lives of people with mental illness.

For some patients, the need for psychotropic medication means that they can no longer deny their symptoms or problems. Others perceive that taking psychotropic medications means that they agree with the label of "crazy" or "psychotic," regardless of whether they experience symptom relief and improved functioning as a result. Other patients fear becoming addicted to medications, especially if they or a family member have a history of drug or alcohol abuse and have received treatment for it. Patients may be influenced by their experiences with medications, including memories from childhood when they witnessed family members receive more primitive forms of psychiatric treatment.

Finally, medications are expensive and patients and families may not be able to afford to pay for regular medication maintenance. They may or may not share this information with their psychiatric caregivers.

Clinicians are urged to treat patients who are having difficulty adhering to their medication regimens with compassion and understanding and avoid an adversarial approach to treatment adherence. For patients who are stopping use because of side-effects, titration of the dose or a change in medication usually can solve this problem. Psychopharmacologist Stephen Stahl urges the "wait, wait, wait" approach with supportive interventions when dealing with side-effects, which are often transient.

When symptoms abate and the patient is feeling better, he or she may stop taking a medication. With many chronic disorders, however, the patient's need for medication is long term. It is essential for patients and their families to understand that many disorders and their management are chronic. Clinicians can play an important role in patients' and their families' understanding that a psychiatric condition is no different in this respect from chronic physical conditions that require ongoing medication (e.g., diabetes, hypertension).

Some methods to assist patients in adhering to medication regimens are given in Box 33.3.

Box 33.3 Assisting Patients in Adhering to Medication Regimens.

- Keep it simple. If a medication can be given once daily rather than in multiple doses it will help treatment adherence. Simple also applies to using the fewest medications possible.
- Keep in close contact with the patient, including performing careful follow-up.
- Respond immediately to patient complaints and change dose, time of administration, and medication if it helps alleviate the difficulty.
- Avoid frequent changes of medication. Allow sufficient time for a medication to result in response and remission.
- Develop a strong therapeutic alliance with the patient.
- Understand community and family supports available to the patient.

33.8 Refractory states

A sizable number of patients suffering from psychiatric disorders experience only partial or no clinical response to conventional treatment. These individuals may be called "treatment resistant" or "treatment refractory." There are a number of strategies available, such as switching agents or classes of medications, combining various pharmaceutical agents, or augmenting medications with a second agent to enhance the efficacy of the first. In some cases, it may involve using electroconvulsive therapy. The evidence supporting many of these approaches is inconsistent and more research is needed comparing different strategies and determining which patients are the best candidates for what treatment. Clinicians should be aware that refractory states are best treated by expert clinicians who have experience in treatment resistance and who have a solid grounding in the empirical clinical literature.

KEY POINTS

- Patients should be thoroughly assessed prior to prescribing medications of any kind.

- Particular psychotropic medications are characterized by specific side-effects and administration guidelines.

- A good rule of thumb when prescribing is to "start low and go slow."

- Medications should be used to treat psychiatric target symptoms at optimized levels for a specified period, allowing sufficient time for remission to occur.

- Specific patient populations requiring psychotropic medication and caution include pregnant and lactating women, older adults, and children and adolescents.

- Families can help to provide essential support to patients receiving psychotropic medication.

- Clinicians must be aware of the specific management issues inherent in polypharmacy.

- Clinicians should blend an understanding of psychosocial needs with specific symptoms to provide optimal care.

Further Reading

Friedman, J.M. and Polifka, J.E. (1998) *The Effects of Drugs on the Fetus and Nursing Infant: A Handbook for Health Professionals*, Johns Hopkins University Press, Baltimore, MA.

Green, W.H. (2007) *Child and Adolescent Clinican Psychopharmacology*, Lippincott, Williams & Wilkins, Philadelphia, PA.

Herrera, J.M. and Sramek, J.J. (1999) *Cross Cultural Psychiatry*, John Wiley, Chichester, UK.

Ng, C.H., Lin, K., Singh, B.S., and Chiu, E. (2008) *Ethno-psychopharmacology: Advances in Current Practice*, Cambridge University Press, Cambridge, UK.

Preston, J.D., Talaga, M.C., and O'Neal, J. (2008) *Handbook of Clinical Psychopharmacology for Therapists*, New Harbinger, Oakland, CA.

Stahl, S. (2008) *Stahl's Essential Psychopharmacology: Neuroscientific Basis and Practical Applications*, 3rd edn, Cambridge University Press, Cambridge, UK.

34 Antidepressants and Mood Stabilizers

34.1 Introduction

The fourth edition of *Diagnostic and Statistical Manual of Mental Disorders,* text revision, categorizes mood disorders into depressive disorders (unipolar depression) and bipolar disorders (see Chapters 13 and 14). The two major subclasses of medications for the treatment of mood disorders are antidepressants and mood stabilizers. The antidepressants are also first-line treatments for anxiety disorders (see Chapter 15). This chapter discusses the major antidepressants and mood stabilizers in current use.

34.2 Antidepressants

The term "antidepressant" is something of a misnomer as medications used to treat mood disorders can also be used to treat the anxiety disorders, as well as pain conditions. Indeed the selective serotonin-reuptake inhibitor class of antidepressant medications is the treatment of choice for most of the anxiety disorders and obsessive–compulsive disorder. In depressive disorders, antidepressant medications are employed to alleviate symptoms such as dysphoric mood, changes in appetite and energy levels, anhedonia, feelings of hopelessness, suicidal ideation, concentration problems, and others.

Antidepressant medications are divided into a number of categories that describe their mode of action. Commonly prescribed antidepressant medications, with their generic and trade names, common dosages, modes of action, and half-lives will be covered here.

34.2.1 The tricyclic and tetracyclic group

Developed in the 1960s, these drugs were the medications first used to combat major depressive disorders, and they were the early precursors to the newer selective serotonin-reuptake inhibitors. They are listed in Table 34.1.

The TCAs inhibit the neuronal uptake of both serotonin and norepinephrine and have high anticholinergic properties, which can be peripheral or central. Some of these properties are listed in Box 34.1. Clinicians should be attuned to these effects as they can be debilitating, especially in susceptible patients such as the elderly.

As a rule, the more sedating the TCA, the more anticholinergic properties it will have. Ways to control side-effects from TCAs include starting the patient with a low dose and raising the dose

Fundamentals of Psychiatry, First Edition. Allan Tasman and Wanda K. Mohr.
© 2011 John Wiley & Sons, Ltd. Published 2011 by John Wiley & Sons, Ltd.
This chapter is based on Chapter 101 (Robert J. Boland, Martin B. Keller) and Chapter 103 (David J. Muzina, David E. Kemp, Joseph R. Calabrese) of *Psychiatry, Third Edition*

Table 34-1   Tricyclic and tetracyclic antidepressants*

Generic Name	Brand Name	Type	Dosing	Half-life	Warnings	Comments
Amoxapine	Asendin	Tricyclic	50 mg b.i.d.; may increase to max 100 mg t.i.d.	8–30 h	Disturbed concentration	Sedating
Amitriptyline	Elavil	Tricyclic	75–100 mg/d in divided doses; max 300 mg/d	10–50 h	Orthostatic hypotension	Sedating
Clomipramine	Anafranil	Tricyclic	75–350 mg/d	17–28 h	Lethal in suicide attempt	Sedating, can cause cognitive impairment
Desipramine	Norpramin, Pertofran	Tricyclic	100–350 mg/d	24 h	Do not administer to patients recovering from MI	Less sedating than others Weight gain; side-effects can be discouraging
Doxepin	Sinequan	Tricyclic	25 mg t.i.d.; divided doses up to 300 mg/d max	8–25 h	Orthostatic hypotension	Sedating
Maprotiline	Ludiomil	Tetracyclic	75–150 mg/d	27–58 h	May cause confusion	Sedating
Imipramine	Tofranil	Tricyclic	100–150 mg in divided doses; 300 mg/d max	8–16 h	Strong anticholinergic effects	Decreased anxiety evident rapidly
Nortriptyline	Pamelor	Tricyclic	25 mg t.i.d. or q.i.d.; 150 mg max dose	18–24 h	Sedation and confusion	Avoid abrupt withdrawal of medication
Proptriptyline	Vivactil	Tricyclic	5–40 mg/d in divided doses; 60 mg/d max	67–89 h	Reported stroke and MI	Activating Make increases in dose in morning
Trimipramine	Surmontil	Tricyclic	100 mg/d in divided doses; may increase to 150 mg/d for maintenance	7–30 h	Confusion	Sedating

*It is urged that this class of medication be avoided in patients who have any cardiac involvement or impairment.

Box 34.1 Potential Adverse Effects of Medications with Anticholinergic Properties.

SERIOUS
Delirium
Vertigo
Respiratory problems or changes
Convulsions
Fever
Increased heart rate
Increased blood pressure
Visual impairment (eye pain, changes in acuity, blurriness, worsening of glaucoma)
Urinary retention
Mental status changes (cognitive decline, confusion or disorientation, hallucinations, memory loss, distress or excitement)

MINOR
Headache
Muscle weakness
Urinary hesitancy
Light sensitivity
Drowsiness
Digestive system changes (bloating, decreased bowel motility, constipation, ileus, nausea or vomiting, dry mouth or nose, dry mucus membranes)
Slurring of speech
Lethargy or fatigue
Dryness or flushing of skin
Decreased sweating

---

slowly, or changing to another antidepressant with less problematic side-effects. Patients taking TCAs frequently do not experience clinical effects for 2–6 weeks because of the secondary messaging system, so they require support and encouragement to get through this time of adjustment.

TCAs should be carefully distributed to suicidal patients, given the high risk and lethality of overdose. The most drastic consequence of this class of medications is the danger that they pose as lethal agents of suicide. Taken together, a 10-day supply of these medications may cause cardiac and cerebral toxicity. With patients beginning antidepressant medication therapy, a good rule of thumb is to limit the amount of medication prescribed at any one time. Moreover, patients beginning any antidepressant therapy should be carefully monitored because research indicates that risk for suicide increases when patients begin to "feel better" or energized.

When TCAs are given in conjunction with oral anticoagulants, patients may be at risk for bleeding. Administration with clonidine may cause severe hypertension. Although monoamine oxidase inhibitors and TCAs can be used together to successfully treat refractory depression, severe adverse reactions (including hyperpyretic crises and hypertensive episodes) may occur.

34.2.2 Selective reuptake inhibitors

These represent the newest class of drugs used to treat depression and anxiety disorders. They are sometimes called the second-generation antidepressants. These medications target the reuptake of serotonin only (SSRIs); dopamine, norepinephrine, or both (SRIs); or norepinephrine only (SNRIs). The medications in each class are structurally different, so people taking these medications will respond better to one than another. Table 34.2 includes these classes of medications.

SSRIs immediately block neuronal transport of serotonin. This blockage stimulates many postsynaptic receptor sites, which probably contributes to the side-effects associated with these

Table 34-2   Second-generation antidepressants

Generic Name	Brand Name	Available as Generic?	Type	Usual Dosing	Half-life	Comments, Cautions or Special Note
Bupropion	Wellbutrin, Wellbutrin XL	Yes	NDRI (NE DA-reuptake inhibitor)	225–450 mg in 3 divided doses XL 150–450 mg	20h +/– 5h Longer for ER: 33–37 h	Low incidence of sexual side-effects; Lowers the seizure threshold; Increased risk of seizures
Citalopram	Celexa	No	SSRI	20–60 mg/d	23–45 h	May increase BP
Desvenlafaxine	Pristiq	No	SNRI	50 mg/d	11 h	Remission rates lower than with others; Higher rates of discontinuation syndrome
Duloxetine	Cymbalta	No	SNRI	40–60 mg/d	12 h	Liver failure
Escitalopram	Lexapro	No	SSRI	10–20 mg/d	27–32 h	May increase BP; May be best tolerated of the SSRIs
Fluoxetine	Prozac, Prozac Weekly, Sarafem	Yes	SSRI	20–80 mg/d in morning	2–9 d	FDA approved for use in children
Fluvoxamine	Luvox, Luvox CR	Yes	SSRI	50–300 mg daily divided doses with larger dose at night	15 h	Not approved for use in depression
Mirtazapine	Remeron	Yes	Alpha-2 antagonist; dual 5-HT and NE agent	15–45 mg at night	20–40 h	High incidence of side-effects; Possible faster onset of action than others; Weight gain and may raise cholesterol
Nefazodone	Unavailable: manufacturer pulled from market in 2003	Yes	Serotoning-2 antagonist/reuptake inhibitor	200 mg/d in 2 divided doses; not to exceed 600 mg/d	2–3 d	Liver failure leading to liver transplant
Paroxetine	Paxil, Paxil CR, Pexeva	Yes	SSRI	20–50 mg/d	1 h	FDA warning; Diaphoresis; High incidence of sexual side-effects; Discontinuation syndrome

Sertraline	Zoloft	Yes	SSRI	50–200 mg/d	26 h	High rate of diahrrea
Trazodone	Desyrel	Yees	Serotoning-2A antagonist/reuptake inhibitor	150 mg daily at night; not to exceed 600 mg in divided doses	First phase 3–6 h; second phase 5–9 h	Not usually employed as antidepressant but as augmenting agent for insomnia associated with depression May cause priapism Sedating
Venlafaxine	Effexor, Effexor XR	Yes	SNRI	75–225 mg/d ER or divided doses	3–7 h	May cause EKG changes High rate of nausea and vomiting May increase BP and HR

drugs. Side-effects include nausea, vomiting, weight loss or gain, and delayed or impaired orgasm. These drugs also may cause agitation or restlessness.

Because these medications have a more tolerable side-effect profile, pose no risk for lethal overdose, and are effective in 70% of cases, they are now the first choice for treating depression. Unfortunately, many individuals complain that these drugs interfere with sexual performance, response, and arousal, a drawback that can affect medication compliance or adherence. The antidepressant response to SSRIs, like TCAs, may take 3–8 weeks. In some cases, a response takes as long as 3 months. Clinicians should explain carefully the need for an adequate medication trial to people beginning this drug therapy and engage family support which may be crucial for the patient who is suffering while waiting for a therapeutic response. They should also avoid ingestion of alcohol and should be counseled to check with their clinicians prior to starting any other medication, whether over the counter or prescription. Cigarette smoking decreases the effectiveness of this class of medications.

Side-effects of the antidepressants occur immediately and can be minimized by beginning with a subtherapeutic dose to improve initial tolerance according to some clinicians, while others opine that the starting dose is usually the same as the maintenance dose. Side-effects of this class of medication appear in Box 34.2.

Box 34.2 Side-Effects of Second-Generation Antidepressants.

SERIOUS
Drowsiness or confusion
Feelings of dread, panic or doom
Increase in suicidal ideation
Loss of libido, anorgasmia
Nervousness, agitation
Weight gain

MINOR OR SHORT-LIVED
Diarrhea
Vertigo
Dry mouth
Headache
Nausea
Sweating
Tremors

34.2.3 Monoamine oxidase inhibitors

The MAOIs are a class of drug that inhibit monamine oxidase A (MAO-A), an enzyme that breaks down amines epinephrine, norepinephrine, and serotonin (Table 34.3). As amines are hypothesized to be deficient in depression, it is thought that this inhibitory effect is responsible for the clinical efficacy of MAOIs as antidepressants. MAOIs are used to treat atypical forms of depression or are prescribed for patients who are unresponsive to other antidepressant regimens. Their use has been replaced largely by the SSRIs.

Side-effects of MAOIs include dizziness, vertigo, headache, overactivity, manic-like behavior, constipation, diarrhea, and nausea. In addition to breaking down amines, MAOIs breaks down tyramine, so *dietary restrictions* are necessary. The most serious risk of MAOI breakdown of tyramine involves hypertensive crises. Examples of foods that should be avoided include dairy products (especially aged cheese), meats (especially processed), and fish (dried, processed, or fermented). Beer, red wine, and certain fruits and vegetables (avocado, figs, raisins, and bananas) are other foods containing significant amounts of tyramine.

Table 34-3   Monoamine oxidase inhibitors

Generic Name	Brand Name	Type	Dosing	Half-life	Warnings	Comments
Phenelzine sulfate	Nardil	MAOI-A	15 mg t.i.d.; increase to at least 60 mg Some may require up to 90 mg	Unknown	Dietary restrictions	Energizing
Tranylcypromine	Parnate	MAOI-A	30 mg/d in divided doses, up to 60 mg/d if needed	Unknown	Dietary restrictions	Stimulating
Isocarboxazid	Marplan	MAOI-A	30–60 mg/d	Unknown	Dietary restrictions	Stimulating
Selegiline transdermal	EmSam	MAOI-B	6–12 mg patch changed daily, rotating sites	10 h	Possible rare cases of reactions with tyramine-containing substances; suggest dietary restrictions	Some patients report irritability

A recent edition to the MAOI armamentarium is the MAOI-B transdermal patch, selegiline, that bypasses the gut. When seligiline was introduced it was marketed as the "dietary-free MAOI," but there have been some rare reports of a kind of hypertensive crisis in some individuals that is hypothesized to have been tyramine-related.

34.2.4 A note on serotonin toxicity

Serotonin toxicity, also known as serotonin syndrome, is a potentially dangerous condition that develops when there is excess serotonergic activity at the central nervous system and peripheral serotonin receptors. This can happen as a result of therapeutic levels of serotonin agonists, inadvertent interactions between certain drugs, overdose of medications, or recreational use of drugs. A partial list of these is contained in Table 34.4. The website http://www.uspharmacist.com/content/t/psychotropic_disorders/c/11467/ contains more information on serotonin toxicity.

The excess serotonin activity results in a number of symptoms that may be mild and barely perceptible or intense and potentially fatal. There is no laboratory test for this condition. Diagnosis is

Table 34-4   Partial list of agents that can cause serotonin toxicity

Antidepressants	MAOIs, TCAs, SSRIs, SNRIs, Any Other Serotonergic Agents
Opiods	Hydrocodone, oxycodone, buprenorphine, meperedine, tramadol, fentanyl
CNS stimulants	Methylphenidte, amphetamines, cocaine, phenteramine, methamphetamine, diethylpropion
Psychdelics	MDMA, MDA, LSD
Herbs	St John's Wort, Syrian rue, panax ginseng, nutmeg
5-HT1 agonists	Triptans

made by history of drug or medication use and observation of the typical cognitive, autonomic, and somatic effects. Signs and symptoms of serotonin syndrome include tachycardia, hypertension, fever, sweating, shivering, confusion, anxiety, restlessness, disorientation, tremors, muscular spasms, and muscle rigidity. The principal differential diagnosis is neuroleptic malignant syndrome (NMS). Common symptoms are alteration of consciousness, diaphoresis, autonomic instability, hyperthermia and elevated creatine kinase levels, but NMS is observed most often following a rapid increase in dosage of a neuroleptic drug. It is crucial for clinicians to know what they are seeing clinically, so interventions are appropriate to the condition. For example, dopamine agonists, such as bromocriptine, are commonly used to treat NMS but may exacerbate the symptoms of serotonin syndrome. Other differentials to consider would be infectious causes, delirium tremens, heat stroke, or intoxication by adrenergic or anticholinergic agents.

If a patient develops serotonin syndrome, temporary withdrawal of serotonergic agents is necessary. Prescription of an antianxiety drug, such as diazepam or propranolol, is likely.

34.3 Mood stabilizers

The term "mood stabilizer" could be applied to any medication that is able to decrease vulnerability to subsequent episodes of mania or depression and not exacerbate the current episode or maintenance phase of treatment. Such a definition does not require absolute antidepressant or antimanic efficacy. The broad class of medications known as mood stabilizers are used primarily to treat bipolar disorders and impulse-control disorders. The predominant treatment of mania at present is lithium carbonate. The other categories of mood stabilizers include anticonvulsants. Owing to its importance in the psychopharmacology toolkit, lithium will be discussed in more depth than other psychotropics dealt with in this chapter.

34.3.1 Lithium

Lithium is an antipsychotic, antimanic medication used with affective disorders including bipolar disorder, bipolar depression, major depression (usually adjunctive), and mania. It is also used for the treatment of impulse-control disorders. Lithium medications may also go by the brand names Eskalith, Eskalith-Cr, Lithane, Lithium, Lithobid, Lithonate, and Lithotabs.

34.3.1.1 Pharmacology and mechanism of action

Lithium is an element of the alkali-metal group. Lithium's mechanism of action as an antimanic mood stabilizer may be related to its interaction with various neurotransmitter systems, much of which is beyond the scope of this text. Little is known about the effects of lithium on noradrenergic neurotransmission in manic individuals, although lithium administration has been reported to be associated with the decreased excretion of norepinephrine and its metabolites in manic patients while increasing this excretion in depressed patients. Lithium may exert antimanic effects via its ability to prevent dopamine receptor supersensitivity. However, just as with its reported effects of increasing acetylcholine synthesis and uptake, these changes in receptor sensitivity have been found to be associated with chronic, but not acute, lithium administration.

A growing body of research has begun to elucidate the complex effects of lithium on various cellular signal transduction pathways, beginning with initial direct targets of lithium, its second messenger roles, and ultimate effects on gene expression and cellular resilience. An established mechanism of lithium's antimanic properties has yet to be determined, although compound effects at different levels and pathways seems most likely. Again, most studies on the effects of lithium on signal transduction mechanisms have explored chronic lithium administration and resultant changes. Lithium has significant inhibitory effects on the cyclic adenosine monophosphate (cAMP)-generating system. Signal transduction may be stabilized by lithium via a balancing effect of increasing basal activity while inhibiting stimulated activity. Studies have suggested that the untreated manic patients may have raised myo-inositol and phosphomonoester (PME) concentrations and that lithium may be clinically effective owing to its normalizing actions on the phosphoinositol second messenger system. Lithium's numerous and varied effects ultimately are believed to alter gene expression and cellular resilience in patients with bipolar disorder.

34.3.1.2 Prescribing lithium

It generally takes 7–10 days to see an initial onset of improvement from lithium and 2–3 weeks of gradually increasing doses for a therapeutic level to develop. The drug has a significant side-effect profile that complicates long-term management (Table 34.5). These effects may be less apparent during acute treatment than during maintenance treatment.

Pretreatment procedures and testing are recommended before beginning therapy with lithium: general medical history, physical exam and weight, blood urea nitrogen and creatinine determination, thyroid function studies, and pregnancy testing for women of child-bearing age. Lithium carries a teratogenicity category D warning. Electrocardiography and complete blood count measurement should be obtained for patients over the age of 40. Some experts recommend more detailed screening to include fasting glucose determination and a dehydration test with vasopressin to determine renal concentrating capacity. Calculation of an estimated creatinine clearance may be more practical and serves to provide a baseline reference value for monitoring of potential renal problems.

In acute mania, lithium generally is prescribed at 600–900 mg three times a day. It is administered orally in slow-release form to produce serum levels between 1 and 1.5 mEq/L. Generally, 300 mg orally three to four times per day produces a serum level of 0.6–1.2 mEq/L. Therapeutic levels in acute mania range from 1 to 1.5 mEq/L. Therapeutic maintenance doses should range from 0.6 to 1.2 mEq/L. Regular serum levels must be drawn to ascertain correct dose. In early weeks of lithium administration, blood should be drawn twice each week before the patient takes the morning dose of the drug. Maintenance therapy requires that the clinician assess blood levels of lithium at least every 2 months.

Lithium has a very narrow therapeutic window, so monitoring for toxicity and educating patients is of utmost importance. Toxicity may be heralded by emergence or aggravation of any of the diverse effects in Table 34.5, progressing to include one or more other symptoms such as coarsening tremor, sluggishness, slurred speech, parkinsonism, hyperreflexia, myoclonic twitches, and mental status changes. Early recognition of toxicity is critical, as is investigation of its cause (Box 34.3). The

Table 34-5 Adverse effects of lithium	
System Affected	**Adverse Effect**
Cardiovascular	Bradycardia, syncope, AV block, EKG changes, sick-sinus syndromes
CNS	Mental dullness, headache, memory troubles, muscle weakness
Dermatologic	Acne, hair loss, psoriasis, skin reactions
Endocrine	Goiter, elevated TSH, hypothyroidism, hyperparathyroidism with hypocalcemia
Gastrointestinal	Nausea, GI pain/distress, vomiting, diarrhea, frequent loose stools
Hematologic	Leukocytosis
Metabolic	Weight gain
Neurologic	Postural tremor, confusion, ataxia
Opthalmic	Blurry vision, nystagmus, eye pain
Renal	Polydipsia, polyuria, reduced concentration capacity

Box 34.3 Some Causes of Lithium Toxicity.

- Excess dose
- Overdose
- Lab error, or less than 10–12 hours between last drug dose and blood sampling
- Increase in lithium absorption
    Diarrhea
    Vomiting
- Drug-interactions reducing renal clearance (NSAIDS, thiazides)
- Dehydration
    Fever/illness
    Hot weather/heat exhaustion
    Intense physical activity/profuse sweating
    Sauna/steam room
- Renal insufficiency or renal disease
- Sodium deficiency (low caloric or low-sodium diet)

possibility of drug interactions with lithium must always be considered, particularly with thiazide (and possibly loop) diuretics, angiotensin converting enzyme (ACE) inhibitors, nonsteroidal anti-inflamatory drugs, and other psychotropics.

34.3.2 Anticonvulsants

34.3.2.1 Overview

Anticonvulsants, or anti-epileptic drugs (AEDs) have been used successfully as mood stabilizers. It does not appear that a distinct class effect for AEDs in the management of bipolar disorder exists since not all anticonvulsants have been able to demonstrate efficacy for this mood disorder. The likely explanation for this variability for AEDs in bipolar disorder relates to the complex differences in the mechanisms of action for these drugs.

Multiple mechanisms of action have been proposed for AEDs as anticonvulsants, including glutamate receptor blockade, enhanced effects of gamma-amino-butyric-acid (GABA), sodium and/or calcium channel blockade, activation of potassium conductance, carbonic anhydrase inhibition, and synaptic vesicle protein modulation. Despite assumed primary modes of anticonvulsant action for any individual AED, each has a dissimilar profile in terms of possessing multiple distinct mechanisms that may confer anticonvulsant properties. These mixed effects may also potentially explain the differential effects among AEDs in terms of treating disordered mood states and why not all AEDs can effectively treat mania. Future exploration of pathophysiologic causes beyond simple catecholamine "imbalances" will better inform our understanding of how AEDs affect mood and direct focused AED drug development that may impact other proposed causes for mood disorders, such as defective G-proteins, altered second-messenger systems, mitochondrial disorders, and excessive methylation of DNA-histone proteins.

This section considers AEDs that may provide antimanic mood stabilization based on randomized, double-blind, placebo-controlled studies with adequate sample size. Other than divalproex and carbamazepine, other AEDs have not demonstrated strong enough evidence to qualify for inclusion although they have been used in clinical practice. Lamotrigine will be mentioned as it has been approved as a first-line treatment for bipolar depression.

34.3.2.2 Divalproex sodium/valproate

Divalproex sodium became the first anticonvulsant approved as a treatment for bipolar mania by the US Food and Drug Administration in 1995, after a large-scale, randomized, double-blind parallel-group study found divalproex equivalent to lithium in superiority over placebo for the management of acute mania. In this study, efficacy of divalproex appeared independent of prior responsiveness to lithium. Both active treatments demonstrated a nearly 50% response rate with monotherapy, while placebo response was only 25%. A new extended release preparation of divalproex received approval for acute manic or mixed episodes of bipolar disorder, with or without psychotic features. Divalproex is recommended as a first-line acute treatment option for mania in most evidence-based practice guidelines, either as monotherapy or in combination with antipsychotics for more severe manic episodes.

Factors associated with acute response to divalproex sodium/valproate are contained in Box 34.4.

Following oral administration of divalproex, its absolute bioavailability quickly approaches 100%; the extended release preparation bioavailability is closer to 90%. This suggests that a slightly higher dose of the ER form is needed in order to reach bioequivalence with the immediate-release preparation (8–20% higher dose for ER). Peak plasma concentrations are achieved within 3–5 hours, although up to 17 hours may be needed to reach peak concentration for the ER form. Mean terminal half-life is about 12–16 hours for either preparation, with steady-state conditions usually being achieved within 3–4 days. This AED is metabolized almost entirely by the liver.

Box 34.4 Factors Associated with Acute Response to Divalproex Sodium/Valproate.

- History of prior poor response to lithium
- Higher number of lifetime episodes of mania or depression
- Eight or more total lifetime episodes
- More than two prior major depressive episodes
  - Mania with depressive features
  - Presence of irritability
  - Atypical manic states
- Later age of illness onset
- Comorbid substance abuse
- Mania associated with neurologic or medical illness

Divalproex can be dosed with either an oral-loading or standard-titration strategy. For acute management of severely ill manic patients, divalproex oral-loading with a therapeutic starting dose of 20–30 mg/kg per day is suggested over standard, gradual titration schedules. Lower, divided doses are initially recommended (250 mg three times a day or 500 mg twice daily) for patients with less severe mania or in elderly patients.

Adverse effects seen during initial therapy with divalproex are usually mild, transient, and easily managed. Gastrointestinal distress and sedation are the most commonly seen side-effects during acute treatment, although other dose-related effects including tremor and benign hepatic transaminase elevations are occasionally encountered. Reduced dosage or slower upwards titration can be helpful, in addition to use of divalproex sodium formulation or ER divalproex instead of valproic acid may also lessen these side-effects. Tremor may be minimized through dose reduction or concomitant beta-blocker medication. During acute treatment with divalproex, clinicians should consider the possibility of rare but potentially serious adverse effects such as irreversible hepatic failure, hemorrhagic pancreatitis, or hyperammonemic encephalopathy when patients experience severe abdominal distress, confusion or delirium.

34.3.2.3 Carbamazepine

Carbamazepine is chemically related to the TCAs, with complex pharmacokinetic characteristics. It is the third most common drug used to treat mania following lithium and valproic acid. In the US, carbamazepine is FDA approved for use as an antiepileptic drug, and for the treatment of mania and mixed episodes of bipolar I disorder. It is also approved for use in controlling the pain of trigeminal neuralgia. Carbamazepine is particularly effective in moderating aggressive or hostile symptoms.

Carbamazepine is 80% bioavailable after oral administration. Nearly 80% is protein bound with the primary route of hepatic metabolism via the cytochrome 3A4 system to its active epoxide form. With initial administration of the extended-release form, half-life averages 35–40 hours, but with repeated administration this falls to 12–17 hours due to auto-induction. Inhibitors of the P450 system will increase carbamazepine levels while inducers can decrease levels.

There is no clear target serum level of carbamazepine for acute mania. Immediate-release carbamazepine therapy may be started at a total divided daily dose of 200–600 mg, with incremental increases of 200–1000 mg/day followed by careful monitoring of blood levels, side-effects, and clinical efficacy. The beaded, ER form may be started at 400 mg/day and increased as tolerated up to 1600 mg/day. Many factors can affect carbamazepine blood levels beyond direct dosing, including auto-induction of metabolism and significant drug interactions.

During acute treatment with carbamazepine, the most commonly observed side-effects are nausea, fatigue, blurred vision, and ataxia. More gradual initial titration of the dose may minimize these effects. Infrequently, liver transaminase elevations, rash, hyponatremia, and blood dyscrasias may complicate acute treatment.

34.3.3 Other mood stabilizing drugs

Lamotrigine is an AED that was approved for use in bipolar disorder I by the FDA in 2003 and is considered to be a first-line treatment and prophylaxis of bipolar depression. While the traditional AEDs are antimanics, lamotrigine is most effective in bipolar depression and lacks the manic, mixed cycling or rapid cycling inducing effects of other medications. The pharmacokinetics of lamotrigine are complex. Proposed mechanisms of action involve effects on sodium channels. The half-life and blood plasma levels are highly variable. Elimination half-life in healthy volunteers is approximately 33 hours after a single dose. It is metabolized through the liver.

Lamotrigine dosing for bipolar depression as a monotherapy is 25 mg/day for the first 2 weeks; at week 3 increase to 50 mg/day; at week 5 increase to 100 mg/day; and at week 6 increase to 200 mg/day (maximum dose). Such slow titration may reduce the incidence of skin rash. Lamotrigine may also be used as an adjunct to valproate, which inhibits its metabolism. Dosing is complex and involves increase in side-effects and possible adverse effects and should not be conducted by neophyte practitioners.

Lamotrigine has been black-boxed for Steven–Johnson syndrome, a life-threatening skin condition in which cell death causes the epidermis to separate from the dermis. Steven–Johnson syndrome usually begins with a fever, sore throat, and fatigue and is sometimes misdiagnosed and treated with antibiotics. Rashes and hyperpigmentation develop, as well as painful ulcers and lesions in the mucous membranes, almost always in the oral cavity affecting the mouth and lips, but theyc also can appear in the genital and anal region. It is a dermatologic emergency. Treatment involves removal of the offending cause (medication) and recovery may take many months.

KEY POINTS

- Antidepressants are medications used to treat mood disorders, as well as the anxiety disorders, and pain conditions.

- The antidepressant class of medications includes tricyclic antidepressants, selective serotonin-reuptake inhibitors, selective serotonin–norepinephrine inhibitors, monoamine oxidase inhibitors (MAOIs), and other atypical agents.

- MAOIs are rarely used as a first-line agent and their administration should be coupled with strict adherence to a tyramine-free diet.

- SSRIs are the treatment of choice for most of the anxiety disorders and obsessive–compulsive disorder.

- In depressive disorders, antidepressant medications are employed to alleviate symptoms such as dysphoric mood, changes in appetite and energy levels, anhedonia, feelings of hopelessness, suicidal ideation, concentration problems, among others.

- Serotonin syndrome is a potentially dangerous condition that develops when there is excess serotonergic activity at the central nervous system and peripheral serotonin receptors which can happen as a result of therapeutic levels of serotonin agonists, inadvertent interactions between certain drugs, overdose of medications, or recreational use of drugs.

- Anticonvulsants have been used successfully as mood stabilizers.

35 Antipsychotic Agents

35.1 Introduction

Antipsychotic medications are agents that are used to treat psychoses, such as that associated with schizophrenia or mania. They are used also for acute and chronic thought disorders and confusion, extreme aggressive behaviors, delirium, and dementia that accompanies conditions such as Alzheimer's disease. Target symptoms for these drugs include disorganized speech and behavior, flat or inappropriate affect, delusions, hallucinations, and catatonic behavior.

Antipsychotic medications are divided into (a) "typical" or first-generation antipsychotic (FGA) drugs, and (b) "atypical" or second-generation antipsychotic (SGA) drugs.

The first generation of antipsychotic medications was developed based on the hypothesis that schizophrenia reflects a disorder of excess dopaminergic activity and that antagonism of the dopamine D2 receptor is most strongly associated with antipsychotic response. For many patients with schizophrenia, the widely used FGAs (phenothiazines, butyrophenones, and others), which are also referred to as "conventional," "traditional," or "typical" antipsychotic drugs, are effective in the treatment of positive symptoms of the illness, and also in preventing psychotic relapse. Accordingly, these agents have permitted many patients to live independently in the community.

However, there are substantial limitations with the use of FGAs. Up to 60% of patients treated with FGAs remain symptomatic and are considered either treatment refractory or only partially responsive. In particular, at best, these drugs only modestly improve negative and cognitive symptoms. FGAs also cause a variety of objective and subjective side-effects, both acutely and with long-term exposure. These side-effects, in many instances, reduce treatment adherence, which leads to relapse and re-hospitalization.

The SGAs were heralded in the 1970s with the development of clozapine. Its advantages over the FGAs included greater efficacy for treatment-refractory schizophrenia, amelioration of some of the negative, cognitive, and mood symptoms of schizophrenia, potential reduction in the likelihood of suicidal behavior, very low liability for acute and chronic extrapyramidal symptoms, and no associated induction of sustained hyperprolactinemia. In the years that followed the introduction of clozapine, concerted research and development efforts were made to replicate the drug's therapeutic profile while avoiding the associated risk of agranulocytosis. Although this goal was never fully realized, the initiative spawned a second generation of atypical antipsychotic medications. Although none of these second-round agents have matched the singular effectiveness of clozapine, they have broadened the therapeutic repertoire available for the treatment of schizophrenia and other psychotic illnesses.

Fundamentals of Psychiatry, First Edition. Allan Tasman and Wanda K. Mohr.
© 2011 John Wiley & Sons, Ltd. Published 2011 by John Wiley & Sons, Ltd.
This chapter is based on Chapter 102 (Seiya Miyamoto, David B. Merrill, Jeffrey A. Lieberman, W. Wolfgang Fleischacker, Stephen R. Marder) of *Psychiatry, Third Edition*

35.2 Mechanism of action

The role of dopamine systems in the pathophysiology and treatment of psychotic disorders has been a subject of intense investigative scrutiny for the past 50 years. Although other systems have since been implicated, the dopamine D2 receptor is still regarded as the primary target associated with antipsychotic effect, as well as with the induction of extrapyramidal syndrome (EPS) and prolactin elevation. All clinically approved, currently used antipsychotic drugs share D2 receptor antagonism properties to some extent.

Differences among antipsychotics in dopamine receptor activity have been proposed to account for the "atypicality" of SGAs; that is, their tendency to produce antipsychotic effects at considerably lower doses than those that induce EPS. Another hypothesized mechanism of SGA atypicality involves regionally selective dopamine receptor binding.

35.3 First-generation antipsychotics

FGAs, as a class, are equally effective in the treatment of psychotic symptoms of schizophrenia, though they vary in potency, side-effect risks, and other pharmacologic properties (Table 35.1). Attributes common to all FGAs are a high affinity for, and full antagonist activity at, dopamine D2 receptors. In addition, all FGAs are capable of producing EPS and increasing serum prolactin concentration, to varying degrees, when used in the usual clinical dosage range. Based on their chemical structure, FGAs may be divided into three groups: butyrophenones, phenothiazines, and others. The butyrophenones, represented by haloperidol, tend to be potent D2 antagonists and to have minimal anticholinergic and autonomic effects. The phenothiazines block D2, acetylcholine, serotonin, histamine, and norepinephrine receptors, each of which is associated with certain adverse effects.

As a class, the FGAs are associated with a high degree of pseudoparkinsonism or EPS due to the blockade of the dopaminergic system, the movement disorder tardive dyskenesia, and a life-threatening condition, neuroleptic malignant syndrome (these are discussed later in the chapter). They may also have the same anticholinergic properties as TCAs, causing the same bothersome symptoms of dry mouth, constipation, blurred vision, and drowsiness.

35.4 Second-generation antipsychotics

The SGAs are a group of unrelated drugs united by the fact that they work differently from the FGAs. Most share a common attribute of working on serotonin as well as dopamine receptors. Amisulpride does not have serotonergic activity, but rather is a partial dopamine agonist. Aripiprazole also displays some partial dopamine agonism, 5-HT_{1A} partial agonism, and 5-HT_{2A} antagonism. In this chapter, SGAs refer to clozapine, risperidone, olanzapine, quetiapine, ziprasidone, sertindole, amisulpride, perospirone, zotepine, aripiprazole, paliperidone, iloperidone, and bifeprunox (Table 35.2).

35.5 Rapid neuroleptization

Rapid neuroleptization was proposed decades ago as a strategy for managing agitation in acutely psychotic patients. This practice involved the use of high doses of intramuscular high-potency FGAs, usually haloperidol, administered repeatedly over a 24-hour period, until the patient demonstrated obvious sedation or other effects. In the years after the introduction of rapid neuroleptization, a number of well-controlled, double-blind studies comparing high-dose strategies

Table 35-1   First-generation antipsychotics

Generic and Brand Names	Usual Dose	Half-life	Cautions	Adverse Effects	Relief of Target Symptom
Chlorpromazine (Thorazine)	200–800 mg/d	8–33 h	NMS	Priapism, seizures, jaundice agranulocytosis	Immediate relief of agitation; psychotic symptoms within 1 wk; several weeks for full effect on behavior
Fluphenazine (Prolixin)	1–20 mg/d maintenance IM generally 30–50% of above dose Decanoate: 12.5 mg/ 0.5 mL to 50 mg/2 mL	Oral formulation 15 h IM formulation 6.8–9.6 d	NMS	Priapism Akathesia	Full therapeutic effect may take 6 wk to 6 mo
Haloperidol (Haldol)	1–40 mg/d orally IM 2–5 mg per dose Decanoate injection 10–20 times the daily oral dose, repeated at 4-wk intervals	Oral 12–38 h Decanoate approximately 3 wk	NMS Cautious use in pts who have respiratory disorders, or Lewy-body dementia Do not use in Parkinson's	Pts with thyrotoxicosis may experience neurotoxicity May precipitate depression if used during manic episode	Immediate relief of symptoms with IM
Perphenazine (Trilafon)	12–24 mg/d in divided doses	9.5 h	NMS Same cautions as haloperidol Potential for weight gain	Same as Fluphenazine	Relief of psychotic symptoms seen within a week; therapeutic effect may take 6 wk or more
Thioridazine (Mellaril)	200–800 mg/d in divided doses	10 h	NMS Dose-dependent QTc prolongation; same as haloperidol Potential for weight gain	Pigmentary retinopathy	Same as Perphenazine
Thiothixene (Navane)	15–30 mg/d in divided doses	3.4 h	NMS Same cautions as haloperidol	Rare fine lenticular pigmentation	Same as Perphenazine
Trifluoperazine (Stelazine)	15–20 mg/d	12.5 h	NMS Same cautions as haloperidol	Rare seizures	Same as Perphenazine

Table 35-2 Second-generation antipsychotics

Generic and Brand Names	Usual Dose	Half-life	Cautions	Adverse Effects/comments	Relief of Target Symptom
Amisulpride (Solian)	400–800 mg/d in divided doses For negative symptoms only: 50–300 mg/d	12 h	Not approved by the US FDA but is used in Europe May increase QTc interval if given with other medications capable of QTc prolongation	Insomnia, anxiety, agitation, weight gain	Psychotic symptoms may improve within 1 wk but full behavioral effects may take up to 20 wk to show good response
Aripiprazole (Abilify)	15–30 mg/d	75–94 h	NMS	Dizziness, insomnia, akathesia, activation	Psychotic symptoms may improve within 1 wk but full behavioral effects may take up to 16–20 wk to show good response
Bifeprunox	20 mg/d	14 h	N/A	In Stage III trials at this writing	N/A
Clozapine (Clozaril)	25 mg twice daily gradually increasing to 450 mg/d Maximum of 900 mg may be given	5–16 h	Agranulocytosis (requires monthly WBC testing) NMS Pulmonary embolus	Sedation, weight gain, drooling seizures	Same as Aripiprazole
Iloperidone (Fanapta)	5 mg/d	18–33 h	NMS	Hypotension, dizziness, somnolence	N/A
Olanzapine (Zyprexa)	10–20 mg/d orally or IM	21–54 h	NMS Life-threatening diabetic ketoacidosis	Sedation, weight gain	Same as Aripiprazole
Paliperidone (Invega)	3–16 mg/d	23 h	NMS Life-threatening diabetic ketoacidosis	Modest increase in QTc interval	Same as Aripiprazole

Drug	Dose	Half-life	Serious adverse effects	Side effects / comments	Notes
Quetiapine (Seroquel, Seroquel SR)	150–750 mg/d in 2 divided doses for schizophrenia; 400–800 mg/d in 2 divided doses for acute bipolar mania	6–7 h	NMS; Life-threatening diabetic ketoacidosis	Weight gain; Somnolence	Same as Aripiprazole
Risperidone (Risperdal, Consta)	4–8 mg/d up to maximum of 16 mg/d; Depot injections 25–50 mg every 2 wk	30 h	NMS; Life threatening diabetic ketoacidosis	Insomnia, agiation	Same as Aripiprazole
Ziprasidone (Geodon)	40–200 mg/d in divided doses for schizophrenia; 80–160 mg/d in divided doses for bipolar disorder; 10–20 mg IM every 2 h as required for maximum dose of 40 mg	6 h	NMS; Life-threatening diabetic ketoacidosis	Highly sedating; Take with food for maximum bioavailability	Same as Aripiprazole; IM formulation can reduce agitation in 15 min
Sertindole (Serdolect, Serlect)	20 mg/d	3 d	May cause dose-dependent QTc prolongation	Recommended for US FDA approval; Available in Europe; ECG monitoring recommended	N/A
Perospirone (Lullan)	8–48 mg/d in 3 divided doses	N/A	Rare NMS	EPS, akathesia, insomnia; Sedation	Same as Aripiprazole
Zotepine (Nipolept, Lodopin, setous)	50–300 mg/d; Maximum of 450 mg/d	12–30 h	NMS	Weight gain; Not FDA approved but used in Europe	N/A

with standard-dosage regimens revealed no significant superiority for high dosage in either degree or rapidity of response in acutely psychotic patients. Moreover, very high doses of FGAs produced a significantly greater incidence of extrapyramidal symptoms, particularly akathisia and akinesia, which can cause significant discomfort and worsen outcome. Thus, rapid neuroleptization has been largely abandoned as a therapeutic strategy.

35.6 Conditions treated with antipsychotic medications

At present, SGAs are prescribed primarily for schizophrenia; however, they are being used increasingly for other psychiatric disorders, as happened with FGAs. A proportion of these uses are empirically well supported, but only preliminary or moderate evidence exists for others. In particular, the prescription of SGAs for nonpsychotic disorders in children and adolescents has become progressively more common, despite limited data regarding the efficacy and safety of this practice.

In common practice, conditions that are treated with antipsychotic medications include adult and childhood schizophrenia, schizoaffective disorder, major depression with psychotic features, bipolar disorder, borderline personality disorder, Tourette's disorder, substance-abuse disorder, delirium, impulse control associated with aggression and violent behavior in youth, dementia, and Huntington's disease.

35.7 Adverse effects of antipsychotics

35.7.1 Neuroleptic malignant syndrome

The most serious and potentially fatal side-effect of the antipsychotic medications is neuroleptic malignant syndrome (NMS), which is characterized by severe muscular rigidity, altered consciousness, disorientation, dysphagia, elevated creatine phosphokinase, stupor, catatonia, hyperpyrexia, and labile pulse and blood pressure. This life-threatening condition can occur after a single dose of a neuroleptic drug, but it is more common during the first two weeks of administration or with an increase in dose. This syndrome can continue for up to two weeks after the discontinuation of medication. Treatment involves immediate cessation of the medication and hospitalization to stabilize acute symptoms.

35.7.2 Tardive dyskenesia

Tardive dyskinesia (TD) is the most serious side-effect of long-term use of these medications because of its often irreversible and severely disabling symptoms, which include involuntary choreoathetotic movements affecting the face, tongue, and perioral, buccal and masticatory muscles. TD also may involve the neck, torso, and extremities. The risk of developing irreversible TD increases with cumulative dose and duration of treatment. Fine wormlike movements of the tongue may be the first signs of TD; discontinuing the medication when this occurs may prevent development of the full-blown syndrome. Whereas decreasing or discontinuing neuroleptic medication is the best treatment for TD, it also can precipitate the development of withdrawal dyskinesia. These symptoms are the same as those of TD, but they tend to resolve within a few weeks. The risk of TD appears to be lower with the SGAs but it has still been reported.

The cause of tardive dyskinesia appears to be related to damage to the dopaminergic system. The most compelling line of evidence suggests that it may result primarily from neuroleptic-induced dopamine supersensitivity in the nigrostiatal pathway with the D2 dopamine receptor being most affected.

Primary prevention of this condition is using the lowest dose of antipsychotic medication for the shortest period of time. This may not always be possible.

35.7.3 Extrapyramidal symptoms

Antipsychotic-induced EPS can occur acutely or after chronic treatment, and all antipsychotic medications are implicated. In general, this liability is more pronounced with FGAs than with SGAs. Among FGAs, agents that possess a high potency with respect to the D2 receptor, such as haloperidol and fluphenazine, carry the highest risk of EPS.

Acute EPS typically develops within hours to weeks of antipsychotic initiation. These movement disorders are dose-dependent and almost always reversible, remitting after the offending agent is discontinued. It has been estimated that more than 60% of patients who receive acute treatment with FGAs develop some form of clinically significant EPS. The increasing use of SGAs is believed to have substantially reduced the burden of acute EPS. Medication-induced parkinsonism is the most common form of EPS caused by FGAs. The disorder usually occurs within days to weeks of antipsychotic treatment initiation, and is characterized by rigidity, tremor, and bradykinesia. Care should be taken to distinguish these patients from those with depression, catatonia, or the negative symptoms of schizophrenia. Medication-induced parkinsonism occurs most commonly with high-potency antipsychotics, especially when anticholinergic medication is not administered concurrently. Other risk factors include older age, higher dose, a history of parkinsonism, and underlying basal ganglia damage.

Dystonia presents as sustained muscular contraction, with contorting, twisting, or abnormal posturing affecting mainly the muscles of the head and neck, but sometimes the trunk or extremities. It tends to be sudden in onset, with 90% of cases occurring in the first 3 days of antipsychotic treatment. Dystonia is often dramatic in presentation and may be extremely disturbing for patients. Laryngeal dystonia is potentially fatal, as it may compromise the airway. Risk factors for acute dystonias include a history of prior dystonia, young age, male gender, use of high-potency antipsychotic agents, higher dose, and IM administration. Mid- and low-potency FGAs pose less risk.

Akathisia is characterized by both subjective and objective somatic restlessness. Patients with akathisia typically experience an inner sensation of restlessness or an irresistible urge to move various parts of their bodies. The disorder appears objectively as psychomotor agitation, such as continuous pacing, rocking from foot to foot, or the inability to sit still. *It is far too often misconstrued as agitation by inexperienced or unknowledgeable staff members, resulting in patients having their antipsychotic dose increased, thereby intensifying the condition.* Clinicians should be on guard against jumping to a conclusion that a patient is agitated if he appears agitated and is being treated by antipsychotics. Akathisia usually begins within hours to days of antipsychotic administration and can occur in as many as 25% of patients treated with FGAs. It can be extremely distressing for patients and may contribute to medication nonadherence or self-injurious behavior.

Patients should be monitored for EPS at weekly intervals during antipsychotic initiation and until their medication dose has been stable for at least 2 weeks. The treatment of acute EPS depends on the specific side-effect. The initial treatment of parkinsonism is to lower the antipsychotic dose, since doses above the EPS threshold are unlikely to yield additional clinical benefit. If symptoms persist, switching to an antipsychotic associated with fewer extrapyramidal symptoms should be considered. Alternatively, adding an anticholinergic agent or dopaminergic medication (e.g., amantadine) may be efficacious, though these drugs carry their own risk of adverse effects and so should be used sparingly. Acute dystonia responds rapidly to treatment with an anticholinergic (e.g., benztropine) or an antihistaminergic agent (e.g., diphenhydramine), especially when administered parenterally. Oral anticholinergic medication should then be continued for a few days to prevent dystonia recurrence. Initial treatment options for akathisia include lowering the antipsychotic dose, or switching to an antipsychotic agent with a lower risk of akathisia. If symptoms persist, or if psychotic symptoms necessitate a higher antipsychotic dose, individual trials of beta-adrenergic antagonists (e.g., 30–90 mg/day of propranolol) or benzodiazepines may be prescribed.

35.7.4 Endocrine and sexual effects

All FGAs can elevate serum prolactin levels by antagonizing the tonic inhibitory actions of dopamine on lactotrophic cells in the pituitary. Among SGAs, risperidone and amisulpride can increase serum prolactin levels to an extent comparable to FGAs, with the others causing less incidence of these side-effects.

Women experience, on average, significantly greater elevation in prolactin than do men during long-term treatment with the same antipsychotic dose. Hyperprolactinemia may manifest differently in men and women, and there is great individual variation in the prolactin level at which symptoms appear. In women, prolactin elevation often leads to menstrual disturbances, including anovulatory cycles and infertility, menses with abnormal luteal phases, or frank amenorrhea and hypoestrogenemia. Women may also experience decreased libido, impaired arousal, anorgasmia, and eventually osteoporosis.

35.7.5 Weight gain and obesity

Obesity can negatively affect self-image, impair social adjustment, and reduce medication compliance. Furthermore, it can have serious deleterious effects on health and life expectancy via a number of disease processes, including hypertension, coronary artery disease, osteoarthritis, diabetes, stroke, sleep apnea, and certain cancers. About 50% of all people with schizophrenia meet criteria for obesity, representing a relative risk of nearly $2:1$ when compared with the general population. Genetic and lifestyle factors may contribute to this phenomenon, but in large measure antipsychotic-induced weight gain is responsible. Recognizing the considerable potential for obesity to impact negatively on morbidity and mortality, expert consensus guidelines recommend frequent monitoring of body mass index in patients taking antipsychotics.

35.7.6 Diabetes

The prevalence of type II diabetes is twice as high among patients with schizophrenia as in the general population, placing these patients at increased risk of coronary artery disease, stroke, peripheral vascular disease, retinopathy, nephropathy, neuropathy, and ketoacidosis. Data are rapidly accumulating that indicate that some SGAs increase this burden.

35.7.7 Dyslipidemia

Elevated lipid levels, particularly low-density lipoprotein and triglyceride, are associated with coronary artery disease and myocardial infarction. Clozapine and olanzapine increase total cholesterol, low-density lipoprotein, and triglyceride levels significantly, as compared with FGAs and other SGAs. Quetiapine and risperidone appear to raise cholesterol levels modestly, whereas ziprasidone and aripiprazole are cholesterol neutral.

35.7.8 Metabolic syndrome

Metabolic syndrome is a common condition in people with schizophrenia and may be mediated by medication, especially SGAs. The syndrome is defined by three or more of the following criteria: abdominal obesity (waist circumference $\geq$35 inches for women or $\geq$40 inches for men); elevated fasting triglycerides ($\geq$150 mg/dL); decreased high-density lipoprotein (<40 mg/dL for men or <50 mg/dL for women); hypertension ($\geq$130/85 mmHg or on antihypertensive medication); and elevated fasting glucose ($\geq$100 mg/dL or on diabetes medication). Patients with this constellation of conditions may be at even greater risk of cardiovascular disease than those with isolated obesity, type II diabetes, or dyslipidemia.

35.7.9 Cardiovascular effects

In addition to coronary artery disease, common cardiovascular effects of antipsychotic agents include orthostatic hypotension, sinus tachycardia, and ECG changes. Abnormalities in cardiac electrophysiology, as reflected in ECG changes, have been observed with most antipsychotic agents. Baseline ECG and yearly monitoring should be standard practice in the comprehensive assessment of patients taking antipsychotic medications.

35.7.10 Gastrointestinal effects

The anticholinergic effects of antipsychotic medications include dry mouth (xerostomia) and constipation. These are relatively commonly encountered with clozapine and low-potency FGAs, and less often with olanzapine and quetiapine. Because they are frequently dose-related, constipation and xerostomia may improve with antipsychotic dose reduction. Elderly patients are particularly susceptible to anticholinergic effects, owing to reduced cholinergic function.

35.7.11 Hepatic effects

Asymptomatic elevations of liver enzyme levels occur with both FGAs and SGAs, usually during the first 3 months of treatment. These abnormalities may be present in more than 20% of patients treated with some antipsychotics, though the relative liabilities of individual agents to cause liver enzyme elevations have yet to be elucidated. More severe antipsychotic-induced hepatic effects are rare. Patients taking an antipsychotic medication who develop nausea, abdominal pain, and jaundice should have their liver function evaluated to exclude hepatotoxicity. Since antipsychotic-induced jaundice is infrequent, other etiologies should be ruled out before the cause is judged to be antipsychotic treatment.

35.7.12 Hematologic effects

Antipsychotic medications may cause blood dyscrasias, including leukopenia, neutropenia, agranulocytosis, and eosinophilia. Clozapine-induced agranulocytosis (defined as an absolute neutrophil count less than 500/mm^3) is a much less common, but potentially fatal, adverse effect. Early agranulocytosis-related fatalities led to the withdrawal of clozapine in some European countries and severe restrictions on its use in others. With the advent of mandatory, systematic blood count monitoring, the reported rate of clozapine-induced agranulocytosis has fallen below 0.4% in the US. Fewer than 2% of these cases now result in mortality, in part because clozapine-induced agranulocytosis is usually reversible if the drug is withdrawn immediately.

35.7.13 Ocular effects

Cataracts are ocular lens opacities that can impair vision. The low-potency FGAs chlorpromazine and thioridazine increase the risk of this condition, especially when used at high doses. There is debate as to whether quetiapine also produces a higher incidence of cataracts. Any vision changes in patients should be cause for ophthalmic consultation.

35.7.14 Other side-effects

Sedation can occur with virtually any antipsychotic, but is particularly common with low-potency FGAs and the SGAs clozapine, olanzapine, quetiapine, and zotepine. This effect is typically most pronounced during dose titration, as the majority of patients develop some tolerance with continued antipsychotic administration.

Antipsychotic medications, in particular clozapine and low-potency FGAs, can lower the seizure threshold in a dose-dependent fashion. Because the seizure rate rises with rapid dose increases, clozapine should be titrated gradually.

Finally, medication cost may be regarded as a kind of adverse effect, present in varying degrees with all antipsychotic treatment, and frequently burdening the healthcare system more than individual patients. Antipsychotic costs can be substantial, especially for SGAs, which may be up to 100-fold more expensive than generic forms of some FGAs.

35.8 The CATIE and CUtLASS studies

The Clinical Antipsychotic Trials of Intervention Effectiveness (CATIE) conducted in the US and the Cost Utility of the Latest Antipsychotic Drugs in Schizophrenia Study (CUtLASS 1) conducted in the UK are important steps in developing a comprehensive understanding of the comparative effects of medications in the treatment of schizophrenia. These two large, noncommercial clinical trials compared first- and second-generation antipsychotic drugs for people with chronic schizophrenia. It is beyond the scope of this chapter to discuss the details of these studies, but they and others have independently demonstrated that SGAs are not necessarily the therapeutic breakthrough they were once hoped, and briefly believed, to be. Rather, SGAs represent an incremental advance in antipsychotic pharmacotherapy, with pharmacologic properties and side-effect profiles that are somewhat different from those of FGAs. The one possible exception is clozapine, which has been found to be the most effective antipsychotic drug in virtually every study in which it has been used. However, more than 30 years after its discovery, we still do not know the pharmacologic basis of clozapine's superiority, or even whether it is qualitatively or quantitatively different fom other antipsychotic drugs.

35.9 Antipsychotics and the elderly patient

In 2005, the US Food and Drug Administration issued a public health advisory to alert healthcare providers, patients, and patient caregivers to safety information concerning an unapproved (off-label) use of SGAs in elderly patients with dementia, warning that these medications have shown a higher death rate associated with their use compared to patients receiving a placebo. In analyses of 17 placebo-controlled studies of four drugs in this class, the rate of death for those elderly patients with dementia was about 1.6–1.7 times that of placebo. Although the causes of death were varied, most seemed to be either heart-related (such as heart failure or sudden death) or from infections (pneumonia). The FDA advisory applied to such antipsychotic drugs as Abilify (aripiprazole), Zyprexa (olanzapine), Seroquel (quetiapine), Risperdal (risperidone), Clozaril (clozapine), and Geodon (ziprasidone). Symbyax, which is approved for treatment of depressive episodes associated with bipolar disorder, was also included in the agency's advisory.

The FDA ordered that the manufacturers of all of this class of drugs add a boxed warning to their drug labeling describing this risk and noting that these drugs are not approved for the treatment of behavioral symptoms in elderly patients with dementia.

KEY POINTS

- Antipsychotic medications are agents that are used to treat psychoses, such as that associated with schizophrenia or mania.

- First-generation antipsychotics are effective in the treatment of positive symptoms of the illness, and in preventing psychotic relapse, but have substantial side-effects.

- Second-generation antipsychotics have advantages that include greater efficacy for treatment-refractory schizophrenia, amelioration of some of the negative, cognitive, and mood symptoms of schizophrenia, and potential reduction in the likelihood of suicidal behavior.

- SGAs have very low liability for acute and chronic extrapyramidal symptoms, and no associated induction of sustained hyperprolactinemia.

- SGAs have the potential to induce metabolic syndrome. This is characterized by abdominal obesity, elevated fasting triglycerides, decreased high-density lipoprotein, hypertension, and elevated fasting glucose. Patients with this constellation of conditions may be at increased risk of cardiovascular disease.

- Other side-effects of antipsychotic medications include cardiovascular, extrapyramidal, ocular, hematologic, hepatic, gastrointestinal, sexual, and weight gain.

- The most serious and potentially fatal side-effect of the antipsychotic medications is neuroleptic malignant syndrome, although it is relatively uncommon.

- CATIE and other similar studies have independently demonstrated that SGAs are not necessarily the therapeutic breakthrough they were once hoped to be.

- Study of SGA use in elderly patients with dementia suggest that these medications have shown a higher death rate associated with their use compared to patients receiving a placebo.

Further Reading

American Diabetes Association, American Psychiatric Association, American Association of Clinical Endocrinologists *et al.* (2004) Consensus development conference on antipsychotic drugs and obesity and diabetes. Diabetes Care, **27**, 596–601.

American Psychiatric Association (2004) *Practice Guideline for the Treatment of Patients with Schizophrenia*, 2nd edn, American Psychiatric Publishing, Washington, DC, pp. 1–184.

Lieberman, J.A. (2006) Comparative effectiveness of antipsychotic drugs: a commentary on "cost utility of the latest antipsychotic drugs in schizophrenia" study (CUtLASS 1) and "clinical antipsychotic trials of intervention effectiveness" (CATIE). *Archives of General Psychiatry*, **63**, 1069–1072.

Lieberman, J.A., Stroup, S., McEvoy, J.P. *et al.* (2005) Effectiveness of antipsychotic drugs in patients with chronic schizophrenia. *New England Journal of Medicine*, **353**, 1209–1223.

36 ● ● ● Anxiolytics, Stimulants, and Cognitive Enhancers

36.1 Anxiolytics

36.1.1 Introduction

The major advancement in the field of anxiolytics in the 1960s was the development and approval of benzodiazepines. These agents were much safer than what had been used until then, had a rapid onset of action (so patients felt better quickly), and had a broad spectrum of efficacy extending from situational anxiety to pathologic anxiety disorders. Many different benzodiazepines, with different absorption times and half-lives, were developed and have been valuable not only for treating anxiety and anxiety disorders but for treating seizure disorders and alcohol withdrawal.

36.1.2 Uses of anxiolytics

Anxiolytic or antianxiety medications are used to treat generalized anxiety disorder and may provide relief for acute anxiety states, social phobia, performance anxiety, and simple phobias. They are used also for short-term relief of insomnia. Anxiolytic medications include the antidepressants, the azopyrones, the benzodiazepines, and beta-blockers. There is research currently being conducted on the use of the antiepileptic medications for the treatment of anxiety as well.

36.1.3 Benzodiazepines

The benzodiazepines as a class work by increasing the relative efficiency of the gamma-amino-butyric acid (GABA) receptor when stimulated by GABA. The benzadiazepines as a group have different affinities for GABA receptors; in fact some agents bind to only one of the two types of GABA receptor.

The pharmacologic effects of the benzodiazepines include anxiolysis, sedation, centrally mediated muscle relaxation, and elevation of the seizure threshold. Benzodiazepines are safe and effective, and their adverse side-effects are extensions of their central actions. They may be excessively sedating. Concurrent use with narcotics or alcohol can potentiate the effects of benzodiazepines. In addition to these effects benzodiazepines can stimulate a mild paradoxical excitatory reaction at the beginning of treatment. Table 36.1 provides a current list of benzodiazepines.

Fundamentals of Psychiatry, First Edition. Allan Tasman and Wanda K. Mohr.
© 2011 John Wiley & Sons, Ltd. Published 2011 by John Wiley & Sons, Ltd.
This chapter is based on Chapter 104 (Deidre M. Edwards, Kathryn L. Hale, Rachel E. Maddux, Mark Hyman Rapaport) of *Psychiatry, Third Edition*

Table 36-1   Benzodiazepines

	Half-life [of Active Metabolite]	Approximately Equivalent Oral Dosages	Market Aim[a]
Benzodiazepines			
Alprazolam (Xanax)	6–12 h	0.5 mg	Anxiolytic
Bromazepam (Lexotan)	10–20 h	5–6 mg	Anxiolytic
Chlordiazepoxide (Librium)	5–30 [36–200] h	25 mg	Anxiolytic
Clobazam (Frisium)[b]	12–60 h	20 mg	Anxiolytic Anticonvulsant
Clonazepam (Klonopin, Rivotril)[b]	18–50 h	0.5 mg	Anxiolytic Anticonvulsant
Clorazepate (Tranxene)	[36–200] h	15 mg	Anxiolytic
Diazepam (Valium)	20–100 [36–200] h	10 mg	Anxiolytic
Estazolam (ProSom)	10–24 h	1–2 mg	Hypnotic
Flunitrazepam (Rohypnol)	18–26 [36–200] h	1 mg	Hypnotic
Flurazepam (Dalmane)	[40–250] h	15–30 mg	Hypnotic
Halazepam (Paxipam)	[30–100] h	20 mg	Anxiolytic
Ketazolam (Anxon)	30–100 [36–200] h	15–30 mg	Anxiolytic
Loprazolam (Dormonoct)	6–12 h	1–2 mg	Hypnotic
Lorazepam (Ativan)	10–20 h	1 mg	Anxiolytic
Lormetazepam (Noctamid)	10–12 h	1–2 mg	Hypnotic
Medazepam (Nobrium)	36–200 h	10 mg	Anxiolytic
Nitrazepam (Mogadon)	15–38 h	10 mg	Hypnotic
Oxazepam (Serax, Serenid D)	4–15 h	20 mg	Anxiolytic
Prazepam (Centrax)	[36–200] h	10–20 mg	Anxiolytic
Quazepam (Doral)	25–100 h	20 mg	Hypnotic
Temazepam (Restoril, Normison, Euhypnos)	8–22 h	20 mg	Hypnotic
Triazolam (Halcion)	2 h	0.5 mg	Hypnotic
"Non-benzodiazepines with similar effects[c]			
Zaleplon (Sonata)	2 h	20 mg	Hypnotic
Zolpidem (Ambien, Stilnoct)	2 h	20 mg	Hypnotic
Zopiclone (Zimovane, Imovane)	5–6 h	15 mg	Hypnotic
Eszopiclone (Lunesta)	6–9 h	3 mg	Hypnotic

[a] Market aim: Although all benzodiazepines have similar actions, they are usually marketed as anxiolytics, hypnotics or anticonvulsants.

[b] In the UK, clobazam (Frisium) and clonazepam (Rivotril) are licenced for use as antiepileptics only.

[c] These drugs are chemically different from benzodiazepines but have the same effects on the body and act by the same mechanisms.

As a class, benzadiazepines are efficacious for the treatment of PD, SAD, GAD, alcohol withdrawal, and situational anxiety. Although OCD falls within the taxonomy of anxiety disorders, benzodiazepines do not seem to be particularly effective in treating these patients.

Benzodiazepines have the potential to lose their efficacy. Patients may begin increasing their dose to achieve the previous response and this may lead to dependence problems.

Benzodiazepines should be used cautiously with older adults, debilitated patients, depressed or suicidal clients, and those with a history of substance abuse. Withdrawal syndrome is possible on discontinuation of the medication and is most common with high dosesused for more than 4 months. Withdrawal symptoms include anxiety, irritability, tremulousness, sweating, lethargy, diarrhea, insomnia, depression, abdominal and muscle cramps, vomiting, and, at its most severe, convulsions. Benzodiazepines should be discontinued gradually with careful monitoring of symptoms during the process. Onset of symptoms related to withdrawal or discontinuation generally reflects the half-life of the medication (1–2 days for short-acting drugs and 2–5 days for longer-acting drugs). Withdrawal symptoms, however, have been known to occur as late as 7–10 days after discontinuation. Symptoms generally peak several days after onset and disappear slowly over 1–3 weeks. Patients must be cautioned not to abruptly discontinue taking these medications.

36.1.4 Buspirone

Buspirone is a member of the group of agents called azaspirodecanediones. It is believed to exert its anxiolytic effect by acting as a partial agonist at the 5-HT$_{1A}$ autoreceptor. Stimulation of the 5-HT$_{1A}$ autoreceptor causes a decreased release of serotonin into the synaptic cleft. It usually takes approximately 4 weeks for the benefit of buspirone therapy to be noticed in patients with GAD. It has not been found to be effective in other anxiety disorders. One major advantage of buspirone is that it does not cross-react with benzodiazepines. The most common side-effects associated with buspirone include dizziness, gastrointestinal distress, headache, numbness, and tingling. Buspirone is contraindicated in patients with marked renal or liver impairment and in lactating women.

Buspirone generally is administered orally in tablet form. Adults usually begin with 15 mg/day in three divided doses. Increases of 5 mg/day are made every 2–3 days, with the maximum dose not to exceed 60 mg daily.

36.1.5 Beta-blockers

Beta-adrenergic blockers competitively antagonize norepinephrine and epinephrine at the beta-adrenergic receptor. It is thought that the majority of positive effects of beta-blockers are due to their peripheral actions. Beta-blockers can decrease many of the peripheral manifestations of anxiety such as tachycardia, diaphoresis, trembling, and blushing. The advent of more selective beta-blockers that block only the beta$_2$-adrenergic receptor has been beneficial since blockade of beta$_1$-adrenergic receptors can be associated with bronchospasm. Beta-blockers may be useful for individuals who have situational anxiety or performance anxiety. They generally have not been effective in treating anxiety disorders such as generalized SAD, PD, or OCD.

36.2 Psychostimulants

36.2.1 Introduction

Psychostimulants are a class of drugs commonly used to treat disruptive behavior disorders, most often attention-deficit hyperactivity disorder. Amphetamines and methylphenidate (MPH), and magnesium pemoline (PEM), are two groups of stimulants that received US Food and Drug Administration approval for ADHD treatment in the pediatric population. They are available in both branded and generic formulations, as well as in long- and short-duration (immediate-release) preparations (Table 36.2).

In the past decade or so there has been a flurry of new stimulant drug approvals by the FDA for pediatric ADHD treatment. Previously, only dextroamphetamine (DEX), MPH, and PEM were sanctioned for use in children. More recently, osmotic-release methylphenidate (OROSMPH), beaded methylphenidate (B-MPH), dexmethylphenidate, long-duration mixed salts of amphetamine (MAS), and several other formulations have been approved. Both DEX and MPH form the active ingredients of these new preparations. Structurally, they are related to the catecholamines, dopamine, and norepinephrine.

The term "psychostimulant" used for these compounds refers to their ability to increase CNS activity in some, but not all, brain regions. As demonstrated by more than 200 placebo-controlled investigations, psychostimulants are highly effective in reducing core symptoms of childhood

Table 36-2 Psychostimulants[*]

Medication	Initial Pediatric Dose	Pediatric Dosage Range and Maximum Dose[a]	Common Pediatric Dose[a]	Preparations
Methylphenidate immediate release (IR) (Ritalin, Methylin, generic)	2.5–5 mg orally	0.1–0.8 mg/kg per dose q.i.d. to 5 times daily Maximum 60 mg/d	0.3–0.5 mg/kg per dose t.i.d./q.i.d.	All preparations available as 5-mg, 10-mg, or 20-mg scored tabs; Methylin also available as 2.5-mg, 5-mg, or 10-mg chewable tab and PO solution
Methylphenidate sustained-release (SR) (Ritalin LA, Metadate CD)	Convert from IR or use 10 mg	0.2–1.4 mg/kg per dose/ dose PO q.i.d/t.i.d. Maximum 60 mg/d	0.6–1 mg/kg per dose PO q.i.d./b.i.d.	10-mg, 20-mg, 30-mg, or 40-mg tabs (Metadate also has 50-mg and 60-mg tabs.) Can be sprinkled into soft food (do not cut, crush, or chew)
Methylphenidate extended release (ER)[c] (Ritalin SR, Methylin ER, Metadate ER, generic SR)	Convert from IR.	0.2–1.4 mg/kg per dose PO q.i.d./t.i.d. Maximum 60 mg/d	0.6–1 mg/kg per dose PO q.i.d./b.i.d.	20-mg Spansules (do not cut, crush, or chew)
Methylphenidate OROS tablets (Concerta)	Convert from IR or use 18 mg	0.3–2 mg/kg PO q.i.d. Maximum 54 mg/d	0.8–1.6 mg/kg PO q.i.d.	18-mg, 27-mg, 36-mg, and 54-mg tabs (do not cut, crush, or chew)
Methylphenidate transdermal patch (Daytrana)[b]	Convert from IR or use 10 mg (12.5 cm² patch) released over 9 h and titrate up p.r.n.	0.3–2 mg/kg released over 9 h Not to exceed one 30-mg patch	10–30 mg released over 9 h	10-mg, 15-mg, 20-mg, 30-mg patches, applied to the ¨hip
Dexmethylphenidate IR (Focalin)	2.5–5 mg	0.1–0.5 mg/kg per dose PO to q.i.d. Maximum 20 mg/d	0.2–0.3 mg/kg per dose PO b.i.d./t.i.d.	2.5-mg, 5-mg, or 10-mg scored tabs (o not cut, crush, or chew)
Dexmethylphenidate extended release (Focalin-XR)	5–10 mg	0.2–1 mg/kg per dose PO b.i.d. to q.i.d. Maximum 20 mg/d	0.4–0.6 mg/kg per dose PO q.i.d./b.i.d.	5-mg, 10-mg, or 20-mg scored tabs Can be sprinkled into soft food (do not cut, crush, or chew)
Dextroamphetamine (Dexedrine, Dextrostat)	2.5–5 mg	0.1–0.7 mg/kg per dose PO q.i.d./b.i.d. Maximum 60 mg/d	0.3–0.5 mg/kg per dose PO q.i.d./t.i.d.	Dexedrine: 5-mg scored tabs Dextrostat: 5-mg and 10-mg scored tabs
Dextroamphetamine Spansules (Dexedrine CR)	5 mg	0.1–0.75 mg/kg per dose PO q.i.d./b.i.d. Maximum 60 mg/d	0.3–0.6 mg/kg per dose PO q.i.d./b.i.d.	5-mg, 10-mg, or 15-mg Spansules Can be sprinkled into soft food (do not cut, crush, or chew)
Mixed amphetamine salts IR (Adderall, generic)	2.5–5 mg	0.1–0.7 mg/kg per dose PO q.i.d./b.i.d.	0.3–0.5 mg/kg per dose PO t.i.d./q.i.d.	5-mg, 7.5-mg, 10-mg, 12.5-mg, 15-mg, 20-mg, or 30-mg scored tabs

Medication	Starting dose	Dose	Dose	Preparations
Mixed amphetamine salt XR (Adderall-XR)	Convert from IR or use 5–10 mg	Maximum 40 mg/d 0.2–1.4 mg/kg per dose PO q.i.d./t.i.d. Maximum 30 mg/d	0.6–1 mg/kg per dose PO q.i.d./b.i.d.	5-mg, 10-mg, 15-mg, 20-mg, 25-mg, or 30-mg Spansules Can be sprinkled into soft food (do not cut, crush, or chew)
Lisdexamfetamine (Vyvanse)	30 mg PO in morning	30–70 mg PO in morning	Data limited (too early to tell)	20-mg, 30-mg, 40-mg, 50-mg, 60-mg, or 70-mg caps Swallow cap whole, sprinkle into soft food, or dissolve contents in glass of water and drink immediately
Methylphenidate immediate release (IR) (Ritalin, Methylin, generic)	2.5–5 mg	0.1–0.8 mg/kg per dose PO q.i.d. to 5 times daily Maximum 60 mg/d	0.3–0.5 mg/kg per dose PO t.i.d./q.i.d.	All preparations available as 5-mg, 10-mg, or 20-mg scored tabs; Methylin also available as 2.5-mg, 5-mg, or 10-mg chewable tab and PO solution
Methylphenidate sustained-release (SR) (Ritalin LA, Metadate CD)	Convert from IR or use 10 mg	0.2–1.4 mg/kg per dose PO q.i.d./t.i.d. Maximum 60 mg/d	0.6–1 mg/kg per dose PO q.i.d./b.i.d.	10-mg, 20-mg, 30-mg, or 40-mg tabs (Metadate also has 50-mg and 60-mg tabs) Can be sprinkled into soft food (do not cut, crush, or chew)
Methylphenidate extended release (ER)[c] (Ritalin SR, Methylin ER, Metadate ER, generic SR)	Convert from IR	0.2–1.4 mg/kg per dose PO q.i.d./t.i.d. Maximum 60 mg/d	0.6–1 mg/kg per dose PO q.i.d./b.i.d.	20-mg Spansules (do not cut, crush, or chew)
Methylphenidate OROS tablets (Concerta)	Convert from IR or use 18 mg	0.3–2 mg/kg PO q.i.d. Maximum 54 mg/d	0.8–1.6 mg/kg PO q.i.d.	18-mg, 27-mg, 36-mg, and 54-mg tabs (do not cut, crush, or chew)
Methylphenidate transdermal patch (Daytrana)[b]	Convert from IR or use 10 mg (12.5-cm² patch) released over 9 h and titrate up p.r.n.	0.3–2 mg/kg released over 9 h Not to exceed one 30-mg patch	10–30 mg released over 9 h	10-mg, 15-mg, 20-mg, 30-mg patches, applied to the hip
Dexmethylphenidate IR (Focalin)	2.5–5 mg	0.1–0.5 mg/kg per dose PO to q.i.d. Maximum 20 mg/d	0.2–0.3 mg/kg per dose PO b.i.d./t.i.d.	2.5-mg, 5-mg, or 10-mg scored tabs (do not cut, crush, or chew)
Dexmethylphenidate extended release (Focalin-XR)	5–10 mg	0.2–1 mg/kg per dose PO q.i.d. to b.i.d. Maximum 20 mg/d	0.4–0.6 mg/kg per dose PO q.i.d./b.i.d.	5-mg, 10-mg, or 20-mg scored tabs Can be sprinkled into soft food (do not cut, crush, or chew)
Dextroamphetamine (Dexedrine, Dextrostat)	2.5–5 mg	0.1–0.7 mg/kg per dose PO to q.i.d. Maximum 60 mg/d	0.3–0.5 mg/kg per dose PO q.i.d./t.i.d.	Dexedrine: 5-mg scored tabs Dextrostat: 5-mg and 10-mg scored tabs

(Continued)

Table 36-2   (*Continued*)

Medication	Initial Pediatric Dose	Pediatric Dosage Range and Maximum Dose[a]	Common Pediatric Dose[a]	Preparations
Dextroamphetamine Spansules (Dexedrine CR)	5 mg	0.1–0.75 mg/kg per dose PO q.i.d./b.i.d. Maximum 60 mg/d	0.3–0.6 mg/kg per dose PO q.i.d./b.i.d.	5-mg, 10-mg, or 15-mg Spansules Can be sprinkled into soft food (do not cut, crush, or chew)
Mixed amphetamine salts IR (Adderall, generic)	2.5–5 mg	0.1–0.7 mg/kg per dose PO to q.i.d. Maximum 40 mg/d	0.3–0.5 mg/kg per dose PO t.i.d./q.i.d.	5-mg, 7.5-mg, 10-mg, 12.5-mg, 15-mg, 20-mg, or 30-mg scored tabs
Mixed amphetamine salt XR (Adderall-XR)	Convert from IR or use 5–10 mg	0.2–1.4 mg/kg per dose PO q.i.d./t.i.d. Maximum 30 mg/d	0.6–1 mg/kg per dose PO q.i.d./b.i.d.	5-mg, 10-mg, 15-mg, 20-mg, 25-mg, or 30-mg Spansules Can be sprinkled into soft food (do not cut, crush, or chew)
Lisdexamfetamine (Vyvanse)	30 mg PO in morning	30–70 mg PO in morning	Data limited (too early to tell)	20-mg, 30-mg, 40-mg, 50-mg, 60-mg, or 70-mg caps Swallow cap whole, sprinkle into soft food, or dissolve contents in glass of water and drink immediately

* In general, when the terms methylphenidate, Dexedrine, and Ritalin are used without abbreviations for extended-release preparations (e.g., continuous release [CR], SR, osmotic-release oral system [OROS]), a short-acting, IR preparation is implied.

[a] Maximum pediatric dose suggested by the US Food and Drug Administration. Although some children benefit greatly from doses greater than these, benefit from use of either the lowest and highest ends of the dose range is uncommon.

[b] The methylphenidate patch contains a different total methylphenidate dose than the name implies because it is designed to last 12 hours (e.g., 10-mg patch [patch size 12.5 cm^2] delivers about 10 mg over 9 h [estimated delivery rate is 1.1 mg/h for this particular patch]). Delivery rate varies depending on patch size.

[c] Many patients describe their experience with methylphenidate SR preparations as erratic and uncomfortable.

ADHD. Short-term efficacy is more pronounced for behavioral rather than cognitive and learning abnormalities.

Use of stimulants requires careful diagnosis of the disorder, the lowest possible effective dose, and careful monitoring of response. Stimulants, when used for illicit purposes, are considered valuable for resale. Like all controlled substances, they should be prescribed in smaller amounts than are other psychotropic medications.

36.2.2 Side-effects of psychostimulants

Side-effects are dose-dependent and range from mild to moderate in most children. These have been described in a placebo-controlled study comparing the baseline and on-medication double-blind parent. Common side-effects include insomnia, decreased appetite, weight loss, headache, heart rate elevation at rest, stomach pain, and minor increases in systolic blood pressure. Many of these side-effects can be managed with temporary dose reduction. Severe insomnia can be alleviated by changing the time of dosing, with most of the medication given early in the day.

Complaints of upset stomach, nausea, or pain may benefit from a change to transdermal MPH, or giving the oral medication in the middle of a meal. Otherwise, the problem can be treated symptomatically with antacid tablets or by switching to sustained-release MPH, which is absorbed more slowly.

Infrequent side-effects include motor tics and reductions in weight velocity. The appearance of minor facial tics is a frequent reason for stopping stimulants in clinical practice. Despite a lack of studies demonstrating a causal link between stimulant treatment and tic disorders, the *Physician's Desk Reference* warns against the use of stimulants in children with pre-existing tic disorders. A history of chronic or episodic involuntary muscle movements or a family history of Tourette's disorder has become a contraindication to MPH use, as it may unmask or exacerbate Tourette's disorder.

36.3 Nonstimulant group of drugs

36.3.1 Atomoxetine and modafinil

Atomoxetine, a nonstimulant selective norepinephrine-reuptake inhibitor (SNRI), has been effective in many people with attention-deficit hyperactivity disorder. This relatively new medication has the advantages of q.i.d.-to-b.i.d. dosing and unscheduled status with the US Drug Enforcement Agency (DEA). However, cases of reversible hepatic failure have been directly attributed to atomoxetine, and an evaluation of other long-term adverse effects has been limited to data from a few years.

Modafinil is a new agent approved by the FDA for promoting wakefulness. It is unclear if it should be classified as a stimulant. It does not have meaningful effects on dopamine release or reuptake, as do amphetamine and methylphenidate, and its mechanism of action is unclear. Nevertheless, modafinil has some stimulant-like properties. Modafinil has been approved by the FDA for the treatment of narcolepsy and disorders of wakefulness. Although it is not approved for Alzheimer's disease and ADHD, Modafinil is being investigated in their treatment.

36.3.2 Nonstimulant cognitive enhancers

Four medications – tacrine, donepezil, rivastigmine, and galantamine – are cholinesterase inhibitors that have been shown to delay to a degree the loss of mental abilities in people with Alzheimer's disease. Cholinesterase is an enzyme that breaks down acetylcholine. The goal of cholinesterase inhibition is to make more acetylcholine available for intrasynaptic cholinergic receptor stimulation, thereby improving executive functioning, attention, memory, language, and behavior.

Cholinesterase inhibitors may not improve a person's ability to do things like plan a meal or decide what to wear, but they do slow down the loss of these skills for some time. These benefits are temporary (they will disappear if treatment is stopped). The improvements peak at 3 months after the drug is started and this is followed by a slow return to the starting point over 9–12 months. After that time, a slower decline is observed compared to people who have not been treated with medication.

Adverse reactions regarding cholinesterase inhibitors are listed in Box 36.1. Adverse event estimates vary widely from study to study, so relative adverse event rates are difficult to estimate. Cholinergic side-effects generally occur early and are related to initiating or increasing medication. They tend to be mild and self-limited. Medications should be restarted at the lowest doses after temporarily stopping.

Box 36.1 Adverse Reactions and Cautions with Cholinesterase Inhibitors.

- **Tacrine**: Nausea, vomiting, diarrhea, dyspepsia, myalgia, anorexia, dizziness, confusion, insomnia, rare agranulocytosis.
  Approximately 50% of patients will develop direct, reversible hepatotoxicity manifested by elevated transaminases.
  Drug interactions may include increased cholinergic effects with bethanacol; increased plasma tacrine levels with cimetidine or fluvoxamine. This may occur by inhibition of P450 1A2. The association of tacrine with haloperidol may increase parkinsonism, and tacrine increases theophylline concentration.
- **Donepezil**: Nausea, diarrhea, insomnia, vomiting, muscle cramps, fatigue, anorexia, dizziness, abdominal pain, myasthenia, rhinitis, weight loss, anxiety, syncope (2 vs. 1%).
- **Rivastigmine**: Nausea, vomiting, anorexia, dizziness, abdominal pain, diarrhea, malaise, fatigue, asthenia, headache, sweating, weight loss, somnolence, syncope (3 vs. 2%).
  Rarely, severe vomiting with esophageal rupture.
- **Galantamine**: Nausea, vomiting, diarrhea, anorexia, weight loss, abdominal pain, dizziness, tremor, syncope (2 vs. 1%).

By increasing the central and peripheral cholinergic stimulation, cholinesterase inhibitors may:

- Increase gastric acid secretion, increasing the risk for GI bleeding especially in patients with ulcer disease or those taking anti-inflammatories

- Produce bradycardia, especially in patients with sick sinus or other supraventricular conduction delay, leading to syncope, falls, and possible injury

- Exacerbate obstructive pulmonary disease

- Cause urinary outflow obstruction

- Increase risk for seizures

- Prolong the effects of succinylcholine-type muscle relaxants.

36.3.2.1 Tacrine

Tacrine is a noncompetitive reversible inhibitor of ChE. It binds near the catalytically active site of the AChE molecule to inhibit enzyme activity, and has other actions as well. Tacrine is no longer actively marketed owing to a high incidence of hepatotoxicity and frequent dosing schedule. The recommended starting dose is 10 mg q.i.d. to be maintained for 6 weeks, while serum transaminase levels are monitored every other week. If the drug is tolerated and transaminase levels do not increase above three times the upper limit of normal, the dose is then increased to 20 mg q.i.d. After

6 weeks, dosage should be increased to 30 mg q.i.d., again with biweekly monitoring and then, if tolerated, to 40 mg q.i.d. for the next 6 weeks.

36.3.2.2 Donepezil

Donepezil is a long-acting piperidine-based highly selective and reversible AChE inhibitor. Donepezil may decrease the rate of hippocampal atrophy in Alzheimer's disease, suggesting a neuroprotective mechanism. Donepezil is initiated at 5 mg/day and then increased to 10 mg/day after 4–6 weeks. Raising the dose earlier increases the risk for cholinergic adverse events. Effective doses are 5–10 mg/day; the higher dose tends to be somewhat more effective and to have more adverse effects than 5 mg.

36.3.2.3 Rivastigmine

Rivastigmine is a pseudo-irreversible, selective AChE subtype inhibitor. The recommended starting dose of rivastigmine is 1.5 mg b.i.d., taken with meals, increasing to 3 mg b.i.d. after a minimum of 2 weeks of treatment if the initial dose is well tolerated. Subsequent increases to 4.5 mg and then 6 mg b.i.d. should be based on good tolerability with the previous dose and may be considered after a minimum 2-week treatment interval. Higher daily doses, averaging about 9–10 mg, were associated with better efficacy than lower doses. It is available as an oral solution. Transdermal rivastigmine is started with an initial 4.6 mg patch per day for at least 4 weeks before the dose is raised to a 9.5 mg patch per day maintenance dose, based on good tolerability with the previous dose.

36.3.2.4 Galantamine

Galantamine, an alkaloid originally extracted from Amaryllidaceae (*Galanthus woronowi*, the Caucasian snowdrop) but now synthesized, is a reversible, competitive inhibitor of AChE with relatively little butyrylcholinesterase activity. Initial dosing of the original formulation of galantamine is 4 mg b.i.d., and should be raised to 8 mg b.i.d. after 2–4 weeks. For patients who are tolerating medication but not responding, the dose can be raised to 12 mg b.i.d. after another 4 weeks.

The FDA approved galantamine in April 2001 under the trade name Reminyl. Owing to confusion with the diabetes medication glimepiride (Amaryl), in 2005 the trade name Reminyl was changed to Razadyne. An extended-release formulation of galantamine (Razadyne ER) was subsequently FDA-approved for once-daily use. The extended-release formulation is started at 8 mg/day and increased to 16 mg/day after 4 weeks. After 4 weeks the dose can be further increased to 24 mg/day based on clinical benefit and tolerability. The Cochrane Database of Systematic Reviews indicates that 16 mg/day showed statistically indistinguishable efficacy from higher doses.

KEY POINTS

- Anxiolytic or antianxiety medications are used to treat generalized anxiety disorder and may provide relief for acute anxiety states, social phobia, performance anxiety, and simple phobias.

- Benzodiazepines are a group of medications that increase the efficiency of the GABA receptor.

- The pharmacologic effects of the benzodiazepines include anxiolysis, sedation, centrally mediated muscle relaxation, and elevation of the seizure threshold.

- As a class, benzadiazepines are efficacious for the treatment of PD, SAD, GAD, alcohol withdrawal, and situational anxiety.

- Benzodiazepines should be used cautiously with older adults, debilitated patients, depressed or suicidal patients, and those with a history of substance abuse.

- Withdrawal syndrome is possible on discontinuation of benzodiazepines and is most common with high doses of medication used for more than 4 months.

- Buspirone is a member of the group of agents called azaspirodecanediones and is a non-sedating, non-habit-forming anxiolytic.

- Beta-blockers can decrease many of the peripheral manifestations of anxiety such as tachycardia, diaphoresis, trembling, and blushing.

- Psychostimulants are a class of drugs commonly used to treat disruptive behavior disorders, most often attention-deficit hyperactivity disorder and narcolepsy.

- Use of stimulants requires careful diagnosis of the disorder, the lowest possible effective dose, and careful monitoring of response.

- Stimulants have been reported to be misused as recreational drugs.

- Atomoxetine, a nonstimulant selective norepinephrine-reuptake inhibitor, has been effective in many people with ADHD.

- Modafinil is a new agent that is approved by the FDA for promoting wakefulness and is not considered to be in the stimulant class.

- Cholinesterase inhibitors are cognitive enhancers that have been shown to delay somewhat the loss of mental abilities in people with Alzheimer's disease. The goal of cholinesterase inhibition is to make more acetylcholine available for intrasynaptic cholinergic receptor stimulation, thereby improving executive functioning, attention, memory, language, and behavior.

Further Reading

Ramchandani, P., Joughin, C., and Zwi, M. (2002) Attention deficit hyperactivity disorder in children. *Clinical Evidence*, **6**, 262–271.

Tasman, A. and Lieberman, J.A. (2006) *Handbook of Psychiatric Drugs*, John Wiley, New York.

Wilens, T.E. (2002) *Straight Talk about Psychiatric Medications for Kids*, Guilford, New York.

CHAPTER 37 ●●● Somatic Therapies

37.1 Introduction

In addition to psychotherapies, which rely on patients working to change dysfunctional thinking and behaviors, somatic (biologic) therapies represent another arsenal of psychiatric tools. Sometimes referred to as "neuromodulation" and "brain-stimulation techniques," somatic therapies include psychopharmacotherapeutics (medications) and nonpharmacological, body-based modalities.

To some extent, differentiating psychotherapies from somatic or biological therapies is incorrect. All therapies in mental health involve biology, in that all human experiences result in biological changes, even if only at the molecular level. As mentioned in Chapter 2, cognitive–behavioral therapy has been shown to result in brain changes, related to the brain's remarkable capacity called *neuroplasticity*. Nevertheless, most texts categorize psychotherapies and somatic therapies in different sections for simplicity and to make content more approachable and containable for readers. This chapter describes nonpharmacologic somatic therapies, their purposes, and their current standing in terms of efficacy and general approval.

37.2 Electroconvulsive therapy

Modern electroconvulsive therapy (ECT), in which electricity is used to induce a convulsion, was introduced into psychiatric practice in the 1930s in Italy. By 1940, ECT had made its way into US psychiatric practice. With the advent of modern psychotropic medications, and because of its indiscriminate use in some state hospitals, ECT began to fall out of favor. ECT overcame its tarnished image and has been reintroduced as an important treatment in the therapeutic toolkit. Approximately 100 000 people in the United States receive ECT treatments annually. It is the most effective treatment available for refractory major depression (i.e., depression that recurs and does not respond to other modalities). Some psychiatric researchers consider ECT as the standard against which other somatic therapies, including medication and other forms of somatic therapies, are compared.

37.2.1 Indications

Generally, ECT is used in patients for whom all other therapeutic interventions have failed and whose lives are at risk. Approximately 85% of patients receiving ECT have major depression as the indication for use, with the remainder having schizoaffective disorders, mania, schizophrenia, and occasionally Parkinson's disease.

Fundamentals of Psychiatry, First Edition. Allan Tasman and Wanda K. Mohr.
© 2011 John Wiley & Sons, Ltd. Published 2011 by John Wiley & Sons, Ltd.
This chapter is based on Chapter 109 (Stefan Rowny, Sarah H. Lisanby) of *Psychiatry, Third Edition*

37.2.2 Pretreatment evaluation

Assessment of patients for whom ECT is a consideration should happen as close to the first treatment with ECT as possible. From a medical standpoint, patients should undergo a complete health history and physical examination. Minimum laboratory and diagnostic tests should include a blood count, evaluation of electrolyte levels, complete metabolic panel, ECG, and chest x-ray. Patients should be evaluated as to their ability to tolerate anesthesia. From a psychiatric standpoint, a baseline of symptoms should be recorded against which the clinician can monitor progress and symptom alleviation. Patients are generally asked to fast after midnight the day of the procedure.

37.2.3 Procedure

Prior to the procedure, the patient undergoes brief general anesthesia with succinylcholine to prevent severe muscle contractions that might result in muscle or bone injuries. Some patients receive anticholinergic medications to dry secretions that might interfere with respiration. Ultrabrief anesthetic agents are used to induce unconsciouness.

ECT itself involves placing an electrode on the temple of the patient and inducing a grand mal seizure. Bilateral stimulation, or placement of electrodes on both temples, has beenused in the past (and sometimes now), but it has more associated adverse side-effects such as memory loss.

An electric current is passed through the electrode for between 100 ms and 1 s, and the patient experiences a convulsion that lasts approximately one minute. During this entire time the patient is oxygenated, and clinicians monitor oxygen saturation and cardiac functioning.

Typically ECT is given twice weekly on nonconsecutive days. Treatments may range from a few to 15 sessions, depending on the patient's response. The entire procedure lasts less than one hour, although each patient's recovery time after the procedure varies. When repeated episodes of depression or serious other life-threatening symptoms occur after a series of treatments with ECT, the physician may opt to taper ECT over several weeks to months. Typically, a tapering schedule will be once a week for 1 month, once every 2 weeks for 2 months, once every 3 weeks for 2 months, and once every month for 2 to 4 months. This kind of tapering may help to prevent rehospitalization. Occasionally, patients relapse and have to return for maintenance treatment.

37.2.4 Mechanism of action

Because the brain is relatively inaccessible for direct study of pathophysiology, the mechanisms by which ECT "works" remain speculative. Several hypotheses have been proposed. One theory is that ECT alters neurotransmitter receptors. Most often, the literature posits that serotonergic levels are increased after ECT treatment but others also mention GABA. Because ECT seems to be effective in conditions with such varying symptoms (i.e., depression, mania, schizophrenia), much simply remains unknown, and more research is needed. Recent work in this area is exploring ECT's effect on neuropeptides and growth factors. Other research includes investigating the effects of the large increases in cerebral blood flow that happen during a grand mal seizure. Yet others are exploring the possible structural changes associated with neuronal plasticity and promotion of neurogenesis.

37.2.5 Side-effects

Following ECT, patients may have a headache, muscle aches, or nausea. Approximately 50% report headaches of a throbbing nature. These can be treated with medications before or after ECT. In addition, some people may exhibit postictal confusion, which typically lasts for 30–60 minutes.

Memory loss is one of the important and legitimate concerns that people have about ECT. The first type is a short-term memory loss limited to the period involving the course of treatment. An example might be the patient forgetting what he or she had for a meal. This situation generally corrects itself, with the patient returning to pretreatment levels of functioning within a few weeks to several months. The second type of memory loss is of past events, with recent past events being more sensitive to ECT. This retrograde amnesia may persevere for several months after treatment. In some instances, it may be permanent. This memory loss is more common with bilateral electrode placement.

ECT is generally considered a low-risk procedure, and is one of the safest procedures performed under anesthesia. Nevertheless, any medical condition involving anesthesia carries some danger. Potential risks include cardiac dysrhythmias and respiratory arrest. Deaths resulting from respiratory or cardiac arrest following ECT are less than 1 in 10 000 cases.

37.3 Phototherapy

Phototherapy (light therapy) was introduced during the 1980s as a treatment for a mood disorder with a seasonal pattern: seasonal affective disorder (SAD). Although competing theories of the etiology of SAD exist, it is generally accepted that it develops in predisposed people as a result of insufficient exposure to sunlight. Hence, the most common treatment for SAD is phototherapy. In this procedure, the person exposes his or her eyes to bright artificial light for approximately 2 hours per day.

Several phototherapy devices are on the market, but the fluorescent light box with a filter to screen out ultraviolet rays is the gold standard. Recommended treatment is exposure in the morning to mimic the natural circadian rhythm. Relief of symptoms generally occurs within 4 days of beginning the treatment, with 50% of patients experiencing relief of symptoms after 1 week. Treatment continues throughout the winter months, because symptoms are likely to return if light exposure stops.

Phototherapy tends to be well tolerated. Some people complain of headaches, eyestrain, nausea, sweating, visual disturbances, and sedation. Ophthalmic damage was reported from the use of earlier, less sophisticated boxes, but newer boxes screen out harmful rays that may damage the eyes. Patients should be instructed to consult an ophthalmologist prior to commencing treatment and not to look directly into the light. As with any other treatment for depression, there is a rare chance that a person may develop mania or hypomania. Patients should be made aware of this possibility.

37.4 Transcranial magnetic stimulation

Transcranial magnetic stimulation (TMS) is a technique in which rapidly changing magnetic fields induce electrical current to the superficial cortex of the brain. The magnetic pulses are roughly the strength of the magnetic scanner used in magnetic resonance imaging, but are considerably more focused. They pass easily through the skull just like the MRI scanner fields do. Because they are short pulses and not a static field, however, they can stimulate the underlying cerebral cortex.

TMS was developed in the 1980s, but not until the last decade or so has it piqued researchers' interest. It is currently being investigated as a potential treatment for major depression, schizophrenia marked by auditory hallucinations, acute and chronic pain, and various other psychiatric and neurologic disorders. TMS is considered the safest and least invasive of the new stimulating techniques now under research. Its advantage is that it has no known side-effects.

TMS has been approved in the US and several other countries for refractory depression.

37.5 Vagus nerve stimulation

Vagus nerve stimulation (VNS) is an FDA-approved treatment that involves implantation of a device under the patient's skin. The action of VNS is on the phrenic nerve, which feeds back to the brain's limbic system. The device emits a steady pulse like a pacemaker. Studies have demonstrated the effectiveness of VNS for medically refractory partial-onset seizures, and it seems to help patients with treatment-refractory depression. Implantation of the VNS device is done under general anesthesia on an outpatient basis.

Side-effects include coughing, hoarseness, voice changes, dyspnea, and irritation at the site of the implant. These results are usually transient.

37.6 Deep brain stimulation

The most invasive form of brain stimulation involves implanting an electrode directly into the brain. The technique, deep brain stimulation (DBS), is used in end-stage Parkinson's disease for relief of distressing tremors. Studies on DBS in the treatment of refractory depression are scant and highly experimental. Most studies have been done in Europe over a long span of years between the 1970s to the 1990s with a subset of people reporting relief. Because of the invasiveness of the procedure, lack of data, and availability of less invasive techniques, DBS is mainly of research interest in psychiatry at this point.

37.7 Psychosurgery

37.7.1 Background

Psychosurgery refers to brain surgery intended to relieve severe and otherwise intractable mental or behavioral problems and is not a new phenomenon. In the recent history of psychiatry, it was recommended for curing or ameliorating schizophrenia, depression, homosexuality, childhood behavior disorders, criminal behavior, and uncontrolled violence. Estimates are that more than 50 000 psychosurgery procedures were performed in the US alone from the 1930s to the 1950s.

Much of the controversy surrounding psychiatric neurosurgery may relate to its overzealous and sometimes indiscriminate application during this period. Although the number of psychosurgical procedures for the purpose of psychiatric intervention performed internationally today is unknown, estimates are that fewer than 25 patients are operated upon annually in the US and the UK.

Outcomes of surgery are an important parameter in terms of improved postoperative functional status. Proponents of psychosurgery have observed that some patients are vastly improved after surgery and they consider it an important therapeutic option when other treatments have failed.

37.7.2 Indications

Psychosurgery remains very controversial, with a theoretical basis of treatment that is not well established. Currently, only patients with chronic, severe, and disabling psychiatric illness that are completely refractory to all conventional therapy are considered for surgery. This implies that well-documented, systematic trials of pharmacologic, psychologic, and – when appropriate – electroconvulsive therapies have been tried both singly and in combination before neurosurgical intervention is considered. Severity and chronicity (of several years' duration) of the patient's illness must be present both in terms of subjective distress and a severe alteration in psychosocial functioning.

37.7.3 Procedures

Psychiatric neurosurgery involves the disconnection of brain tissue (referred to as ablation) with the intent of altering affective and behavioral states caused by mental illnesses. The goal is to restore patients to a better level of functioning. Several of these procedures have differing targets, such as the cerebral cortex, nuclei, or other pathways that display abnormal physiologic activity. The temporal lobe may be the target in intractable epilepsy. Surgical treatment of Parkinson's disease may involve making lesions in the basal ganglia.

Four procedures are most commonly employed and regarded as the safest and most effective: anterior cingulotomy, subcaudate tractotomy, limbic leucotomy, and anterior capsulotomy. All are performed bilaterally, and all involve creating lesions of limbic or paralimbic structures and interruptions of their connections with deeper brain structures.

KEY POINTS

- Somatic therapies are biologically based interventions that include pharmacologic and nonpharmacologic modalities.

- ECT is a treatment employed when other treatment modalities have failed to improve a patient's condition. It involves placement of an electrode on the patient's temple under general anesthesia so as to induce a grand mal seizure.

- ECT is very safe. Side-effects include short-term memory loss and any other effects of a procedure requiring general anesthesia.

- Phototherapy involves exposure of a patient to a light source during fall and winter months in order to treat seasonal affective disorder. Side-effects can include hypomania.

- Transcranial magnetic stimulation, deep brain stimulation, and vagus nerve stimulation are promising modalities that have not yet been approved in the US by regulatory authorities.

- Psychosurgery is a relatively rare treatment modality and indicated only when a patient has chronic, severe, and intractable mental illness.

Further Reading

Abrams, R. (2002) *Electroconvulsive Therapy*, Oxford University Press, New York.

George, M.S. and Belmaker, R.H. (2006) *TMS in Clinical Psychiatry*, American Psychiatric Press, Washington, DC.

Greenberg, M.S. (2005) *Handbook of Neurosurgery*, Thieme Medical, New York.

Starr, P.A., Vitek, J.L., and Bakay, R.A. (1998) Deep brain stimulation. *Neurosurgery Clinics of North America*, **9**, 381–402.

Unit 5
Special Topics

38 Psychiatric Emergencies

38.1 Introduction

The Task Force on Psychiatric Emergency Care Issues of the American Psychiatric Association in collaboration with the American College of Emergency Physicians Committee on Behavioral Emergencies provides a summary of the essential components defining psychiatric emergencies. The definition states that a psychiatric emergency is an acute disturbance of thought, mood, behavior or social relationship that requires an immediate intervention as defined by the patient, family or community.

Disturbances of this nature have differential diagnoses and, like all psychiatric conditions, should be comprehensively evaluated. A biopsychosocial model should place the cause for a psychiatric emergency into its biologic, social, and psychologic contexts, recognizing the unique interplay of these factors in each patient and applying evaluations on an individual basis. Thus, a major behavioral disturbance should be identified, its intensity quantified, its accompanying symptoms enumerated, and a search for etiologies commenced so that intervention can be targeted to causes and contexts.

This chapter discusses three commonly encountered psychiatric emergencies: acute delirium, suicidality, and violent and aggressive behavior.

38.2 Delirium

Delirium is the superordinate term for a syndrome characterized by a *rapid* onset of cognitive dysfunction and disruption in consciousness. Delirium is also referred to as intensive care or critical care psychosis, acute brain syndrome, acute confusion, and acute toxic psychosis.

Certain patients are at increased risk for delirium, specifically older adults and cognitively impaired older adults recovering from surgery. Older adults are especially susceptible to delirium disorders because the aging neurologic system is vulnerable to insults caused by underlying systemic conditions. Delirium often predicts or accompanies physical illness in older adults.

38.2.1 Etiology

Delirium is the most common psychiatric syndrome found in general medical hospitals. It can be induced by any process, disorder, or agent that disrupts the integrity of the central nervous system and diffusely impairs its functioning at a cellular level. Risk factors for delirium are generally:

- Postoperative conditions or metabolic disorders
- Withdrawal of drugs and substances such as alcohol or cocaine

Fundamentals of Psychiatry, First Edition. Allan Tasman and Wanda K. Mohr.
© 2011 John Wiley & Sons, Ltd. Published 2011 by John Wiley & Sons, Ltd.
This chapter is based on Chapter 116 (Glenn A. Melvin, Kelly Posner, Barbara H. Stanley, Maria A. Oquendo) and Chapter 117 (Wanda K. Mohr. Kevin Ann Huckshorn, Kim J. Masters) of *Psychiatry, Third Edition*

Table 38-1 Causes of delirium	
Primary Brain Disease/disorder	**Head Injury, Tumor**
Systemic diseases	Disrupted acid–base balance, cerebral vascular accident, dehydration, endocrine disorders, epilepsy, fever, electrolyte imbalance, hypoperfusion of the brain, hypo- or hyperthermia, hypoproteinemia, hypoxia, hypotension, infection, malnutrition, organ failure, postoperative state, trauma, uremia, vitamin deficiencies
Withdrawal of exogenous substances of abuse	Alcohol, sedatives
Toxic exogenous substances	Anticholinergics, antidepressants, antidysrhythmic drugs, antihypertensives, antiparkinson agents, antipsychotics, cimetadine, corticosteroids, diuretics, narcotic analgesics, nonsteroidal anti-inflammatory agents, over-the-counter cough medicines, diet aids, xanthines

- Toxicity secondary to drugs or other exogenous substances

- Impaired respiratory functioning.

Any disturbance in any organ or system that affects the brain can disrupt metabolism and neurotransmission, leading to a decline in cognition and function. Infections, fluid and electrolyte imbalances, and drugs are the most frequent causes of delirium. An often overlooked form of delirium is hypoxia, which can cause agitation and confusion. Medications are the primary exogenous offenders, especially in older adults. Table 38.1 delineates some specific causes of delirium and conditions that can disrupt brain homeostasis.

38.2.2 Signs, symptoms, and diagnostic criteria

Although delirium presents a mixed clinical picture, three salient features are usually present:

- Disordered cognition

- Attention deficit

- Disturbance of consciousness.

Cognition includes the aspects of thinking, perception, and memory. In delirium, the thinking aspect of cognition becomes disorganized, and affected patients appear confused and cannot reason, handle complex tasks, or solve problems. Speech reflects disordered thinking and may be pressured, rambling, bizarre, incoherent, or nearly absent. Patients often cannot distinguish reality from imagery and dreams, as orientation and spatial ability are impaired. Suspiciousness with persecutory delusions is fairly common.

Patients experience perceptual disturbances, such as hallucinations and illusions. If present, hallucinations – which can be auditory, tactile, or visual – are often graphic and can induce a state of anxiety verging on panic. Patients can become agitated and combative. Mood alterations can exhibit great lability, from irritability and dysphoria to euphoria.

Memory becomes impaired, with short-term memory being especially affected. Inability to focus or shift attention is another feature of delirium. In addition, patients experience difficulty attending to environmental stimuli. This diminished ability to control focus of attention and attention span fluctuates during the day and is more pronounced at night. Patients are frequently disoriented to time and sometimes to place and person. In more severe cases of delirium, patients mistake the unfamiliar for the familiar.

Additional features of delirium may include a reduced level of consciousness, a disrupted sleep–wake cycle, and an abnormality of psychomotor behavior. Change in level of consciousness may fluctuate between alertness and somnolence. The patient may reverse the sleep–wake cycle, appearing drowsy throughout the day and napping sporadically at night, awakening to become extremely agitated.

The patient's psychomotor activity may range from hypoalert and hypoactive (more typically observed in metabolic dysfunction) to hyperalert and hyperactive (which typically occur during drug withdrawal), or any combination thereof. The hypoalert, hypoactive patient exhibits minimal activity, appears stuporous, and is slow to respond to requests. This person is often mistakenly judged to be depressed and the delirium may be missed. The patient in a hyperalert, hyperactive state is animated to the point of agitation and frequently has loud and pressured speech. The patient in this agitated state often will try to remove intravenous lines and other tubes, "pick" at the air or the bed sheet, and try (often successfully) to climb over side rails or the end of the bed. In addition, the patient often will exhibit the classic, autonomic response symptoms of dilated pupils, elevated pulse, and diaphoresis.

38.2.3 Implications and prognosis

Delirium indicates the existence of a medical illness and should be considered a medically urgent condition. The prognosis for recovery from delirium is good if recognition and management of the underlying cause are attended to early. Depending on early recognition and management, the acute state of delirium can last for 3–5 days or, rarely, up to 3 weeks. *Failure to deal with the underlying factors causing the delirium may result in irreversible brain damage or even death.*

38.2.4 Treatments

The goal is to identify patients who are vulnerable to the development of delirium, recognize early signs of delirium, and quickly institute measures to correct underlying causes. In addition to early diagnosis and prompt medical treatment, therapeutic goals include managing the acute confusion to maximize cognitive functioning and prevent injury or further cognitive decline.

Medical interventions include treatment of the underlying cause. Therefore, treatment varies according to each patient's physical condition. In cases of hypoperfusion or cerebral hypoxia, supplemental oxygen may significantly improve acute symptoms. Identifying and withdrawal of medication or a toxin causing the delirium and treatment of infections will result in improvement. The use of an antipsychotic or sedating agent may be necessary; but owing to the confusion and clouding of consciousness associated with delirium, they should be used prudently and judiciously and the entire medical condition should be taken into account prior to administering them. For example, benzodiazepines may depress respiration and disinhibit patients and may not be optimal in cases of COPD. The same medications discussed later in this chapter on the pharmacologic treatment of aggression and violence are normally those used to treat delirium.

Both physical restraints and chemical restraints must be avoided or, when absolutely necessary, used with utmost caution. The impetus for the use of chemical or physical restraints clearly must be to protect the patient from harm rather than for staff convenience. Indeed, either chemical or physical restraints are a risk factor for, and may compound, the delirium.

The patient's environment should be structured to ensure safety as well as to maximize cognitive abilities and psychological comfort. A fine balance exists between environmental over-stimulation and under-stimulation. Tailoring the environment to enhance the patient's cognitive capability is essential. Providing a private room is beneficial so that staff can minimize noxious and confusing environmental stimuli and maximize the use of a sitter or supportive family members. Adequate lighting during both the day and evening is essential to promote the patient's realistic perception of the environment. The patient should use any other sensory aides (e.g., eyeglasses, hearing aids) that he or she normally requires.

The patient's safety during an acute episode of delirium must not be compromised. House staff must be alerted if the patient is considered a candidate to leave the institution's premises. The patient's propensity to pull tubes, climb over side rails, or fall may require the staff to institute a one-on-one observation or encourage the family to stay with the patient. Consistency on the part of the staff in terms of an unhurried, daily routine, repeatedly assigned staff, and continuous visits by family members is helpful. Family members must be kept informed and included in the plans taken to resolve the delirium. They need to understand the biologic basis for the behavior that they are witnessing in their loved one.

38.3 Suicidality

Management of the suicidal patient is challenging. A clear and thorough approach to risk assessment and a comprehensive, yet focused management plan is required. Accurately predicting which patients will eventually commit suicide is not currently possible. However, factors that raise and protect against risk have been identified.

38.3.1 Suicidal ideation and behavior

Suicidal ideation is the occurrence of passive thoughts about wanting to be dead or active thoughts about killing oneself. Suicidal thoughts may range from the occasional and fleeting to the ruminative and omnipresent. Typically, they fluctuate and are ambivalent, countered by the will to live. A suicide attempt is defined as a potentially self-injurious behavior with at least some intent to die as a consequence of the act.

The intention of suicidal behavior is to end one's own life. Suicidal intent is necessary for a potentially self-injurious behavior to be labeled an attempt; however, other motivations may also be present, for example, to influence another. Attempting suicide may or may not cause actual injury.

38.3.2 Scope of the problem

According to the World Health Organization, in 2000, suicide accounted for up to 1 million deaths worldwide including approximately 30 000 in the US. Globally, suicide is among the top three leading causes of death for ages 15–44 years. Suicide rates vary by country. National rates may be influenced by religion, socioeconomic factors, access to means, and mental illness. The quality and type of data collection and classification varies between countries, limiting the utility of the data. Suicidal behavior may be more significant than is actually accounted for by reported numbers.

38.3.3 Risk and protective factors

While suicide is responsible for a substantial number of preventable deaths, it accounts for only a small percentage of all deaths. The relatively infrequent nature of suicide and its complex etiology contribute to the difficulty in identifying predictors that have reasonable levels of sensitivity and specificity. Typically, risk factors have a low level of specificity, in that they produce a high proportion of false positives. For example, psychiatric diagnosis is highly associated with suicide but the majority of people with a psychiatric diagnosis do not attempt suicide. Factors that protect against suicidal behavior have also been identified. Like risk factors, knowledge of protective factors, such as employment and social support, in some cases, can provide targets for treatment. Hence, knowledge of risk and protective factors for suicidality are important for the clinician managing a suicidal patient. The following is a summary of those factors.

38.3.3.1 Gender
Males are almost four times as likely to die by suicide. Females are twice to three times more likely to think about suicide and almost twice as likely to make an attempt.

38.3.3.2 Age
In the US, completed suicide increases markedly from childhood, where it is a very rare event (6–11 years, 0.13 per 100 000), to early adolescence (1.34 per 100 000) and mid-late adolescence (8.2 per 100 000), before stabilizing in early adulthood (20–24 years, 12.47 per 100 000) to adult levels. While frequency of completed suicide is generally stable throughout adult life, there is a sharp, dramatic increase in completed suicide in elderly populations. In contrast, suicidal ideation and attempts have been noted to decline with age. Apart from the possibility that risk of suicidal ideation indeed decreases with age, this could imply that attempts become more lethal and/or better planned, resulting in fewer remaining potential victims, or that, as the population ages, more of the at-risk individuals have died by suicide or other causes.

38.3.3.3 Religiosity
Religious belief or affiliation is associated with a reduced risk of suicide, but not always. The protective effect of religion may be due to the deterrent effect of religious beliefs, such that suicide is a sin or is morally wrong, or social support from family or a religious group. The protective effect of religion may not be universal because some religions having beliefs that are congruent with suicide; for example, condoning suicide as an honorable way of dealing with problems, or that death may be a way of being reunited with loved ones. Considering this variability, clinicians ought to query patients about their religiosity and the likely impact of religious beliefs on suicidality.

38.3.3.4 Family and social factors
Separated, divorced, and widowed individuals have been found to be at twice the risk of attempted suicide. Another study has shown that risk varies with gender and is only elevated in divorced males. The relative protective effects of marriage may be gained from companionship, social support, and a sense of responsibility. Having children appears to attenuate risk and number of children has been negatively associated with suicide risk in women. Suicidal patients may require encouragement and assistance in establishing or connecting with their social network, particularly given the impact of psychiatric disorders on social functioning.

38.3.3.5 Familial association
A family history of suicide raises the risk of suicidal behavior. Suicide attempts have been found to be six times more likely in the offspring of depressed suicide attempters compared with depressed nonattempters. Further, suicide attempters with a family history of suicide were more likely to have made multiple attempts than those without a family history. Evidence suggests that risk is transmitted via an impulsive–aggressive trait. A family history of suicidality should be taken during the assessment of an individual for suicide risk.

38.3.3.6 Employment
Suicide attempts and completed suicide are more prevalent in unemployed populations. Unemployment has been found to place women at greater risk of suicide relative to males.

38.3.3.7 Past suicidality
A history of suicidal ideation and behavior are consistently identified as predicting further suicidality and completed suicide. Suicidal ideation prospectively predicts completed suicide and suicide attempt while ideation with a plan was found to be a stronger predictor of suicide attempt than ideation without. Suicide attempts have been found to be a marker of future suicidal acts and completed suicide. A thorough assessment of the patient's past history of suicidal behavior or ideation is critical.

38.3.3.8 Psychiatric disorders
Prevalence of a psychiatric diagnosis in completed suicide populations is as high as 90% in both child and adolescent and adult samples. Those with more disorders, regardless of type of disorder, were more likely to attempt suicide in all age groups.

Individuals with schizophrenia are at high risk of suicide attempt and completion. A recent estimate suggests that the lifetime suicide rate for individuals with schizophrenia is 5%. Younger age and the initial years after onset of illness have been identified as the times of greatest risk. Other risk factors in schizophrenia include the presence of depression, substance abuse, and poor adherence to treatment.

Anxiety disorders have been suggested to increase risk of suicidal ideation and attempt. Comorbid depression and substance abuse compounds the risk. Alcohol and substance-use disorders raise risk of suicide attempts and completed suicide. Alcohol-related disorders are less common in females but have been shown to be more highly associated with suicide attempts in females compared with males. Comorbidity between alcohol-use disorders and other psychiatric disorders, depression in particular, raises the risk of suicide. Risk of suicide associated with opiate and mixed substance abuse has been associated with even greater risk of suicide than alcohol.

Given the common comorbidity and increased risk, it is essential that patients are screened for the presence of alcohol and substance-use disorders.

The diagnostic criteria for borderline personality disorder include multiple risk factors for suicide, including recurrent suicidal behavior, gestures, or threats, or self-mutilating behavior as well as impulsivity. In clinical populations, it is estimated that up to 10% of those with borderline personality disorder complete suicide and approximately 75% attempt suicide.

38.3.3.9 Other factors
Impulsivity has been linked with suicide attempts in a variety of psychiatric populations. Impulsivity may relate to behavioral disinhibition and therefore increase risk of suicidal behavior. A patient's history of impulsivity and aggression should be assessed and might be elucidated by inquiring about previous trouble with the police for assault or violence, fighting, hostile behavior, agitation, conflict in relationships, domestic violence, actions lacking forethought, and disinhibited behavior.

Hopelessness increases the risk of suicidality independently of psychiatric illness and is often stable over time, making it an important factor to assess.

Physically abused children have been found to be more likely to exhibit suicidality and depressive symptoms than children who had experienced neglect or those who experienced neither abuse nor neglect. In addition, childhood sexual abuse significantly increases the risk of a suicide attempt in females and even more so in males.

Chronic medical illness is associated with increased risk of suicide attempt and completion. Illnesses identified as having suicide rates greater than the normal population include epilepsy, human immunodeficiency virus and acquired immune deficiency syndrome, multiple sclerosis, and Huntington's disease.

38.3.4 Assessment of the suicidal patient

Establishing a therapeutic relationship is the first task for the clinician managing the suicidal patient and comes before assessing risk. Engaging the patient may be a challenging task given ambivalence about life, possible previous negative experiences in therapy, severity of illness, and the clinician's competing need to establish an assessment of risk.

Although there are no definitive empirically based approaches to predicting suicide risk, the aim of the assessment of a patient is to evaluate the patient's current suicidal risk by determining diagnosis as well as demographic and clinical suicide risk and protective factors. Table 38.2 contains some warning signs of suicide.

Interviewing a patient about current suicidality requires the asking of direct and indirect questions about thoughts and behaviors in a sensitive manner. Table 38.3 contains a number of questions that are designed to elicit suicidal ideation.

Valuable details about suicidality include time of onset, course (e.g., episodic, escalating), levels of suicidal intent associated with attempts, precipitants (e.g., conflict with spouse, isolation, unemployment, command hallucinations), probability of rescue from attempt (i.e., remote location with low chance of rescue versus in a populated or public area), medical seriousness, need for medical attention, actual lethality of the attempt, and the patient's understanding of lethality. These details may provide insight into the risk of future attempts and provide information about targets for intervention. A brief tool to assess and track both suicidal ideation and behavior during management of a patient, such as the Columbia Suicide Severity Rating Scale (C-SSRS; http://www.maps.org/mdma/mt1_docs/c-ssrs_1-14-09_sincelastvisit.pdf), may enhance clinical practice.

Interviewing other caregivers, if possible, as well as the patient or involved family members about family history of mental illness (particularly depression, bipolar disorder, schizophrenia, alcohol, and substance abuse) is indicated.

38.3.5 Management

Upon completion of a risk assessment a clinician is not expected to be able to predict the future, but will develop a judgment about a patient's current level of risk and respond accordingly in the interest of the patient's safety. This may include referral for inpatient treatment, increased monitoring as an outpatient, engagement of the support group or family to provide more intensive supervision,

Table 38-2   Some warning signs of suicide

Emotional/psychological	Behavioral
Hopelessness and helplessness	Making a will
Frequent mood changes	Putting one's life in order
	Giving away prized possessions
Tiredness and fatigue	Making suicidal threat or verbalizing wanting to harm oneself
Feelings of being a burden to others	Talking about death or dying
Lack of enjoyment in anything	Previous suicide attempt
Anxiety and agitation	Changing in eating or sleeping habits
Sadness and/or depression	Increase in alcohol or substance use
Feelings of worthlessness, guilt, failure	Engaging in reckless behavior
	Skipping school or running away from home
Feelings of isolation	Withdrawing from others

Table 38-3	Eliciting information about suicidality
Eliciting passive thoughts	• Have you had any thoughts of wanting to be dead or of ending your life? • Has it gotten more serious, where you had thought about killing yourself? • Tell me about your hopes for the future. • Have things been so bad that you don't feel like going on? • Are you feeling so badly that it would be a relief to no longer go on?
Asking about plan	• Have you thought about how you would kill yourself? • Do you have a plan? • When having these thoughts, have you had an intention to act upon them? • Are there means available for you to kill yourself? • Have you actually rehearsed or practiced how you would kill yourself? • What would keep you from carrying out a plan?
Asking about self-harm	• Have you ever hurt yourself in any way on purpose? • What did you intend to happen? • Did you intend to kill yourself ?
Asking about a recent suicide attempt	• How did you try to commit suicide? • Where was the attempt made? • Did anyone else know about what you were going to do? • Who found you? • How many times have you tried to commit suicide? • Was the attempt an impulsive act or one that had a plan? • Did you have any harm or permanent impairment from the attempt? • How did you get treated?

development of a plan regarding procedures to institute if the patient becomes more suicidal (e.g., go to the local emergency department, contact the clinician). Above all, the uppermost goal is that patients should be kept safe.

There are two common approaches to treating the suicidal patient. The primary approach is to address the disorder underlying the suicidality. The second approach is to directly treat the suicidality, which is the focus of some psychotherapeutic approaches. Treatment might also be useful to stabilize additional risk factors for suicide while enhancing any protective factors. Treatment planning should be informed by results of risk assessment, while also considering the patient's capacity to self-care particularly in a crisis and understanding of treatment options.

Provision of psychoeducation about mental illness being a disease rather than a personal flaw or inadequacy and suicidal behavior as being related to mental illness may reduce self-blame and misperceptions within the family. Treatment options and setting should be discussed with the patient and family, where appropriate, and written consent gained.

When the risk of a suicide attempt is highly elevated, and/or confidence in a patient's ability to refrain from acting on suicidal thoughts is low, inpatient hospitalization may be required on a voluntary or involuntary basis. Both psychopharmacologic and psychosocial treatments have a role in the management. In the absence of comprehensive efficacy evidence for the treatment of suicidality, clinicians are advised to aggressively treat the underlying psychopathology following current treatment guidelines.

38.4 Aggressive and violent behavior

Aggressive behavior is generally considered to include anger and physical or verbal aggression. Aggression may manifest itself as verbal aggression and/or physical aggression against objects, other people, or the self with a potential toward destructiveness or an intent to cause harm. Aggression toward oneself may include self-mutilation and suicidal acts. Violence refers to human behaviors and responses that are destructive and denotes physical aggression by one person against another.

38.4.1 Contributors to aggressive or violent behavior

38.4.1.1 Endogenous factors

Studies on violence and age generally support the idea that violence rates peak in the late teens and early twenties. A study of violence in emergency departments found that young patients (mean age younger than 28 years) were nearly twice as violent (57% vs. 30%) as older patients.

In terms of gender, most research findings indicate that men have a greater tendency to behave violently than do women. In women with a serious psychiatric diagnosis, however, the rate of violence is similar to that of men.

Though most people with mental illness will not become violent, people with untreated mental disorder have a higher incidence of violence and aggression in their lives. This association may be especially significant for those who require psychiatric hospitalization in adolescence. Incidents of aggressive behavior, including physical violence, occur in all clinical diagnostic categories and are not exclusively manifested by patients with a diagnosed psychiatric disorder. Psychiatric diagnoses associated with patterns of aggression and violence are listed in Box 38.1.

An often overlooked factor that can increase the risk for aggression and violence is a medical condition that might lead to psychiatric symptoms. Patients who experience anxiety, irritability, agitation, and thought problems and have a predilection to injure themselves or others present a complicated diagnostic and treatment dilemma. They require a differential evaluation for any contributing medical condition, treatment of the condition, while at the same time keeping them and others around them safe. Some selected medical conditions associated with aggression and violence are presented in Box 38.2.

38.4.1.2 Exogenous factors

Incidents of violence toward healthcare providers, in the form of threats and verbal and physical assaults, have escalated in inpatient mental-health care facilities and in emergency care, long-term care, and home care. Factors such as postoperative confusion, receiving unwanted treatment, and delayed treatment have been found to be precursors of patient aggression in general hospitals. A common approach involving a "show of force" by way of calling hospital security staff has been found to exacerbate the problem.

Box 38.1 Psychiatric Diagnoses and Patterns of Aggression or Violence.

- Antisocial personality disorder
- Attention-deficit hyperactivity disorder
- Bipolar disorders (especially bipolar 1 manic episodes)
- Conduct disorder in children
- Delusional disorder (persecutory type)
- Dementia
- Dissociative identity disorder
- Impulse-control disorder
- Oppositional defiant disorder
- Paranoid personality disorder
- Post-traumatic stress disorder
- Schizophrenia (paranoid type)
- Substance-related disorder

Box 38.2 Medical Conditions Associated with Aggression and Violence.

- **Pain**: chronic or acute.
- **Neurological conditions**: brain tumor, seizure disorder, multiple sclerosis, Parkinson's disease, Huntington's disease, dementia, traumatic brain injury.
- **Infectious disease**: neurosyphilis, meningitis, HIV encephalopathy, herpes simplex encephalitis
- **Metabolic disorder**: hyponatremia, systemic lupus erethymatosus, porphyria, hepatic encephalopathy, chronic renal failure, hypernatremia.
- **Endocrine disorder**: hyperthyroidism, hypothyroidism, hyperparathyroidism, adrenal disorders, diabetes mellitus, pancreatic tumors, progressive hypoglycemia.
- **Exogenous toxin**: alcoholic hallucinosis, hallucinogens, illicit stimulants, amphetamine-induced psychosis, heavy metals, any medications, inhalants, withdrawal from substances of abuse.
- **Vitamin deficiency**: Wernicke's encephalopathy, pernicious anemia, folate deficiency.

There has been research on the importance of staff members' interaction styles with patients as related to violent incidents on psychiatric units. These have been shown to be important precipitants to patient aggression and in escalating aggressive behavior. Clinicians who make every effort to show respect and empathy for a violent-prone patient's situation and suffering are more likely to be successful in defusing a patient's anger than are clinicians who interact with the patient in an authoritarian manner. Interpersonal precursor events that have been linked with escalating patient violence include occasions when patients are angered or frustrated by the behavior of other patients, such as disputes over cigarettes or food, or by some type of aversive stimulation of the patient by staff or the environment. Examples of such staff behavior include preventing the patient from leaving the ward, engaging in disputes over medication, generally enforcing rules or denying requests, physically restraining the patient, taking something from the patient, ignoring the patient, or requesting the patient to do or refrain from doing something. In addition, either over-stimulation on a psychiatric unit due to ward turmoil, or under-stimulation due to a lack of engaging activities, may promote aggressive patient responses.

38.4.2 Nonpharmacologic interventions

Although pharmacologic treatments may ultimately be required, in the absence of immediate danger, a combination of one or more of the following de-escalation strategies should be initiated when managing acute aggression. These can include interventions such as verbal de-escalation by talking to the patient, asking family members to assist, and avoidance of over-stimulation.

If attempts to calm an acutely aggressive patient fail to yield the desired outcome, the use of physical or mechanical restraint and/or seclusion may become necessary. However, caution should be used when resorting to such measures because they have been associated with death and injuries. Death typically occurs from asphyxia, but can also occur from aspiration, blunt trauma to the chest, cardiac arrhythmia from catecholamine rush, severe metabolic acidosis, and in the case of substance abusers, sudden death from a form of delirium associated with cocaine abuse. Cases of death associated with physical or mechanical restraint use and questions of misuse of these procedures have resulted in comprehensive legislation governing their use as measures of last resort by the Center for Medicare and Medicaid Services (CMS) and standards by the Joint Commission (JC). A synopsis of the regulations regarding restraint orders are provided in Box 38.3.The final rules can be accessed at the CMS (Hospital Conditions of Participation: Patients' Rights, 42 CFR Part 482. Baltimore, MD, US Department of Health and Human Services). Current US legislation and national standards require that behavioral restraint use should be an option of last resort after less restrictive alternatives have been tried.

Box 38.3 Regulations Regarding Restraint Orders.

1. MD/LIP * to order [CMS].
2. Qualified trained staff may initiate restraint before order obtained [Joint Commission].
3. MD/LIP to see patient:
   a. within 1 h [CMS]
   b. within 4 h (or less for a child) [JC]
4. Re-evaluation and renewed order by primary treating MD/LIP [CMS/JC]:
   a. every 4 h for adults
   b. every 2 h for 9- to 17-year-olds
   c. every 1 h for those under 9 years.
5. MD/LIP in person, re-evaluation every 24 h thereafter [CMS].
6. MD/LIP in person, re-evaluation thereafter [JC]:
   a. every 8 h for adults
   b. every 4 h for those under 18 years.
7. No PRNs or standing orders [CMS/JC].
8. Can "reuse" existing order if has not expired [JC].

LIP = licensed independent professional, including nurses and physicians' assistants.

Contraindications to restraint use include any medical condition that might increase the likelihood of injury or death from a restraint procedure. They should never be used for staff convenience or in lieu of adequate staffing. Patients' airways should never be obstructed with a towel or any other article that would preclude them from breathing.

Restraints and seclusion should be avoided with patients who have a history of sexual or physical abuse. Likewise they should be used cautiously with those who are confused and combative as they may increase agitation.

Chronic management of the violent or aggressive patient can also include a number of nonpharmacologic strategies either alone or in combination with psychopharmacologic approaches. The specific psychopathology and treatment needs of patients with chronic violence will dictate appropriate interventions. For example, treatment of aggression related to psychosis may require supportive therapy and social skills training as well as psychotropic medications. Potential nonpharmacologic interventions are summarized in Box 38.4.

38.4.3 Emergency pharmacologic interventions

The clinical use of forced medication is distasteful to many clinicians who see it as a departure from the usual ideal of collaborative relationship between clinician and patient. Some well-known scholars have opined that involuntary medication is more invasive than physical restraint.

The terminology used to describe forced medication used to control behavior or restrict movement is known as chemical restraint. The indication for this is to protect the patient from

Box 38.4 Selected Nonpharmacologic Interventions for Treatment of Violence.

- Anger management
- Dialectical behavioral therapy
- Victim empathy training
- Social skills training
- Behavioral therapy
- Marital/family therapy
- Substance-abuse counseling
- Occupational therapy

Table 38-4   Medications employed for control of aggressive/violent behavior

Medication	Route	Dose	Onset of Efficacy	Contraindications[a]	Adverse Reactions[b,c]
Lorazepam	IM	Initial 4 mg After 10–15 min may administer again Maximum generally 10 mg/d	5–10 min	Acute narrow glaucoma, respiratory insufficiency, sleep apnea syndrome	Sedation, dizziness, weakness, unsteadiness, respiratory depression
Haloperidol	IM	2–5 mg every 30–60 min until sedation achieved	10 min	Parkinson's disease, caution in severe cardiovascular disease	Extrapyramidal symptoms, hypotension, angina pain
Ziprasidone	IM	10–20 mg Doses of 10 mg may be given every 2 h Doses of 20 mg may be given every 4 h Maximum dose of 40 mg/d	15 min	Known history of QT prolongation, recent MI, uncompensated CHF	Somnolence, nausea, headache, asthenia, orthostatic hypotension, seizures (rare), sudden death
Olanzapine	IM	Initial dose of 10 mg, second dose of 5–10 mg 2 h later No more than 3 injections per 24 h	15–30 min	Any unstable medical condition (e.g., acute MI, sick sinus syndrome, recent cardiac surgery), prostatic hypertrophy, narrow-angle closure glaucoma, paralytic ileus	Somnolence, dry mouth, dysphagia, dizziness, asthenia, joint pain
Risperidone	PO Liquid 1 mg/mL Orally disintegrating tabs: 0.5-mg, 1-mg, and 2-mg	1 mg initially Increase as tolerated up to 3 mg b.i.d. Manufacturer recommends dose increases in no less than 24 h period	Peak concentration achieved in 1 h	Oral solution incompatible with cola or tea	Extrapyramidal symptoms, somnolence, nausea, hyperkinesias, orthostatic hypotension

| Aripiprazole | IM single-dose vials ready-to-use, 9.75 mg/1.3 mL | Efficacy of IM demonstrated in a dosage range from 5.25 to 15 mg IM (no additional benefit with a 15 mg dose vs. a 9.75 mg dose) | 30 min to 1 h | Caution in patients with a history of seizures | Dizziness, insomnia, possible activation |
| | Available in oral solution: 1 mg/mL | Repeat injections should not be given in less than 2 h Maximum daily dose 30 mg | | | |

[a]Hypersensitivity to the drug is always a contradiction.
[b]Increased risk of death from CVA reported with SGA antipsychotic use in elderly.
[c]Neuroleptic malignant syndrome (rare) is always a consideration with antipsychotic medications; hyperglycemia in some cases extreme and associated with ketoacidosis or hyperosmolar coma and death has been reported in patients taking antipsychotic medications.

harm to self or from hurting others when there is impending danger and measures to de-escalate have failed. Medications can be given orally or intramuscularly. In most cases the latter is preferred owing to the more rapid onset of action. The selection of route depends on, among other factors, the cause of the agitation and the emergent situation. Medications can be used at a patient's request and ideally should be taken voluntarily as opposed to forced.

The American Association of Child and Adolescent Psychiatry practice parameter prohibits the use of *pro re nata* use of chemical restraint.

Clinicians must devote care to obtaining a good medical history and documenting the patient's most recent list of medications. They should ideally be aware of the patient's possible overdose on unknown medications (prescribed or over-the-counter) or intoxication with illicit drugs or alcohol. The incidence of drug interactions can be a risk and potential problem in emergency room populations, so clinicians should be vigilant, especially among patients taking multiple medications. They also should be aware of what medications may be contraindicated with a patient's comorbid medical conditions. As with all restraints, constant monitoring should be done that includes vital signs and neurologic checks until the patient is fully awake and ambulatory.

Table 38.4 summarizes the most common medications employed in acute agitation. It should be noted that haloperidol is not available in an intravenous preparation, although it has been used in this way off-label by some who advocate rapid tranquilization. However, in 2006 the US FDA issued a warning against the use of IV haloperidol, citing the danger of sudden death resulting from QT prolongation and Torsades de pointes (see Chapter 35).

KEY POINTS

- When a severe behavioral disturbance is identified, the clinician should quantify its intensity, enumerate its accompanying symptoms, and search for etiologies so that intervention can be targeted to causes and contexts.

- Delirium is a syndrome that can have many causes and is characterized by a *rapid* onset of disordered cognition, attention deficit, and disturbance of consciousness. The prognosis for recovery from delirium is good if recognition and management of the underlying cause are attended to early.

- Suicidal ideation is the occurrence of passive thoughts about wanting to be dead or active thoughts about killing oneself. Such thoughts may range from the occasional and fleeting to the ruminative and omnipresent.

- Prevalence of a psychiatric diagnosis in completed suicide populations is as high as 90% in both child/adolescent and adult samples.

- Treatment planning for the suicidal patient should be informed by results of risk assessment, while also considering the patient's capacity to self-care particularly in a crisis and understanding of treatment options.

- When risk of suicide attempt is highly elevated, and/or confidence in a patient's ability to refrain from acting on suicidal thoughts is low, inpatient hospitalization may be required on a voluntary or involuntary basis.

- Aggressive behavior generally is considered to include anger and physical or verbal aggression, and violence refers to human behaviors and responses that are destructive and denotes physical aggression by one person against another.

- If attempts to calm an acutely aggressive patient fail to yield the desired outcome, the use of physical or mechanical restraint and/or seclusion may become necessary. However, caution should be used when resorting to such measures in that they have been associated with death and injury.

- The indication for chemical restraint is to protect patients from harm to self or from hurting others when there is impending danger and measures to de-escalate have failed.

Further Reading

Allen, M.H., Oldham, J.M., and Riba, M.B. (2002) *Emergency Psychiatry*, American Psychiatric Association, Washington, DC.

Allen, M.H., Carpenter, D., Sheets, J.L. *et al.* (2003) What do consumers say they want and need during a psychiatric emergency. *Journal of Psychiatric Practice*, **9** (1), 39–58.

American Academy of Child and Adolescent Psychiatry (2002) Practice parameter for the prevention and management of aggressive behavior in child and adolescent psychiatric institutions, with special reference to seclusion and restraint. *Journal of American Academy of Child and Adolescent Psychiatry*, **41** (2), 4–24.

Kleespies, P.M. (2008) *Behavioral Emergencies: An Evidence-based Resource for Evaluating and Managing Suicidal Behavior, Violence, and Victimization*, American Psychological Association, Washington, DC.

Morrison, E.F. (1992) A coercive interactional style as an antecedent to aggression in psychiatric patients. *Research in Nursing Health*, **15**, 421–431.

National Alliance for the Mentally Ill (2003) *Seclusion and Restraints: Task Force Report*, NAMI, Arlington, VA.

Simon, R.I. (2008) Behavioral risk assessment of the guarded suicidal patient. *Suicide and Life Threatening Behavior*, **38** (5), 517–522.

39   Violence

39.1 Introduction

This chapter briefly describes issues related to violence which the clinician interested in understanding mental health and illness and providing treatment will encounter. These include intimate partner violence, child maltreatment, elder abuse, and rape/sexual assault. Because of space considerations these will be summarized. Treatment of aggressive and violent behavior *per se* can be found in Chapter 38 on psychiatric emergencies.

39.2 Intimate partner violence

The World Health Organization has declared violence a major public health problem, with intimate partner violence (IPV) being one of the most common types against women. It has reached epidemic proportions in US society and is the single major cause of injury to women in the United States, more common than rapes, muggings, and automobile accidents combined. Approximately 1.5 million women are raped or assaulted annually by an intimate partner. IPV does occur against males; however, women are significantly more likely to be a victim.

Intimate partners are current or former spouses or current or former nonmarital partners (dating or same-sex partners). Violent acts include both physical and sexual violence, as well as threats and psychological/emotional abuse. Physical violence includes acts used with enough force to have the potential to cause death, disability, or injury – actions such as scratching, pushing, shoving, burning, or use of restraint on another's body. These uniform definitions are important for researchers but also for clinicians charged with detecting IPV.

IPV exacts a heavy toll, not only on the direct victim, but on the children who are exposed to it. Children who live in homes where partner violence occurs are at risk for developing a range of emotional, physical, and behavioral symptoms. Research suggests that they are at serious risk of developing a host of trauma symptoms and delinquency problems. Children who witness domestic violence demonstrate higher levels of depression and lower levels of self-esteem; these effects are especially pronounced in boys. In addition, children from families with domestic violence are at risk for experiencing physical violence themselves.

Screening for domestic violence needs to be systematic and direct. The inclusion of questions that identify IPV in triage and entry-point protocols significantly increases the identification of abused women. Screening for domestic violence also is critically important because the way in which the immediate aftermath of violence is handled is an important determinant of the survivor's psychologic response.

Fundamentals of Psychiatry, First Edition. Allan Tasman and Wanda K. Mohr.
© 2011 John Wiley & Sons, Ltd. Published 2011 by John Wiley & Sons, Ltd.
This chapter is based on Chapter 127 (Fabian M. Saleh, John P. Federoff, Adekunle G. Ahmed, Debra A. Pinals) of *Psychiatry, Third Edition*

The American College of Emergency Physicians' policy statement on this emphasizes the need for evaluating patients presenting to an emergency department for IPV; develops multidisciplinary approaches for identification, treatment, and referral; and recognizes the special services and resources necessary for victims. The Joint Commission has mandated that hospitals have objective criteria for identifying and assessing possible victims of abuse and neglect and that these standards be uniform throughout the organization.

39.3 Child maltreatment

Child maltreatment is a major public health crisis. Neglect is the most common form, followed by physical abuse, and then sexual abuse, emotional maltreatment, and medical neglect.

Child neglect is the presence of certain deficiencies in caretaker obligation that harm the child's psychological or physical health, or both. Child neglect covers a range of behaviors including educational, supervisory, medical, physical, and emotional neglect and abandonment, often complicated by cultural and contextual factors. *Physical abuse* includes scalding, beatings with an object, severe physical punishment, and Münchhausen syndrome by proxy. *Sexual abuse* includes incest, sexual assault by a relative or stranger, fondling of genital areas, exposure to indecent acts, sexual rituals, or involvement in pornography. *Emotional maltreatment* includes acts such as verbal abuse and belittlement, acts designed to terrorize a child, and lack of nurturance or emotional availability by caregivers. It is difficult to unpack emotional maltreatment from the other forms of abuse insofar as it can be argued that it may be an integral component of all other forms of maltreatment.

Children who are maltreated evidence both physical and behavioral symptoms. Any verbal report or suspicion of child maltreatment must be acted upon. Box 39.1 lists some symptoms to which the

---

Box 39.1 Symptoms of Maltreatment.

General symptoms

- Developmental delays in which the child does not reach developmental milestones as expected.
- Regression in development or losing skills already mastered and moving back to a earlier state of development.
- Failure to thrive in which the child's growth pattern is not in a healthy range. Both weight and height can be affected, but low weight for height and head circumference is the most common symptom. Most cases of failure to thrive are the result of problems with the immediate care of the child, the interaction between the child and the caregiver (usually the mother), or the social and emotional health of the caregiver.
- Unusual parent/child interaction. The parent may be uninterested in the child, or a child may be especially sensitive to or fearful about to the parent's moods and may attempt to smooth over any potential conflict.
- Low self-esteem, anxiety, depression, or suicidal tendencies.
- Sudden decline in academic performance.
- Inappropriate or problem behavior, for example, unusual fussiness, fear, or lack of interest in activities, sudden disruptive behaviors such as violence or sexual activity. Older children may act out by being promiscuous or running away.

Symptoms of physical abuse

- Physical abuse often results in cuts, bruises, burns, broken bones, head injuries, and abdominal injuries.
- Clinicians should be suspicious if injuries are unlikely to have been caused by an accident, especially for the child's developmental stage.
- Geometric patterns or mirror (symmetrical) injuries are suspicious, as are those located on areas of the body that usually are protected, such as the inside of the legs and arms, the back, the genitalia, and the buttocks.
- Explanations may change or not adequately account for how an injury occurred. The history of the injury does not match the actual type of injury, its location, or how long ago it occurred.
- Evidence may show that serious injuries have occurred previously.
- Medical care for the injury might have been delayed.

Symptoms of psychological abuse

An emotionally abused child may:

- Be apathetic and amotivational; have little interest in what is going on around him.
- Have inappropriate responses to pain, other people, or changes in his or her environment.
- Be avoidant of parent or caregiver.
- Act overly fearful, angry, depressed, or anxious.
- Perform poorly in school.
- Inflict self-injury or be self-destructive.

Symptoms of sexual abuse

- Children with symptoms of recent sexual abuse may be reluctant to go to the bathroom; may show signs of discomfort or pain while sitting, urinating, or passing stools; may have discharge from the vagina or penis; or blood on their underwear.
- Certain behaviors may also indicate sexual abuse. These include:
  - Age-inappropriate knowledge of sex or sexual behavior.
  - Promiscuity or seductiveness.
  - Running away from home.
  - Suicide attempts.
  - Involvement with drugs or prostitution.

clinician should be attuned. Certain symptoms can occur with all types of maltreatment, while others are specific to certain forms of maltreatment.

According to evidence, maltreated children tend to be attached less securely to their mothers or primary caregivers than are children who are not maltreated. Interactions with caregivers occur less frequently for maltreated children, and those interactions that do occur are characterized by more negative effects. In addition to problems in caregiver relationships, maltreated children have been shown to have more difficulties with peers. They generate lower quality solutions to interpersonal problems and have more difficulty understanding complex social roles. Moreover, maltreated children tend to display less social involvement and lower sophistication in play. They display fewer socially competent behaviors in interactions, initiate fewer positive interactions with peers, are both withdrawn and aggressive with other children, and show more inappropriate responses to peer distress. Because of these difficulties in peer interactions, maltreated children are not popular with peers; they have fewer friends, and their peer group is more likely to reject them.

39.4 Rape and sexual assault

Rape is a crime of forced or coerced unwanted sexual penetration (oral, anal, or vaginal) of a nonconsenting person. In victims younger than the age of consent, such penetration – whether wanted or not – is considered statutory rape (the age of minors varies from state to state). Physical injuries resulting from rape may include tears in the upper part of the vagina and injuries to other parts of the body, such as bruises, black eyes, cuts, and scratches.

Sexual assault is a broader term, including the use of force and threats to coerce any sexual contact and unwanted touching, grabbing, or kissing.

The emotional effects of a rape are often more devastating than the physical. Shortly after a rape occurs, almost all women have symptoms of post-traumatic stress disorder. Women feel fearful, anxious, and irritable. They may feel angry, depressed, embarrassed, ashamed, or guilty (wondering whether they may have done something to provoke the rape or could have done something to avoid it). They may have intrusive, upsetting thoughts about, or mental images of, the assault, and they may relive the rape. Or they may stifle thoughts and feelings about the act. They may avoid situations that remind them of it. Difficulty sleeping and nightmares are common. These symptoms may last for months, interfering with social activities and work. However, for most women, symptoms lessen substantially over a period of months.

Clinicians should be aware that, after a rape, there is a risk of infection with a sexually transmitted disease and this should be assessed and treated. Rarely, a woman becomes pregnant.

39.5 Elder abuse

Elder abuse may include one or a combination of the following: physical abuse, physical neglect, sexual abuse, psychological abuse or neglect, financial abuse, and violation of personal rights.

Physical abuse is the intentional infliction of bodily harm. The older adult who has been physically abused may present with physical signs such as bruises, burns, lacerations, dislocations, sprains, or fractures. Victims of physical abuse may have frequent visits to emergency rooms with unexplained traumatic injuries. Individuals who have experienced physical abuse may give unreasonable descriptions of how the injury happened. Patients who have been physically abused often appear depressed, anxious, withdrawn, or confused.

Physical neglect is the intended or unintended failure of the caregiver to meet the basic needs of the older adult. Unmet needs may be physical or psychological. Patients may present with malnourishment, dehydration, poor hygiene, pressure ulcers, contractures, perineal excoriation, fecal impaction, signs of over- or under-medication, and untreated health problems. Older adults who have been physically neglected may present with depression and apathy.

Sexual abuse is sexual activity without consent or the ability to provide consent. The older adult who has been sexually abused may present with physical signs of reddened or traumatized genitals, genital pain, a sexually transmitted disease, and bruises, scratches, or abrasions. Seniors who have been sexually abused may be depressed, anxious, and withdrawn.

Psychologic abuse is the infliction of mental anguish by yelling, verbally assaulting, or threatening, humiliating, and intimidating the person. The older adult who has been psychologically abused may present with restlessness, insomnia, hand tremors, or worsening in chronic health conditions. Behaviors associated with psychologic abuse may include depression, anxiety, paranoia, and confusion. The victim of psychologic abuse may demonstrate fear of strangers in his or her home environment.

Psychologic neglect is the failure of the caregiver to meet the emotional needs of older adults. This type of mistreatment includes isolating the elder from contact with other people or not providing a stimulating environment, socially and cognitively. Behaviors seen in victims of psychologic neglect are the same as those seen in psychologic abuse.

Financial abuse or *material exploitation* involves the use of, or taking the possessions of, an older adult for personal or monetary gain without consent or by using unwarranted power. This abuse may include theft, mismanagement of funds, such as giving improper financial advice, or use of the older adult's money for personal benefit.

Theories on the causes of elder abuse vary. They suggest that elder abuse is a result of complex interactions among the older adult victims, caregiver characteristics, life stresses, and the social system. Families provide most of the care to older adults and thus are most likely to be the perpetrators of elder abuse.

KEY POINTS

- Community violence includes numerous forms of aggression that individuals inflict on one another. It includes phenomena such as youth violence, IPV, child maltreatment, elder abuse, and rape and sexual assault.

- IPV affects the lives of 2–4 million women a year, yet health professionals often fail to adequately screen for IPV.

- Maltreatment affects every aspect of a child including his or her social, behavioral, emotional, intellectual, and physical development.

- Rape and sexual assault are acts of violence in the form of sexual behaviors that are forcefully perpetrated on others.

- Older adults are increasingly victims of abuse (i.e., physical, sexual, psychological, or neglect) that may occur at the hands of their caregiver.

Further Reading

American College of Emergency Physicians (ACEP) (1996) ACEP policy statement: Emergency medicine and domestic violence. (On-line). Available at: http://www.acep.org/policy/p0004163.htm.

Brown, E.J. (2003) Child physical abuse: risk for psychopathology and efficacy of interventions. *Current Psychiatry Reports*, **5** (2), 87–94.

De Bellis, M.D. and Thomas, L.A. (2003) Biologic findings of post-traumatic stress disorder and child maltreatment. *Current Psychiatry Reports*, **5** (2), 108–117.

Frick, P.J., Cornell, A.H., Bodin, S.D. *et al.* (2003) Callous–unemotional traits and developmental pathways to severe conduct problems. *Developmental Psychopathology*, **39**, 2246–2260.

Kitzman, K.M., Gaylord, N.K., Holt, A.R., and Kenny, E.D. (2003) Child witnesses to domestic violence: a meta-analytic review. *Journal of Clinical and Consulting Psychology*, **71** 339–352.

National Research Council (1993) *Understanding Child Abuse and Neglect*, National Academy of Sciences, Washington, DC.

Thurston, W. and McLeod, L. (1997) Teaching second-year medical students about wife battering. *Women's Health Issues*, **7**, 92–97.

Index

Fundamentals of Psychiatry, First Edition. Allan Tasman and Wanda K. Mohr.
© 2011 John Wiley & Sons, Ltd. Published 2011 by John Wiley & Sons, Ltd.